Introduction to

GLOBAL HEALTH

SECOND EDITION

Kathryn H. Jacobsen, MPH, PhD

Department of Global and Community Health
George Mason University
Fairfax, VA

JONES & BARTLETT
LEARNING

World Headquarters
Jones & Bartlett Learning
5 Wall Street
Burlington, MA 01803
978-443-5000
info@jblearning.com
www.jblearning.com

Jones & Bartlett Learning books and products are available through most bookstores and online booksellers. To contact Jones & Bartlett Learning directly, call 800-832-0034, fax 978-443-8000, or visit our website, www.jblearning.com.

Production Credits
Publisher: Michael Brown
Managing Editor: Maro Gartside
Editorial Assistant: Chloe Falivene
Production Assistant: Alyssa Lawrence
Senior Marketing Manager: Sophie Fleck Teague
Manufacturing and Inventory Control Supervisor: Amy Bacus
Composition: Lapiz
Cover Design: Michael O'Donnell
Cover Image: © Marie Docher/age fotostock
Printing and Binding: Edwards Brothers Malloy
Cover Printing: Edwards Brothers Malloy

To order this product, use ISBN: 978-1-4496-8834-9

Library of Congress Cataloging-in-Publication Data
Jacobsen, Kathryn H.
  Introduction to global health / Kathryn H. Jacobsen. -- 2nd ed.
    p. ; cm.
  Includes bibliographical references and index.
  ISBN 978-1-4496-4825-1 (pbk.) -- ISBN1-4496-4825-8 (pbk.)
  I. Title.
  [DNLM: 1. World Health. 2. Communicable Disease Control. 3. Health Transition.
4. Internationality. WA 530.1]
  362.1--dc23

                                                             2012039129

6048

Printed in the United States of America
17 16 15 14 13   10 9 8 7 6 5 4 3 2

CONTENTS

PREFACE

On June 16, 2006, Bill Gates, founder of Microsoft and the richest man in the world, made headlines when he announced his intention to scale back his work at Microsoft to devote more time to the charitable foundation he had co-founded with his wife, Melinda.[1] Ten days later, even bigger headlines were made when Warren Buffett, the second wealthiest man in the world, made a surprising announcement—he was handing over most of his fortune to Bill Gates.[2] More precisely, the bulk of his accumulated wealth was going to the Bill & Melinda Gates Foundation, which focuses primarily on improving global health. As a result, the Bill & Melinda Gates Foundation, the largest philanthropic foundation in the world even prior to Buffett's generous donation, doubled in value to more than $60 billion.

What would inspire the wealthiest men in the world to develop such a passion for one cause? They had become aware of an awful reality: Every year, several million children die of diseases that are completely preventable. In an address to the World Health Assembly, the governing body of the World Health Organization, Bill Gates described the awakening of his philanthropic impulse:

> I first learned about these tragic health inequities some years ago when I was reading an article about diseases in the developing world. It showed that more than half a million children die every year from "rotavirus." I thought, "'Rotavirus?'—I've never even heard of it. How could I never have heard of something that kills half a million children every year!?"
>
> I read further and learned that millions of children were dying from diseases that had essentially been eliminated in the United States. Melinda and I had assumed that if there were vaccines and

xi

treatments that could save lives, governments would be doing everything they could to get them to the people who needed them. But they weren't. We couldn't escape the brutal conclusion that—in our world today—some lives are seen as worth saving and others are not. We said to ourselves: "This can't be true. But if it is true, it deserves to be the priority of our giving."[3]

Gates ended his speech with a call to action:

I am optimistic that in the next decade, people's thinking will evolve on the question of health inequity. People will finally accept that the death of a child in the developing world is just as tragic as the death of a child in the developed world. And the expanding capacities of science will give us the power to act on that conviction. When we do, we have a chance to make sure that all people, no matter what country they live in, will have the preventive care, vaccines, and treatments they need to live a healthy life. I believe we can do this—and if we do, it will be the best thing humanity has ever done.

Since global health has become the object of attention for Bill Gates, Warren Buffet, and other influential world leaders, it has, not surprisingly, also developed rapidly as an academic and professional field. The Consortium of Universities for Global Health (CUGH), founded in 2009, reports that the number of undergraduate and graduate students at large universities majoring in global health studies doubled in just the 3 years from 2006 to 2009.[4] By 2009, all of the top 50 liberal arts colleges ranked by *U.S. News & World Report* were offering at least one course in global health or public health, and nearly half offer a major, concentration, or other program of study in global or public health.[5] The American Association of Medical Colleges reports that nearly one-third of medical students graduating in 2011 completed a global health experience during medical school,[6] up from only about 15% of medical students in the 1990s and less than 10% in the 1980s.[7] The trend toward higher enrollment in global health courses, programs, and experiences is expected to continue in the coming years.

Global health is not just about health in low-income countries; it is about common health problems faced by the human population as a whole. In today's interconnected world, our own experiences of health and well-being are literally inseparable from everyone else's. We cannot prevent the birds and insects that carry influenza, West Nile virus, and other infectious agents from flying over national borders, just as we cannot inspect every imported banana or bean sprout for possible contaminants. The complexities of infectious disease, mental health, injuries, reproductive health, aging, nutrition, and other health-related issues require us to think beyond our households and immediate communities to regional, national, and global levels. Global health is relevant in the workplace too. No matter what the occupation— business, public service, education, medicine, religion, engineering, social work, community development, agriculture, manufacturing, or anything else—workers are involved in activities that intentionally or unintentionally impact human and environmental health close to home and around the world.

The study of global health helps us to make a positive difference in the world. It helps us to understand the causes and consequences of health concerns; to make connections between economics, politics, biology, medicine, sociology, psychology, and a host of other fields; to learn from others about effective and ineffective responses to critical problems; and, more generally, to make sense of the complexities of 21st-century life. A solid foundation in global health allows global citizens to assess their own vulnerabilities and health risks, to make informed choices about their career paths, and to make wise decisions about how to use their time and resources. Studying global health is an opportunity to explore important questions about how the world works, to develop intellectual and practical skills, and to engage with real-world challenges close to home and across the planet. This second edition of *Introduction to Global Health* provides a starting point for achieving those educational and personal goals.

REFERENCES

1. Markoff J, Lohr S. Gates to cede software reins. *New York Times*. 2006 Jun 16.
2. O'Brien TL, Saul S. Buffett to give bulk of his fortune to Gates charity. *New York Times*. 2006 Jun 26.
3. Gates B. Address to the 2005 World Health Assembly. Geneva; 2005 May 16.
4. *Saving lives: Universities transforming global health*. CUGH; 2009.
5. Hill DR, Ainsworth RM, Partap U. Teaching global public health in the undergraduate liberal arts: a survey of 50 colleges. *Am J Trop Med Hyg*. 2012;87:11–15.
6. *Medical school graduation questionnaire: 2011 all schools summary report*. Washington, DC: AAMC; 2011.
7. Drain PK, Primack A, Hunt DD, Fawzi WW, Holmes KK, Gardner P. Global health in medical education: a call for more training and opportunities. *Acad Med*. 2007;82: 226–230.

New to This Edition

Global health as a field of study has matured a great deal since the first edition of this textbook was published, and the second edition of *Introduction to Global Health* has been updated to reflect the current state of the field (including, of course, all new statistics).

The first unit of the book focuses on the foundations of global health as an academic and professional discipline.

- Chapter 1 has a new emphasis on health transitions, which are the demographic, epidemiologic, and nutritional changes that occur in populations undergoing socioeconomic development.
- Chapter 2 is a new overview of global health metrics, the numbers that form the basis for evidence-based policy and practice. Chapter 2 also introduces the eight countries that are highlighted throughout the book as examples of the health profiles in different world regions and income strata: the United States, South Korea (the Republic of Korea), Poland, Brazil, China, India, Kenya, and Sierra Leone.
- Chapter 3 provides a brief overview of global health research methods. This chapter gives readers the tools to find, read, understand, and apply health research articles and reports, including the more than 550 sources cited in the textbook. Research skills allow readers to peruse the most up-to-date primary source material, an essential skill for a field as dynamic as global health.
- Chapter 4 is about the social determinants of health—the social, cultural, economic, political, and related factors that influence health status.

The second unit is about global health across the lifespan.

- Chapter 5 is an expanded chapter on infant and child health that emphasizes ways to prevent the most common causes of neonatal and pediatric death worldwide.
- Chapter 6 is a new chapter on the health of young adults that discusses mental health, injuries, maternal mortality, family planning, and other important global issues.
- Chapter 7 is a new chapter on chronic noncommunicable diseases (NCDs) and aging that highlights the diseases that are the most common causes of death and disability among older adults in every region of the world. These include cardiovascular diseases, cancer, chronic lung disease, diabetes, and sensory impairments.

The third unit is about global health biology and the environmental context of health.

- Chapter 8 focuses on drinking water, sanitation, energy, occupational health, and other aspects of environmental health.
- Chapter 9 has a new focus on infectious disease prevention and control. Behavior change, environmental control, vaccination, drug therapy, and other methods for preventing and treating diarrheal, respiratory, vectorborne, and other infections are described.
- Chapter 10 provides an in-depth look at HIV/AIDS, tuberculosis, malaria, and influenza, with new coverage of the major initiatives working to address these global concerns.
- Chapter 11 covers the complex issues of global nutrition.

The fourth unit is about global health policy and practice.

- Chapter 12 describes the various entities that pay for and implement public health programs, highlighting the many different career paths and volunteer opportunities for those with interests in global health.
- Chapter 13 is an expanded chapter that highlights several of the key emerging issues of globalization and global health, such as urbanization, emerging infectious diseases, nutrition and food safety, bioterrorism, and global environmental change.

- Chapter 14 is a new chapter focusing on health and human rights, access to health, health during disasters and humanitarian emergencies, and emergency preparedness and response.
- Chapter 15 summarizes the successes in global health to date and examines priority areas for global health in the 21st century.

A transition guide showing how the first and second editions of *Introduction to Global Health* relate is available from the publisher.

ABOUT THE AUTHOR

Kathryn H. Jacobsen is an associate professor of epidemiology at George Mason University. She earned an MPH in International Health and a PhD in Epidemiology from the University of Michigan. Her research portfolio includes analyses of the global burden of disease and field projects in Africa, Asia, and the Americas. Dr. Jacobsen's work has been published by the World Health Organization and in dozens of international peer-reviewed journals. She is also the author of *Introduction to Health Research Methods: A Practical Guide*, published by Jones & Bartlett Learning.

CHAPTER 1

Global Health and Health Transitions

One hundred years ago, most populations around the world had similar disease profiles, with a high burden from infectious diseases. Modern medical technologies like antibiotics and vaccines have enabled many people to live longer, healthier lives. But modern lifestyles put a large number of people at risk for serious chronic diseases, and the disparities in health between the rich and the poor have increased. Global health draws on a wide variety of disciplines in order to understand and improve the health of people around the world.

1.1 DEFINING HEALTH

Health is often defined as the absence of disease (or the absence of illness, injury, infection, pain, tumors, or other physical disorders), but this is an incomplete explanation because it focuses on what health is *not* rather than on what health *is*. Some definitions of health try to capture its essence by emphasizing health as the ability to conduct normal daily activities. But that kind of statement is also limited, because the definition of "normal" varies from person to person. For example, some people assume that it is normal for an older person to have limited mobility and forgetfulness, but this is not true. Many older people are very active and mentally sharp, and many of those who have joint pain or memory loss could be helped by therapy and medication. Similarly, in many parts of the world parents think it is normal for their children to have intestinal worms. This is also not true, and untreated worm infections significantly reduce the health, growth, and school performance of millions of children around the world.

A more comprehensive definition of health addresses both physical and mental health as well as the presence of a social system that facilitates health. The Constitution of the World Health Organization (WHO), written

1

in 1948, defines **health** as "*a state of complete physical, mental, and social well-being and not merely the absence of disease or infirmity.*" This definition recognizes that health is not just a function of biology. Health stems from biology, psychology, sociology, and a host of other factors.

Although there is almost no one in the world today who would be classified as having "complete" health according to the WHO statement,[1] this definition provides a target for medical and public health systems to aim for as they work together to promote the improved health status of individuals and communities.

1.2 MEDICINE AND PUBLIC HEALTH

Medicine is concerned with the health of individuals, and clinical health practitioners like physicians, surgeons, dentists, nurses, and physical therapists are instrumental in helping individuals and families reach and maintain health by providing preventive, diagnostic, and therapeutic health services.

But because individual health is often the result of socioeconomic, environmental, and other factors, medicine by itself is a limited approach to health. Clinicians, other health workers, social workers and counselors, spiritual advisors, government officials, trash collectors, farmers, and many other people in many other professions all make important contributions to the social, economic, policy, and physical environments that promote or inhibit the health of communities and nations and, by extension, the health of individuals and families.

Public health focuses on the health of populations, whether small villages or entire world regions. The public health system, which addresses health at local, state and provincial, national, and international levels, also works to keep individuals safe and healthy. The goals of public health include preventing illnesses, injuries, and deaths at the population level, identifying and mitigating environmental hazards, promoting healthy behaviors, ensuring access to essential health services, and providing health education targeted toward at-risk groups of people (**Table 1–1**).[2] Both public health and medicine make important contributions to global health, but public health plays an especially important role because of its population focus (**Figure 1–1**). (The line between medicine and public health is also fairly blurry, with community health nurses and preventive medicine physicians working in both domains.)

Table 1–1 Essential public health services.

1	Monitor health status to identify community health problems.
2	Diagnose and investigate health problems and health hazards in the community.
3	Inform, educate, and empower people about health issues.
4	Mobilize community partnerships to identify and solve health problems.
5	Develop policies and plans that support individual and community health efforts.
6	Enforce laws and regulations that protect health and ensure safety.
7	Link people to needed personal health services and ensure the provision of health care when otherwise unavailable.
8	Ensure a competent public health and personal healthcare workforce.
9	Evaluate effectiveness, accessibility, and quality of personal and population-based health services.
10	Research for new insights and innovative solutions to health problems.

Source: Reproduced from the Centers for Disease Control and Prevention (2010). National Public Health Performance Standards Program (NPHPSP): 10 Essential Public Health Services. http://www.cdc.gov/nphpsp/essentialservices.html. Last updated December 9, 2010. Accessed August 31, 2012.

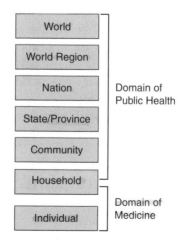

Figure 1–1 The domains of medicine and public health.

1.3 THE EMERGENCE OF GLOBAL HEALTH

Global health refers to *transnational health*, health concerns that cross national borders. The term *global health* is sometimes used interchangeably with *international health*, but **international health** is now more often used to describe a focus on the health issues of people who live in lower-income countries.[3,4]

Global health is not new. Infectious diseases have long been spread by migration and trade. By the mid-1800s, European countries had cooperation agreements in place to help control the spread of cholera, plague, yellow fever, and other epidemic diseases, and by the early 1900s international regulations addressed drugs and alcohol sales, occupational health and safety, and water pollution.[5]

In recent decades, global health as a field of work and study has expanded in scope and recognition as modernization and globalization have occurred. Modern transportation allows infectious diseases to spread across the world at an alarming rate. Advances in medical technology and pharmaceuticals are curing diseases that used to be untreatable, but new technologies have also created superbugs that are resistant to current antibiotic therapies. And the threat of bioterrorism requires coordination of public health responses from many nations. The increasing attention on global health also arises from the continued and growing disparities in health status between nations and within nations, which raise human rights concerns and may contribute to insecurity.

Although the main health concerns of communities in rural Africa (often HIV/AIDS and malaria) are very different from the key health concerns of urban Americans (often heart disease and cancer), there are important commonalities across the globe. Emerging infections such as multidrug-resistant tuberculosis (MDR-TB), rising cancer rates, and the high prevalence of mental health disorders are concerns for everyone. Global health helps communities, nations, and the world prepare to respond appropriately to emergent health concerns.

1.4 HEALTH TRANSITIONS IN THE 20TH CENTURY

One hundred years ago, most populations across the world had similar health profiles: high birth rates, high death rates, short life expectancies, and a lot of disease and death due to infections and undernutrition. During the 20th century, most high-income nations made a transition to a lower birth rate, a lower death rate, longer life expectancies, and a higher burden from the chronic diseases often associated with overnutrition. Low-income countries have not experienced such dramatic changes, but the health profiles of middle-income areas are currently shifting. These demographic, epidemiologic, and nutrition transitions are summarized in **Table 1–2**.

In the United States, the leading causes of death in 1800 and 1900 were pneumonia (including pneumonia caused by influenza), tuberculosis, and diarrhea—all infectious diseases.[6] By 1950 the death rate had dropped significantly, life expectancy had increased, and the most common causes of death had shifted to heart disease, cancer, and stroke, the same noncommunicable diseases that are the most frequent causes of death today.[7] These changes in population health status were due to a variety of factors, including new health technologies (such as new

Table 1–2 Health transitions.

Category	Low-Income Areas (and most of the world 100 years ago)	Middle-Income Areas	High-Income Areas
Demographic Transition	High fertility rate	Intermediate fertility rate	Low fertility rate
	Relatively high child mortality rate	Low child mortality rate	Very low child mortality rate
	Relatively high mortality rate	Intermediate mortality rate	Relatively low mortality rate
	Relatively low life expectancy	Intermediate life expectancy	Relatively high life expectancy
	Children are a large proportion of the population	Intermediate aging profile	Older adults are a sizeable proportion of the population
Epidemiologic Transition	High burden from diseases of poverty (infectious diseases)	Dual burden of infectious and chronic diseases	High burden from diseases of affluence (chronic diseases)
Nutrition Transition	Underweight is a major concern	Concerns about underweight in some populations and obesity in others	Overweight and obesity are major concerns

vaccines, new antibiotics, and new contraceptives), improved nutrition, increased education, and economic growth.[8]

1.4.A Demographic Transitions

The **demographic transition** describes a shift toward lower birth and death rates that often occurs as populations move from being low-income economies (often referred to as developing countries) to being high-income economies (often called developed countries) (**Figure 1–2**).[9] Pre-transition populations have high birth rates and high death rates, and the population maintains a stable, but relatively small, number of people. During the early stages of the demographic transition, increased food security and improved health care reduce the death rate, but the birth rate stays high and the population size increases, possibly drastically. In later stages, education, technology, economic growth, and other factors reduce the birth rates—a process called the

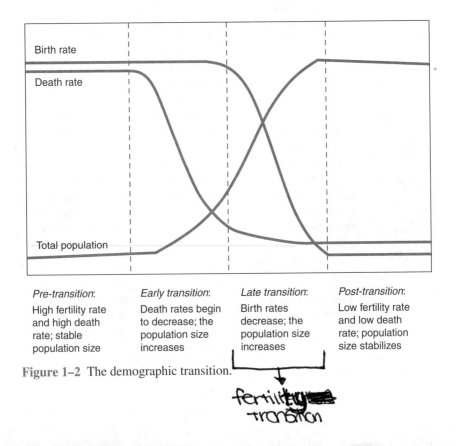

Pre-transition:	Early transition:	Late transition:	Post-transition:
High fertility rate and high death rate; stable population size	Death rates begin to decrease; the population size increases	Birth rates decrease; the population size increases	Low fertility rate and low death rate; population size stabilizes

Figure 1–2 The demographic transition.

fertility transition

fertility transition—and the population begins to stabilize at its larger size. Eventually, prolonged low birth rates may lead to a slow decline in population size.

1.4.B Epidemiologic Transitions

The **epidemiologic transition**, a shift from infectious diseases to chronic, noncommunicable diseases (NCDs) being the primary health problem in a population, often follows the demographic transition as the economic status of a population improves (**Figure 1–3**).[10] The epidemiologic transitions that occurred in many high-income countries in the past century are now being seen in many middle-income areas.[11] During the years of transition, many of these countries are experiencing a **dual burden** of disease, as some population groups continue to suffer from diseases of poverty (such as infections, undernutrition, and complications of childbirth), while other population groups bear a considerable burden from diseases of affluence (NCDs).

The complex epidemiologic profile of middle-income countries highlights two key points. One is that socioeconomic conditions have a huge

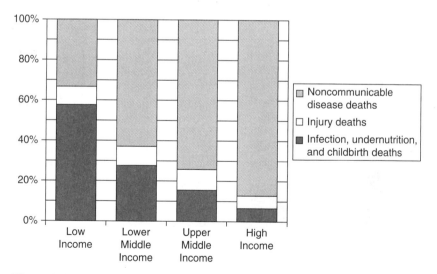

Figure 1–3 Proportion of deaths from various causes by country income level in 2008.

Source: Data from *The global burden of disease: 2004 update (May 2011 update).* Geneva: WHO; 2011.

influence on the diseases experienced by individuals and populations. There is heterogeneity in the disease profile within every country, with urban professionals in every part of the world having a very different health profile than the urban poor and rural residents surviving by subsistence farming. The other key observation is that every population at every income level has health concerns. Reducing deaths from infections and childbirth is an excellent public health achievement, especially because these conditions tend to kill young people. But those averted deaths will be replaced with other causes of death, often deaths from heart disease and cancer.

Thus, the goal of public health is not to prevent death, because everyone will eventually die of something. The goal of public health is to prevent *premature* death, and to promote long and healthy lives. By this standard, shifting the burden of disease from children and young adults to older adults is a good outcome, and that is what happens during the epidemiologic transition. The burden of disease in pre-transition populations falls heavily on the young, while the burden of disease in post-transition populations falls mostly on the elderly. This can be seen in the age distributions of deaths in low- and high-income countries. In some low-income countries, more than one-third of the deaths that occur are of children; in high-income countries, nearly all deaths occur in older adults (**Figure 1–4**).[12]

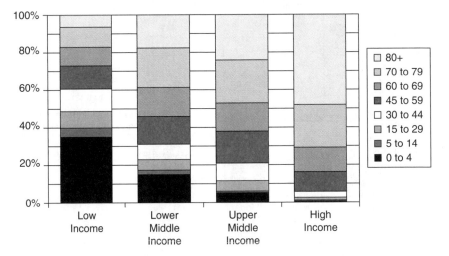

Figure 1–4 Proportion of deaths by age group and country income level in 2008.
Source: Data from *The global burden of disease: 2004 update (May 2011 update)*. Geneva: WHO; 2011.

It is also important to note that while the epidemiologic transition is a helpful model for understanding the differences in health status between higher- and lower-income countries and regions, the health changes that occur with economic development are much less predictable than the model implies.[13] Although many illnesses and deaths in low-income nations are due to infection and undernutrition and most illnesses and deaths in high-income nations are due to NCDs, globalization is reintroducing infectious diseases into industrialized nations and introducing new chronic diseases into developing nations. Every country in the world experiences a mix of deaths from infection, noncommunicable conditions, injuries, and other causes, even though the relative proportion of these causes of deaths differs by the country's income level.

1.4.C Nutrition Transitions

The **nutrition transition** describes a population shift from a stage in which undernutrition and nutrient deficiencies are prevalent to an intermediate stage in which undernutrition and obesity are both problems in the population to a stage in which overweight and obesity are the dominant nutritional disorders.[14] Pre-transition populations are concerned about having too little food and may consume primarily energy-dense foods that have a lot of calories but are low in nutrients. Children are at high risk of vitamin and mineral deficiencies because starchy staple foods form the bulk of the diet, and many children have stunted growth because they eat too few calories or too little protein. Few convenience foods are available, and a lot of effort goes into acquiring and preparing foods for consumption. Post-transition populations consume a greater variety of nutritious foods, but also eat more refined and processed foods, foods of animal origin, and fats. Most of these populations have shifted toward an industrialized economy that demands less physical labor from its workers, which exacerbates rising rates of obesity.

The nutrition transition provides a helpful framework for understanding the changing nutritional status of populations around the world, but an important new trend has emerged with the globalization of the food supply and with increasing urbanization in low-income countries: **lifestyle diseases** related to obesity and physical inactivity are now found among some populations even in pre-transition countries where the majority of families are food insecure and famine is a potential threat.[15]

1.5 RISK FACTORS

A first step toward improving population health is identifying major health problems and conducting research to identify the characteristics of the people most likely to be affected by those conditions. After data about a population have been collected, statistics are used to see if an exposure or characteristic is associated with an increased likelihood of having a particular disease. If a statistically significant **association** is present, then the next step is to try to determine whether the exposure causes the disease. A causal factor is an exposure that has been scientifically tested and shown to occur before the disease outcome and to contribute directly to its occurrence. Identifying **causation** requires more than just statistics. It also requires logical thinking (**Table 1–3**).[16,17] For example, there may be a statistical association between hot weather and the number of shark attacks, but that does not prove that hot weather causes sharks to fall into a frenzy. A more likely explanation is that hot weather increases the number of humans in the water, which increases the number of humans attacked. For that matter, there may be an association between ice cream sales and shark attacks. Removing the "risky" exposure by banning ice cream sales at the beach would probably not do much to prevent shark attacks, unless people stopped going to beaches because of the absence of ice cream.

A **risk factor** is an exposure or characteristic that increases the likelihood of developing a particular disease. Age, ethnicity, and genetic markers for certain diseases are examples of **unmodifiable risk factors** that cannot be changed. **Behavioral risk factors**, such as tobacco smoking and exercise habits, and other **modifiable risk factors** can be altered, even if making lifestyle changes is challenging for the individuals and the communities who are trying to adopt healthier behaviors. The goal of public health is not merely to identify problems, but to use that information to promote health and prevent disease. Once a major risk factor for a disease has been found, policy or programmatic interventions to reduce exposure to the risk factor (or to promote a protective factor) can be designed and implemented.

Some diseases have no currently known modifiable risk factors. It is not always possible to identify the **etiology**, or cause, of a particular disease or the risk factors for it, at least not with current technology. For example, the etiology of many neurological conditions like Parkinson's disease and epilepsy are unknown in most cases, as are the causes of many mental illnesses, autoimmune diseases, and other conditions. For these disorders, the

Table 1–3 Criteria for causation.

Criterion	Explanations/Examples
Is the association strong?	If smokers are 15 times more likely to develop lung cancer than nonsmokers, that is stronger evidence of causality than if smokers are 1.1 times more likely to develop lung cancer. Prevalence of the disease (the total amount of disease in a population) should be significantly higher in those exposed to the risk factor than those not. In studies that follow people over time (longitudinal studies), the incidence of the disease (number of new cases in a population) should be significantly higher in those exposed to the risk factor than those not exposed.
Is there clear temporality (time sequence)?	Exposure to the agent or risk factor must precede development of the disease, and the disease should follow exposure to the risk factor within a predictable time frame.
Is there a dose–response effect?	If exercising for 3 hours a week is slightly protective against breast cancer and exercising for 6 hours a week is more protective, it is more likely that exercise is protective than if the extra hours of exercise are not associated with increased protection. If exposure to radiation is harmful, then people with higher radiation exposure should be sicker than people with minimal exposure.
If an experiment removes the risk factor does that reduce the risk of the disease?	People who are exposed to the risk factor should develop the disease more frequently than those who do not have the exposure, and exposure to the risk factor should be more frequent among those with the disease than those without. Reducing or eliminating the risk factor should reduce the risk of the disease.
Other criteria	Is the link between the exposure and the outcome specific, biologically plausible, and consistent with existing knowledge? Have alternate explanations for the apparent causation been considered? Have different studies in different populations made consistent conclusions?

Source: Causal criteria from Hill AB. The environment and disease: association or causation? *Proc R Soc Med.* 1965;58:295–300; and Evans AS. Causation and disease: the Henle-Koch postulates revisited. *Yale J Biol Med.* 1976;49:175–195.

public health focus is on research to identify causal factors and on support for the individuals and families affected by the conditions.

But most diseases do have known risk factors and known protective factors. Many diseases are **multifactorial**, which means that they have many different causes and multiple risk factors. A risk factor is said to be a **necessary** part of the disease pathway if it must be present for a person to develop a disease. A risk factor is **sufficient** if that exposure or characteristic by itself can cause disease. Some exposures are necessary but not sufficient on their own to cause disease. Some exposures are sufficient but not necessary. Few risk factors are both necessary and sufficient. However, when several risk factors are present together they can create a situation in which disease can develop.

For example, heart disease is caused by the build-up of plaque on the walls of the arteries that supply blood to the heart. This build-up is associated with high cholesterol levels in the blood, inflammation, infection, and genetics. Diet, stress, and physical inactivity also contribute to the development of cardiovascular disease. Thus, there are many risk factors for heart disease and many targets for prevention. A broken hip may directly result from a fall, but the underlying cause of the fracture might be osteoporosis (loss of bone density) caused by genetics, inactivity, lack of calcium in the diet during childhood, endocrine disorders, or one of many other medical conditions, and the fall itself may have occurred because of a loss of balance due to a nervous system disorder like Parkinson's disease or multiple sclerosis, or because of vision problems, or because of not living in a barrier-free home or with someone who can assist with tasks that require reaching or balancing. Addressing any one of these contributing factors may prevent a negative health outcome.

Public health considers personal biology, psychology, behavior, and other characteristics to be only a starting point for understanding the risk factors for disease. A person's friends, family, and coworkers also contribute to the health problems that an individual is likely to encounter, whether that is an increased risk of knee injuries in a person whose closest friends are avid basketball players or an increased risk of obesity in a person whose family gatherings are built around high-calorie foods. Living and working conditions, such as the quality of housing available in a person's neighborhood and whether local employers provide health insurance, add another layer of factors that affect health. And broader social, cultural, economic, political, environmental, and policy considerations also influence individual and community health.[18] Targeting a risk factor at any one of these levels can improve personal and public health (**Figure 1–5**).

Individual characteristics and behavior	Social networks (friends, family, coworkers)	Living and working conditions (including access to health services)	Broader social, cultural, economic, political, environmental, and policy conditions

Figure 1–5 Contributors to individual and population health.

Source: Adapted from the Committee on Assuring the Health of the Public in the 21st Century. *The future of the public's health in the 21st century.* Washington DC: National Academies Press; 2002.

1.6 PREVENTION

A **causal web** can be used to display the relationships among the many different biological, behavioral, social, economic, political, and environmental exposures that might have a causal relationship with a particular health outcome. Causal webs indicate the immediate causes of disease and also show more distant causes. For example, **Figure 1–6** shows the

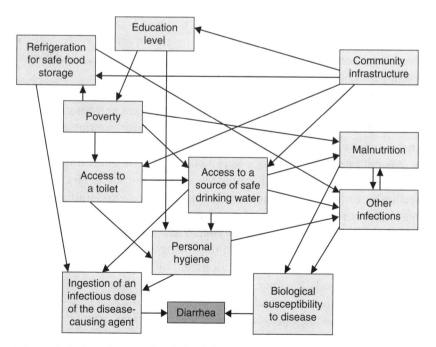

Figure 1–6 Sample causal web for infectious diarrhea.

relationships between both direct and less direct causes of infectious diarrhea, which is usually acquired through the ingestion of fecally contaminated food or water.

When a complex set of characteristics contribute to causing disease, there are also multiple paths to a solution. Interrupting any of the pathways shown on a causal diagram may prevent the disease outcome for at least some members of a population. An intervention that removes any one of the arrows in Figure 1–6, whether by introducing electricity to a rural community to allow for refrigeration, teaching illiterate mothers to read, or bringing low-cost water filters to an urban slum, could be successful in preventing at least some cases of childhood diarrhea. Solutions to community and global health concerns often must address broad socioeconomic and environmental issues and not just household problems.

There are three levels of prevention (Table 1–4). When modifiable risk factors for a disease have been identified, the goal is **primary prevention**, preventing the disease from ever occurring. Primary prevention methods include immunizations, improved nutrition, adequate sleep, safety devices, health education, and any interventions that reduce susceptibility to infection, injury, or disease. The goal of **secondary prevention** is to diagnose disease at an early stage when it has not yet caused significant damage to the body and can be treated more easily. The aim of **tertiary prevention** is to reduce complications in those with symptomatic disease in order to prevent death or minimize disability.

Given the three levels of prevention, there is almost always some intervention that could improve the health of those who are vulnerable to a particular disease or are already sick. Most public health campaigns focus on primary prevention, such as the promotion of handwashing, breastfeeding, mosquito net use, family planning methods, and immunizations. Some prevention work focuses on changing the health environment by spraying insecticides to kill the mosquitoes that spread infections, implementing clean delivery room practices to prevent infections of new mothers and newborns, and increasing access to improved sanitation facilities to prevent diarrhea. Other efforts focus on improving access to health care and health insurance, to essential medications and micronutrient supplements, and to healthy foods through community-building and policy changes. These are in addition to secondary prevention activities such as screening promotions and tertiary prevention methods that treat existing diseases and disabilities.

Table 1–4 Levels of prevention.

Level	Also Called...	Target Population	Goal	Examples
Primary Prevention	Prevention	People without disease	Prevent disease from ever occurring	• Giving vitamin A capsules to at-risk children to prevent blindness • Giving tetanus shots to pregnant women to prevent tetanus
Secondary Prevention	Early diagnosis	People with early, non-symptomatic disease	Reduce the severity of disease and prevent disability and death	• Screening with mammography to detect cases of breast cancer in early stages • Checking blood pressure routinely to detect early hypertension
Tertiary Prevention	Treatment and rehabilitation	People with symptomatic disease	Reduce impairment and minimize suffering	• Detecting cases of acute respiratory infections in children early so they can be treated with antibiotics • Checking for foot problems among diabetic persons so they do not develop into severe ulcers • Providing physical therapy to people who have been injured in a vehicle accident in order to prevent long-term disability

1.7 CAREERS IN GLOBAL HEALTH

Global health professionals work in a variety of fields to promote population health. Among other roles, global health workers track outbreaks of infectious diseases, develop new vaccines, monitor the safety of medications, assess environmental risk factors for disease, educate communities about diabetes care, and promote HIV/AIDS awareness and prevention. Public health geneticists determine which genes are associated with an increased risk of cancer. Public health educators and nutritionists work with schools and communities to reduce risky behaviors, such as unsafe sex, drug use, and reckless driving, and to promote healthy behaviors such as wearing bicycle helmets, getting screened for cervical cancer, and eating vegetables. Environmental public health experts develop plans for communities that want to reduce the spread of infections caused by insect bites. Public health administrators work with hospitals and physicians, elected officials and lawyers, biomedical researchers, the pharmaceutical industry, and others to promote health.

People who want to work in global health need to understand the social and environmental contributors to disease and the biological causes of disease. They must be familiar with the traditional areas of international health, such as infectious disease, nutrition, child health, reproductive health, and water and sanitation. They must also be knowledgeable about emerging global public health concerns, such as aging, mental health, injury prevention, and food safety. An understanding of the impact of poverty, culture, and economic globalization on health is also essential.

The diversity of work within global health means that there are many pathways to getting started in a global health career. Many professionals working in the field have training in at least one of the core disciplines of public health, which include health education and health behavior; epidemiology and biostatistics (the fields that focus on measuring health status in populations); environmental health; and health policy, health economics, and health administration and management. Global health professionals may also specialize in areas such as public health nutrition, maternal and child health, emergency preparedness and response, and public health research. Common undergraduate majors for those preparing for global health careers include biology, psychology, sociology, and the health sciences, and majors in fields like business, communications, economics, political science, international relations, and statistics can also offer excellent preparation. Every area of study provides tools that can be applied to improving public health as a professional or as a volunteer.

1.8 DISCUSSION QUESTIONS

1. How has the medical system contributed to your health? Based on the list of public health services in Table 1–1, how has the public health system contributed to your health? What are the differences in how medicine and public health influence your health?

2. What are some of the most significant health concerns in your community? Are these concerns that are likely to be shared by other communities in your country and in other parts of the world? Could these problems be considered global health issues?

3. Do you agree that shifting the burden of disease and death from the young to the old is a successful public health outcome?

4. Choose one relatively common disease affecting health in your community, then list as many risk factors for that disease as you can think of in 2 minutes. How many of the risk factors on your list are modifiable? How many are necessary? How many are sufficient? What interventions would reduce the number of people in your community who develop the disease?

5. Sketch out a causal web for a relatively common disease in your country, adding at least 10 risk factors to the figure. Based on the arrows on your web, what interventions might prevent the disease from occurring?

6. What are some examples of primary prevention, secondary prevention, and tertiary prevention activities you have engaged in during the past year?

7. How does global health relate to your major field of study and/or the field you are working in?

REFERENCES

1. Huber M, Knottnerus JA, Green L, et al. How should we define health? *BMJ.* 2011;343:d4163.
2. Harrell JA, Baker EL; Essential Services Work Group. The essential services of public health. *Leadersh Public Health.* 1994;3:27–30.
3. Koplan JP, Bond TC, Merson MH, et al.; Consortium of Universities for Global Health Executive Board. Towards a common definition of global health. *Lancet.* 2009;373:1993–1995.
4. Brown TM, Cueto M, Fee E. The World Health Organization and the transition from "international" to "global" public health. *Am J Public Health.* 2006;96:62–72.
5. Fidler DP. The globalization of public health: the first 100 years of international health diplomacy. *Bull World Health Organ.* 2001;79:842–849.
6. Jones DS, Podolsky SH, Greene JA. The burden of disease and the changing task of medicine. *New Engl J Med.* 2012;366:2333–2338.
7. Guyer B, Freedman MA, Strobino DM, Sondik EJ. Annual summary of vital statistics: trends in the health of Americans during the 20th century. *Pediatrics.* 2000;106:1307–1317.
8. Martens P. Health transitions in a globalising world: towards more disease or sustained health? *Futures.* 2002:34:635–648.
9. Kirk D. Demographic transition theory. *Pop Studies.* 1996;50:361–387.

10. Omran AR. The epidemiologic transition: a theory of the epidemiology of population change. *Milbank Mem Fund Q.* 1971;29:509–538.

11. *The global burden of disease: 2004 update (May 2011 update).* Geneva: WHO; 2011.

12. Lopez AD, Mathers CD, Ezzati M, Jamison DT, Murray CJL. *Global burden of disease and risk factors.* Washington DC: Oxford University Press and IBRD/World Bank; 2006.

13. Caldwell JC. Population health in transition. *Bull World Health Organ.* 2001;79:159–170.

14. Popkin BM. Global nutrition dynamics: the world is shifting rapidly toward a diet linked with noncommunicable diseases. *Am J Clin Nutr.* 2006;84:289–298.

15. Caballero B. The global epidemic of obesity: an overview. *Epidemiol Rev.* 2007;29:1–5.

16. Hill AB. The environment and disease: association or causation? *Proc R Soc Med.* 1965;58:295–300.

17. Evans AS. Causation and disease: the Henle-Koch postulates revisited. *Yale J Biol Med.* 1976;49:175–195.

18. Committee on Assuring the Health of the Public in the 21st Century. *The future of the public's health in the 21st century.* Washington DC: National Academies Press; 2002.

CHAPTER 2

Measuring the Global Burden of Disease

The burden of disease, disability, and death caused by infections, malnutrition, chronic diseases, mental health conditions, and injuries varies between countries and within countries. Quantifying the health problems that affect populations and the individuals who make up those populations provides a foundation for making prudent policy and funding decisions at local, national, and global levels.

2.1 THE IMPORTANCE OF HEALTH METRICS

As more resources are being devoted to global health efforts, it is becoming increasingly important to quantify the health needs in various parts of the world, to identify major modifiable risk factors for common diseases, to assess the impact of new public health interventions, and to monitor changes in the health status of populations over time. All of these measures provide an evidence base for making policy and funding decisions.[1] This chapter describes the key measures of health and disease used in global health, the major categories of disease, and several helpful sources of reliable health information.

In order to highlight key measures of global health throughout the book, eight countries representing a range of world regions and economic statuses will be highlighted in most chapters (**Table 2–1**).[2–4] These countries also represent a range of population sizes, including the three most populous countries in the world (China, India, and the United States), but also Sierra Leone, which is not among the 100 most populous countries. Statistics for nearly all of the other countries in the world are available from the same sources provided for each data table and graph in the book.

Table 2–1 Basic information for featured countries in 2011.

Country	USA	South Korea	Poland	Brazil	China	India	Kenya	Sierra Leone
World region	North America	East Asia	Europe	South America	East Asia	South Asia	East Africa	West Africa
Income group	High	High	High	Upper Middle	Upper Middle	Lower Middle	Low	Low
Income group 5 years before (in 2006)	High	High	Upper Middle	Lower Middle	Lower Middle	Low	Low	Low
Human development ranking (out of 187 ranked countries)	4	15	39	84	101	134	143	180
Population size	313 million	48 million	38 million	197 million	1348 million	1242 million	42 million	6 million

Source: Data from *Human development report 2012*. New York: UNDP; 2012; and *World development report 2011*. Washington DC: World Bank; 2011; and *World development report 2006*. Washington DC: World Bank; 2005.

2.2 MEASURING HEALTH AND DISEASE

The key measures of health and disease in a population include information about population size, the birth rate and death rate, the causes of death, the frequency and causes of disease and disability, and the rate at which members of the population engage in risky behaviors.

2.2.A Vital Statistics and Demography

Demography is the study of the size and composition of human populations. Most countries maintain **vital statistics** on their residents, which are collected from birth and death certificates, from marriage and divorce certificates, and from census records. Demographers use these statistics to understand the current population distribution and to predict the size and characteristics of the population in future years.

The **birth rate** is the annual number of births per 1000 people in the total population and the **death rate** (or **mortality rate**) is the annual number of deaths per 1000 total population. The death rate is usually higher in populations with a large percentage of older adults than in populations with lots of children, so an **age-adjusted rate** that accounts for differences in the age structures of populations is usually used to compare mortality rates in two or more populations.

2.2.B Measuring Mortality

Identifying when an individual has died is fairly uncomplicated, but measuring **mortality** at the population level can be challenging for two principal reasons. The first is that in many parts of the world there is no system for reliably registering vital statistics. In places where most births and deaths occur in homes instead of in hospitals, few births and deaths are documented by government officials. The most disadvantaged populations—often the ones with the highest mortality rates—are the least likely to have their life events accurately counted. Thus, while very precise mortality statistics are available from high-income countries, death rates in low-income countries often have to be estimated based on limited data. The second key challenge is assigning one cause of death to each deceased individual. Should a person with HIV/AIDS who dies of tuberculosis be recorded as an AIDS death or a TB death? Should a person with advanced-stage cancer who dies of pneumonia be counted as a cancer death or an infectious disease death? These decisions about how to assign causes of death can have a significant impact on which diseases appear to be the most common causes of mortality in a population. Even with these limitations, epidemiologists using standardized estimation methods and the best available data are able to make reasonably accurate assessments of the annual number and causes of death by age group and sex in every region of the world.

Another common way of examining mortality and survival at the population level is through the estimation of life expectancy. **Life expectancy at birth** is the median expected age at death of all babies born alive. Some estimates of life expectancy instead focus on **healthy life expectancy**, which is the number of years the average individual born into the population can expect to live without disability (**Figure 2–1**).[5] Life expectancy captures the

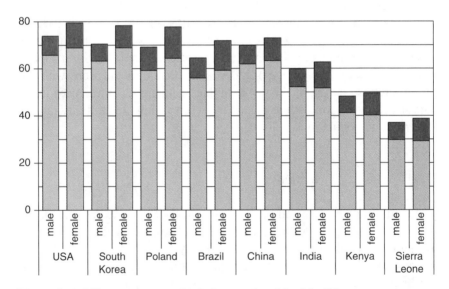

Figure 2–1 Life expectancy at birth (in years) and healthy life expectancy at birth in 2000. The total height of each bar represents total life expectancy at birth. The lighter portion of the bar represents the number of years the average person in the region is expected to live a healthy life, and the darker portion of the bar represents years the average person is expected to live with disability.

Source: Data from Mathers CD, Murray CJL, Lopez AD, et al. *Estimates of healthy life expectancy countries for 191 countries in the year 2000: methods and results.* WHO Global Programme on Evidence for Health Policy Working Paper No. 38. Geneva: World Health Organization; 2001.

burden from infant and child deaths in addition to the average age at death of adults. In places with high infant mortality rates, the median age at death is often in middle adulthood, which represents an age somewhere between a large number of child deaths and an even larger number of deaths in older adults.

While there are considerable differences in life expectancy at birth between various countries and world regions, the life expectancy of people who have already survived to adulthood is relatively similar across nations (**Table 2–2**).[6] In most parts of the world an adult who has survived to age 50 can expect to live into his or her 70s or beyond and a person who has survived to age 70 can expect to live until about age 80. This is one of the reasons why aging is a concern in all countries, even those with a relatively low life expectancy at birth.

Table 2–2 Life expectancy by age in 2009.

Country	USA	South Korea	Poland	Brazil	China	India	Kenya	Sierra Leone
At least half of **newborns** will live until age…	76	77	72	70	72	63	58	48
At least half of **5-year-old children** will live to age…	77	77	72	72	73	67	63	60
At least half of **50-year-old adults** will live to age…	80	79	75	76	76	73	72	70
At least half of **70-year-old adults** will live to age…	84	83	82	83	81	80	80	79
At least half of **85-year-old adults** will live to age…	91	90	90	91	90	89	89	89

Source: Data from *World health statistics 2011*. Geneva: WHO; 2011.

2.2.C Measuring Morbidity

Morbidity refers to the presence of illness or disease, whether that disease is relatively mild, like the common cold, or quite severe. The two most common terms used to describe the morbidity rate for a particular disease in a population are incidence and prevalence. **Incidence** is the number of *new* cases of the disease occurring in a time period divided by the total number of people at risk for that disease in that time period. Incidence is usually used to study infectious diseases, acute diseases (diseases that occur suddenly), and outbreaks. **Prevalence** is the number of *total* existing cases, both newly diagnosed cases and cases diagnosed in the past, divided by the total number of people in the population at the time the prevalence is measured. Prevalence is usually used to describe the amount of chronic (long-lasting) disease in population, such as the proportion of a population with diabetes, asthma, or schizophrenia. The difference between the two terms is illustrated in **Figure 2–2**.

One of the goals of public health is to decrease the incidence and prevalence of diseases and disabilities. For example, the incidence of a

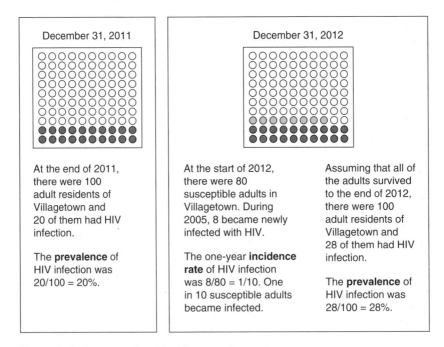

Figure 2–2 An example of incidence and prevalence.

disease may decrease if a new vaccine or other preventive measure becomes available, and the prevalence of a disease usually decreases if a new therapy cures lots of cases of the disease. These successful interventions are said to increase the number of **quality-adjusted life years (QALYs)** for recipients by adding to the duration and quality of life. However, there are some times when an increased prevalence is considered to be a public health success. For example, the reported prevalence of a disease may increase when a new diagnostic test allows more people with the disease to be properly diagnosed or when a new therapy allows people to live longer after developing the disease, even if the treatment does not cure the disease.

Health researchers measuring the **burden of disease** in a population must have a clear **case definition** that spells out exactly what characteristics indicate that a person has the disease of interest. They must also specify a well-defined population of interest, especially if the researchers are tracking changes in the health status of a population over time. (Because the prevalence of disease in a community may change due to the migration of sick people into the community or the migration of healthy people out of the community, some studies track individuals rather than just whole towns or cities.) Age-adjustment can be used to standardize two populations with different age structures before their morbidity rates are compared.

2.2.D Measuring Disability

The **disability-adjusted life year (DALY)** is a way of estimating the burden of disease in a population by combining the burden from premature deaths, measured as **years of life lost (YLLs)**, plus the burden from disability, measured as **years of life with disability (YLDs)**. Weights are assigned to the level of disability caused by each type of physical or mental health condition. Diseases that kill children, who would have had decades of productive life remaining had they survived, and chronic conditions that limit productivity for lengthy periods of time result in many YLLs and YLDs.

One of the key benefits of the DALY is that it highlights the high burden of disability caused by mental health disorders. Neuropsychiatric conditions (including conditions like Alzheimer's disease, epilepsy, and Parkinson's disease as well as depression, anxiety disorders, schizophrenia, and other mental health issues) and self-inflicted injuries are estimated to account for 3.5% of deaths worldwide each year, but they contribute more than 14% of DALYs.[7]

The main criticism of DALYs is the difficulty in assigning weights to the amount of disability caused by various illnesses and impairments. It will never be possible to assign an accurate weight to the decrease in quality of life caused by blindness, loss of a limb, depression, a brain tumor, or asthma, because the experience of disability varies so much based on the individual, living conditions, the level of community support, access to health care, and other individual factors. For example, the amount of disability caused by an amputated foot would be much higher for a manual laborer in a low-resource setting where prosthetics are not available than it would be for an office worker in a place where high-tech prosthetics are common.

2.2.E Quantifying Risk Factors

Health metrics also seek to identify risk factors for death, disease, and disability, and to measure the number of people worldwide who are exposed to these risks. The focus is usually on modifiable risk factors, because the prevalence of these exposures can be reduced with public health interventions. Some of the most common preventable risk factors are listed in **Table 2–3**. Different countries have different risk profiles, and in many places men and women have somewhat different sets of risks (**Table 2–4**).

Table 2–3 Common risk factors for morbidity and mortality.

Health-related Behaviors	Nutritional Exposures	Environmental Exposures	Untreated Medical Conditions
• Tobacco use • Physical inactivity • Unsafe sex • Alcohol abuse • Lack of contraception • Illicit drug use	• Overweight and obesity • Child underweight • Low fruit and vegetable intake • High fat intake • Suboptimal breastfeeding • Vitamin A deficiency • Zinc deficiency • Iron deficiency	• Indoor smoke from solid fuels • Unsafe water, sanitation, hygiene • Urban outdoor air pollution • Occupational risks • Lead exposure	• High blood pressure (hypertension) • High blood glucose (hyperglycemia, which is a risk factor for diabetes) • High cholesterol (hypercholesterolemia) • Chronic cancer-associated infections

Source: Information from *Global status report on noncommunicable diseases 2010*. Geneva: WHO; 2011; and *Global health risks: mortality and burden of disease attributable to selected major risks*. Geneva: WHO; 2009.

Table 2–4 Prevalence of selected risk factors in 2008.

Country	Age Group (years)	Sex	USA	South Korea	Poland	Brazil	China	India	Kenya	Sierra Leone
Prevalence (%) of tobacco use	≥25	Male	33	49	36	22	51	26	26	39
		Female	25	7	25	13	2	4	1	8
Physical inactivity (%)	≥15	Male	34	–	24	47	30	13	15	16
		Female	47	–	32	52	32	18	18	24
Alcohol consumption per person per year (liters)	≥15	Both	10	15	14	10	6	3	4	10
Prevalence (%) of high blood pressure (≥ 140/90 mm Hg)	≥25	Male	17	18	41	39	30	23	37	42
		Female	14	13	33	27	26	23	33	41
Mean blood pressure (mm Hg)*	≥25	Male	123	124	135	133	128	124	132	135
		Female	118	117	130	125	124	123	130	135
Prevalence (%) of high fasting blood glucose*	≥25	Male	13	7	8	10	11	11	8	9
		Female	9	5	7	10	10	11	8	10
Prevalence (%) of obesity	≥20	Male	30	7	23	17	5	1	3	4
		Female	33	8	23	22	7	3	7	10
Mean blood cholesterol level (mmol/L)*	≥25	Male	5.1	4.8	5.3	4.8	4.5	4.3	4.3	3.8
		Female	5.2	4.9	5.2	4.9	4.6	4.5	4.4	4.1

*These values are age-standardized so that the countries' values can be compared. SBP ≥ 140 mm Hg is considered to be hypertension and cholesterol ≥ 5.0 mmol/L is considered to be hypercholesterolemia. Medication can be used to lower both of these values.

Source: Data from Global Burden of Metabolic Risk Factors of Chronic Diseases Collaborating Group. *Country trends in metabolic risk factors.* London: Imperial College London; 2011; and Hallal PC, Andersen LB, Bull FC, Guthold R, Haskell W, Ekelund U; Lancet Physical Activity Series Working Group. *Global physical activity levels: surveillance progress, pitfalls, and prospects.* Lancet. 2012;380:247–257; and *World health statistics 2012.* Geneva: WHO; 2012.

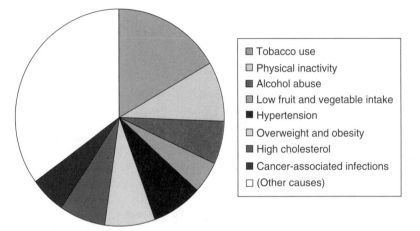

Figure 2–3 The proportion of *noncommunicable disease* deaths worldwide in 2008 attributable to various risk factors.

Source: Data from *Global status report on noncommunicable diseases 2010.* Geneva: WHO; 2011.

A few of these preventable risk factors are responsible for a sizeable proportion of all global deaths each year. For example, more than 10% of adult deaths worldwide are attributable to tobacco use,[8] alcohol consumption is the cause of about 4% of deaths worldwide every year,[9] and vitamin and mineral deficiencies contribute to more than 10% of the annual deaths of young children.[10] Together, modifiable risk factors are thought to be responsible for at least two-thirds of all worldwide deaths from noncommunicable diseases like heart disease, stroke, diabetes, cancer, and chronic lung disease[11] (**Figure 2–3**). Other exposures increase the risk of morbidity or mortality from particular diseases.[12–14] For example, outdoor air pollution may be the cause of 5% of lung cancer deaths worldwide,[15] more than half of all strokes are attributed to high blood pressure,[16] and more than 70% of cases of cervical cancer are associated with chronic infection with human papillomavirus (HPV).[17] Identifying common contributors to reduced individual and population health allows health scientists, clinicians, educators, and individuals to prioritize actions that lessen exposure to these hazards.[18]

2.2.F Health Systems Performance

In addition to measuring health outcomes like mortality and disability, it is important to track the performance of health systems, the financers and providers of health care and public health services, because the health of a population is often a function of the access of its members to essential health services. Health systems metrics may involve quantifying the coverage rates for various interventions, tallying the financial, human, and material resources put into health systems, evaluating the satisfaction of clients with health service providers and public health programs, determining which interventions are cost-effective, and tracking the inequalities that may remain within a health system.[1] This information provides a foundation for priority setting and for evidence-based policy and practice.

2.3 CLASSIFYING DISEASE

The World Health Organization and most of the Global Burden of Disease studies use three main classifications for causes of death and disability: (1) communicable (infectious) diseases (a category often grouped with pregnancy-related conditions, diseases of newborns, and nutritional deficiencies), (2) noncommunicable conditions (including mental health disorders), and (3) injuries. The proportion of deaths (**Figure 2–4**) and DALYs (**Figure 2–5**) due to each of these categories varies significantly between countries in different income strata.[7]

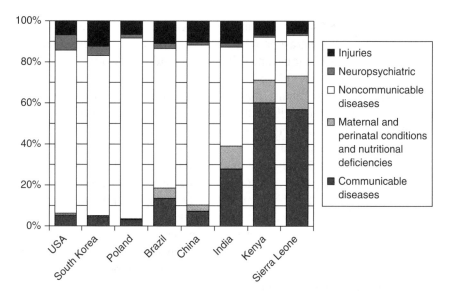

Figure 2–4 Estimated proportion of deaths due to communicable diseases, noncommunicable diseases, and injuries in 2004.

Source: Data from *The global burden of disease: 2004 update*. Geneva: WHO; 2008.

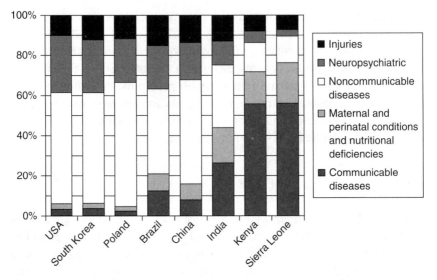

Figure 2–5 Estimated proportion of DALYs due to communicable diseases, noncommunicable diseases, and injuries in 2004.

Source: Data from *The global burden of disease: 2004 update.* Geneva: WHO; 2008.

2.3.A Infectious and Parasitic Diseases

Communicable diseases are caused by infectious agents such as bacteria, viruses, fungi, and parasites (such as protozoa and helminths/worms). Tuberculosis, sexually transmitted infections, intestinal worms, meningitis, malaria, and respiratory infections are all in this category. In the early and middle part of the 20th century, the use of microscopes and the development of new laboratory techniques led to the identification of many specific microbes and the development of vaccines and antibiotics like penicillin. These discoveries generated a great deal of optimism and confidence about the ability of humans to control and eradicate communicable diseases. However, although modern science has provided a good understanding of the infectious disease process and allowed for the development of therapies and cures for many types of infection, scientists now recognize that microbes continue to adapt and to emerge. Even with improved prevention and therapeutic techniques, infectious diseases continue to be a health risk in all populations in every part of the world. Developing new vaccines, treatments, and prevention methods remains an important part of global health.

This disease category is often grouped with other conditions that primarily affect lower-income populations: perinatal conditions (diseases of newborns), maternal conditions, and nutritional deficiencies. Perinatal conditions include low birthweight, premature (early) birth, birth asphyxia, and birth trauma. Maternal conditions are those related to pregnancy, childbirth, and the hours after giving birth. Malnutrition may result when a person does not consume nutrients in the right quantities and combination. Taking in too few, or too many, calories or nutrients can be a cause of poor health. In addition to under-weight- and obesity-related conditions, malnutrition includes deficiencies of particular vitamins and minerals, such as iron, vitamin A, zinc, and iodine.

2.3.B Noncommunicable Diseases

Noncommunicable diseases (often shortened to "**NCDs**") are conditions that are not contagious, such as heart disease and other cardiovascular diseases, cancers, chronic respiratory diseases, endocrine and metabolic disorders, digestive diseases, kidney diseases, musculoskeletal and skin diseases, and neurological and psychiatric disorders (**Table 2–5**). Most noncommunicable conditions are chronic diseases that develop gradually and last for a long time.

Noncommunicable conditions result from a variety of etiologic processes. Some NCDs are caused by inflammation and by immune system dysfunctions. The immune system helps the body to fight disease by recognizing and attacking invaders like infectious agents and allergens. Autoimmune disorders like lupus and rheumatoid arthritis occur when the body has trouble distinguishing between "self" and "nonself" and begins to attack its own cells. Allergies are another type of immune dysfunction in which the body is hypersensitive to substances that are usually not harmful. And although the process is not yet well understood, inflammation appears to play a role not just in arthritis and other conditions in which swelling is easily observed, but also in heart disease and possibly in diabetes, cognitive disorders, and many other conditions. Poor nutrition and some infections (like HIV) can also cause immune system suppression and lead to other illnesses.

Some noncommunicable conditions are caused by genetic disorders present at birth. Genes are sequences of nucleic acids that are part of the chromosomes that are found in the nucleus of every cell in the human body.

Table 2–5 Examples of noncommunicable conditions.

Cardiovascular Diseases	• Ischemic heart disease (heart attacks)	• Cerebrovascular disease (strokes) • Hypertension	• Rheumatic heart disease • Congestive heart failure
Blood Disorders	• Anemia • Hemophilia	• Sickle cell • Thalassemia	• Hemochromatosis
Cancers	• Lung cancer • Stomach cancer • Colorectal cancer • Liver cancer • Breast cancer • Esophageal cancer	• Lymphoma • Mouth and throat cancer • Prostate cancer • Leukemia • Cervical cancer	• Pancreatic cancer • Bladder cancer • Ovarian cancer • Uterine cancer • Melanoma and other skin cancers
Respiratory Diseases	• Chronic obstructive pulmonary disease (COPD)	• Asthma	• Cystic fibrosis
Endocrine and Metabolic Disorders	• Diabetes	• Thyroid disease	• Adrenal disorders (like Addison's disease and Cushing's syndrome)
Digestive Diseases	• Cirrhosis of the liver • Gallstones	• Hernias • Peptic ulcer disease	• Inflammatory bowel disease • Hemorrhoids
Genitourinary Diseases	• Kidney disease	• Benign prostatic hypertrophy (BPH)	• Pelvic inflammatory disease (PID)
Musculoskeletal Diseases	• Muscular dystrophy	• Osteoarthritis • Rheumatoid arthritis	• Osteoporosis
Skin Diseases	• Acne	• Eczema	• Psoriasis
Oral Diseases	• Dental caries (cavities)	• Periodontal disease	• Edentulism (toothlessness)
Sense Organ Disorders	• Blindness • Deafness	• Cataracts • Glaucoma	• Macular degeneration

This genetic material directs every function of the body, including cell replication, which is important for healing as well as for growth and development. Each cell contains identical DNA (deoxyribonucleic acid), although only some parts of the code are active in certain cells, which is why cells in a person's heart form different kinds of tissue than the cells that line the intestine. A **genotype** is the version of a gene a person carries and a **phenotype** is the way a characteristic that results from having a particular **allele**, or version of a gene, is expressed—perhaps in physical appearance, the way a person develops or functions physiologically, or disease status. Some alleles are **dominant**, which means that inheriting a copy of that allele from either parent will cause a person to display the phenotype associated with that allele. For example, Huntington's disease, which causes a progressive degeneration of brain cells, is an autosomal dominant genetic disorder. Some alleles are **recessive**, which means that a person must inherit a copy of the allele from both parents to display the phenotype associated with the allele. Cystic fibrosis, sickle cell disease, and hemophilia are examples of autosomal recessive disorders. Some conditions are caused by the presence of an extra chromosome or a missing part of a chromosome. For example, Down syndrome (trisomy 21) is the result of an extra 21st chromosome. Other conditions are caused by genetic **mutations**, permanent changes in the sequence of bases that make up DNA that occur after birth. These mutations may result from exposure to radiation, chemicals, pollutants, or other substances. Cancers generally involve a series of mutations that lead to tumor development.

The causes of many NCDs are not yet clear. However, all of the most common causes of NCD death—heart disease, cancer, stroke, chronic obstructive pulmonary disease (COPD), and diabetes—are linked to unhealthy behaviors such as tobacco use, physical inactivity, overconsumption of alcohol, and diets that are low in fruits and vegetables and high in fats.[11] NCDs are the leading cause of death of adults in every part of the world (**Figure 2–6**).

2.3.C Neuropsychiatric Disorders

The neuropsychiatric conditions category includes mental illnesses as well as developmental disorders (such as mental retardation), autism spectrum disorders, neurological disorders (such as Parkinson's disease, multiple sclerosis, cerebral palsy, and migraines), seizure disorders such as epilepsy, and dementias like Alzheimer's disease. There are a wide variety

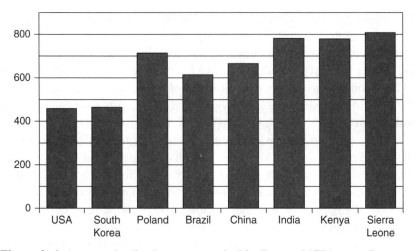

Figure 2–6 Age-standardized noncommunicable disease (NCD) mortality rate per 100,000 people in 2008.

Source: Data from *Global status report on noncommunicable diseases 2010*. Geneva: WHO; 2011.

of recognized mental illnesses, including anxiety disorders, mood disorders, impulse-control disorders, substance abuse, and schizophrenia and other delusional disorders (**Table 2–6**).[19] One challenge when trying to assess the impact of neuropsychiatric conditions on population health and disability is that the diagnosis of mental health disorders is in part dependent on culture,[20] and many disorders exist as part of a spectrum where the distinction between what is classified as "normal" and what is classified as a "disorder" is blurry. Mental health disorders are known to be significantly underdiagnosed and undertreated worldwide.[21]

2.3.D Injuries

An **injury** is physical damage to the body. An injury may be a fracture of a bone, a strain or sprain of a joint, a brain or spinal cord injury, wounds to the skin, or damage to internal organs. Injuries may be unintentional, such as a traffic accident, fall, burn, or drowning, or intentional. Intentional acts are further classified as self-directed violence (self-mutilation or suicide), interpersonal violence by family members, intimate partners, or community members, or collective violence such as war, mob violence, gang violence,

Table 2–6 Types of mental health disorders.

Type of Disorder	Examples
Disorders usually first diagnosed in infancy, childhood, or adolescence	• Developmental disorders such as mental retardation • Learning, motor skills, and communication disorders • Pervasive developmental disorders like autism and Asperger's • Attention-deficit and disruptive behavior disorders like attention-deficit hyperactivity disorder (ADHD), conduct disorder, and oppositional-defiant disorder • Tic disorders like Tourette's
Cognitive disorders	• Alzheimer's and other dementias
Substance abuse disorders	• Alcohol abuse • Drug abuse with amphetamines, caffeine, cannabis, cocaine, hallucinogens, inhalants, nicotine, opioids, phencyclidines, sedatives, hypnotics, or anxiolytics
Schizophrenia and other psychotic disorders	• Schizophrenia • Delusional disorder
Mood disorders	• Major depressive disorder (unipolar depressive disorders) • Bipolar disorder
Anxiety disorders	• Panic disorder • Obsessive-compulsive disorder (OCD) • Posttraumatic stress disorder (PTSD)
Impulse-control disorders	• Anorexia nervosa • Bulimia nervosa • Pathological gambling

Source: Information from *Diagnostic and statistical manual of mental disorders*, 4th edition (DSM-IV-TR). Arlington VA: American Psychiatric Association; 2000.

or terrorist acts (**Table 2–7**).[22] About two-thirds of injury deaths worldwide each year are from unintentional injuries and one-third from intentional injuries, with some variation between regions and countries (**Figure 2–7**).[7,23]

    People living in poverty are at increased risk of injury because they are more likely than others to live, work, and go to school in unsafe environments. For example, low-income individuals are more likely to use

Table 2–7 Examples of types of injuries.

Unintentional Injuries	Intentional Injuries
• Road-traffic injuries	*Self-directed violence*
• Falls	• Suicide
• Burns	• Cutting
• Drowning	*Interpersonal violence*
• Poisoning	• Spousal/intimate partner abuse
	• Child abuse
	• Elder abuse
	Collective violence
	• War
	• Terrorist acts
	• Gang violence

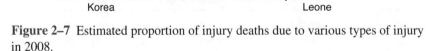

Figure 2–7 Estimated proportion of injury deaths due to various types of injury in 2008.

Source: Data from *The global burden of disease: 2004 update (May 2011 update)*. Geneva: WHO; 2011.

overcrowded and poorly maintained vehicles for transportation, to be pedestrians on crowded streets, to live in homes that are vulnerable to fire, and to have limited access to preventive health tools.[24] Environmental exposures to chemicals, like poisons, alcohol, smoke, and heavy metals, or to physical trauma, radiation, heat, cold, or allergens can also cause illness and injury, and some of these exposures are more common in low-income nations where there is limited access to clean water and trash removal, where food must be prepared over a fire, and where enforcement of safety laws is minimal. These injuries and exposures can cause immediate health problems, and they can also cause long-term disability and lead to the development of other health problems. For example, radiation from an industrial accident can cause cancer to occur years after the initial exposure.

Many injuries that are the result of accidents could have been prevented by the use of safety belts and child car seats in motor vehicles, helmets for cyclists, designated drivers who have not consumed alcohol, flame-resistant clothing, smoke detectors, fencing around bodies of water, swimming lessons, protective eyewear, safety harnesses when working at dangerous heights, and locked storage of weapons and ammunition, or any of the hundreds of other preventive safety measures that can be implemented by individuals, families, workplaces, and communities.[25] One goal of global health is to increase access to safety tools and encourage behaviors that reduce the risk of injuries.

2.4 SOURCES OF HEALTH INFORMATION

Health information comes from a wide variety of sources: census data, vital statistics registries, surveillance systems, household surveys, health services records such as hospital patient files and insurance claims, and maps of the locations of health facilities.[26] Many types of data gathered as part of **health information systems** are available online. That makes it possible for everyone to read, interpret, critique, and use the scientific research that informs global public health. These findings are most often disseminated through the websites and annual reports of major governmental and nongovernmental health organizations and through academic journal articles.

Three of the best sources for basic disease information are the websites of the World Health Organization (WHO), the U.S. Centers for Disease Control and Prevention (CDC), and the U.S. National Institutes of Health (NIH). All three of these organizations provide easy-to-read and regularly updated fact sheets about hundreds of diseases. They also provide resources like health glossaries and image databanks. The websites of these and other trusted organizations are an excellent first place to go for information about disease symptoms, prevention methods, diagnostic techniques, and treatments.

Table 2–8 Selected annual publications with global public health information.

Report	Source
Human Development Report	United Nations Development Programme (UNDP)
State of World Population	United Nations Population Fund (UNFPA)
State of the World's Children	United Nations Children's Fund (UNICEF)
World Development Report	World Bank
World Health Statistics	World Health Organization (WHO)

For global health statistics, the best sources are often the annual reports of United Nations agencies (**Table 2–8**). These usually focus on a particular theme but provide a variety of country-level health and development indicators in statistical appendices. For disease-specific statistics, the reports of specialty organizations may be the best references. For example, the American Cancer Society (ACS) reports some global cancer statistics every year, as does the International Agency for Research on Cancer (IARC), which is part of the United Nations system. For critical health issues, such as new outbreaks of serious infections, the CDC's Morbidity and Mortality Weekly Report (MMWR) and the WHO's Weekly Epidemiological Record may be helpful.

Fact sheets, annual reports, and other summaries of research findings are called **secondary sources** because they provide "second-hand" information about a topic. The best way to find more detailed information about particular research studies is to read **primary sources** such as original research reports published in academic journals. An **abstract** is a one-paragraph summary of the methods, results, and conclusions of a scientific investigation. Abstract databases, including PubMed, which is freely available on the Internet, and subscription services purchased by libraries, can be used to find abstracts summarizing journal articles related to medicine and public health. The full reports that are summarized by these abstracts can then be found online or in a library. The articles from journals indexed in academic databases are **peer-reviewed**, which means that before the paper was published the manuscript was sent to experts in the field, who scrutinized the methodology and reviewed the results to make sure they seem reasonable.

The ability to find and understand relevant primary and secondary information is a critical tool for anyone working in or studying global health. Ideally, access to a variety of high-quality resources provides an evidence-based foundation for anyone seeking to create, implement, evaluate, or improve global public health policies and practices.

2.5 DISCUSSION QUESTIONS

1. Look up the human development ranking and the population size of a country not listed in Table 2–1 using the same references listed for the table. What do these two numbers alone tell you about the likely public health profile of the country?
2. How long do you expect to live? What factors did you consider when estimating your life expectancy? What events might occur that would cause you to significantly lower or raise your life expectancy?
3. When is incidence the best measure to use for assessing disease burden? When is prevalence a better measure to use?
4. Which of the risk factors listed in Table 2–2 are ones that affect a large proportion of your home community? What public health interventions might help reduce the burden of disease attributable to these risk factors in your home community?
5. What do you think will be the cause of your death? What would your likely cause of death have been if you had been born 100 years ago? How would your likely cause of death differ if you lived in a different part of the world today?
6. Create a brief disease profile for one of the many infections, diseases, or disabilities introduced in this chapter. What sources provide trusted background information about the symptoms of the disease and ways to prevent and treat it? What sources provide good statistical information about how many people worldwide are affected by the condition? What can academic publications contribute to your profile?

REFERENCES

1. Murray CJ, Frenk J. Health metrics and evaluation: strengthening the science. *Lancet.* 2008;371:1191–1199.
2. *Human development report 2012.* New York: UNDP; 2012.
3. *World development report 2011.* Washington DC: World Bank; 2011.
4. *World development report 2006.* Washington DC: World Bank; 2005.

5. Mathers CD, Murray CJL, Lopez AD, et al. *Estimates of healthy life expectancy countries for 191 countries in the year 2000: methods and results.* WHO Global Programme on Evidence for Health Policy Working Paper No. 38. Geneva: WHO; 2001.

6. *World health statistics 2011.* Geneva: WHO; 2011.

7. *The global burden of disease: 2004 update.* Geneva: WHO; 2008.

8. Jha P. Avoidable global cancer deaths and total deaths from smoking. *Nat Rev Cancer.* 2009;9:655–664.

9. Rehm J, Mathers C, Popova S, Thavorncharoensap M, Teerawattananon Y, Patra J. Global burden of disease and injury and economic cost attributable to alcohol use and alcohol-use disorders. *Lancet.* 2009;373:2223–2233.

10. Bhutta ZA, Ahmed T, Black RE, et al.; Maternal and Child Undernutrition Study Group. What works? Interventions for maternal and child undernutrition and survival. *Lancet.* 2008;371:417–440.

11. *Global status report on noncommunicable diseases 2010.* Geneva: WHO; 2011.

12. Global Burden of Metabolic Risk Factors of Chronic Diseases Collaborating Group. *Country trends in metabolic risk factors.* London: Imperial College London; 2011.

13. Hallal PC, Andersen LB, Bull FC, Guthold R, Haskell W, Ekelund U; Lancet Physical Activity Series Working Group. Global physical activity levels: surveillance progress, pitfalls, and prospects. *Lancet.* 2012;380:247–257.

14. *World health statistics 2012.* Geneva: WHO; 2012.

15. Cohen AJ, Ross Anderson H, Ostro B, et al. The global burden of disease due to outdoor air pollution. *J Toxicol Environ Health A.* 2005;68:1301–1307.

16. Lawes CMM, Vander Hoorn S, Rodgers A; International Society of Hypertension. Global burden of blood-pressure-related disease, 2001. *Lancet.* 2008;371:1513–1518.

17. Smith JS, Lindsay L, Hoots B, Keys J, Franceschi S, Winer R, Clifford GM. Human papillomavirus type distribution in invasive cervical cancer and high-grade cervical lesions: a meta-analysis update. *Int J Cancer.* 2007;121:621–632.

18. *Global health risks: mortality and burden of disease attributable to selected major risks.* Geneva: WHO; 2009.

19. *Diagnostic and statistical manual of mental disorders*, 4th edition (DSM-IV-TR). Arlington VA: American Psychiatric Association; 2000.

20. Summerfield D. How scientifically valid is the knowledge base of global mental health? *BMJ.* 2008;336:992–924.

21. Demyttenaere K, Bruffaerts R, Posada-Villa J, et al.; WHO World Mental Health Survey Consortium. Prevalence, severity, and unmet need for treatment of mental disorders in the World Health Organization World Mental Health Surveys. *JAMA.* 2004;291:2581–2590.

22. *Injury: a leading cause of the global burden of disease, 2000.* Geneva: WHO; 2002.

23. *The global burden of disease: 2004 update (May 2011 update).* Geneva: WHO; 2011.

24. Laflamme L, Burrows S, Hasselberg M. Socioeconomic differences in injury risks: a review of findings and a discussion of potential countermeasures. Copenhagen: WHO-EURO; 2009.

25. *World report on child injury prevention.* Geneva: WHO/UNICEF; 2008.

26. AbouZahr C, Boerma T. Health information systems: the foundations of public health. *Bull World Health Organ.* 2005;83:578–583.

CHAPTER 3

Research and Global Health

Population health research provides essential information about the prevalence of diseases around the world, risk factors for those diseases, and the effectiveness of interventions. A basic knowledge of the methods used to collect, analyze, and synthesize global health data allows anyone to read and understand a vast array of resources for evidence-based global health practice and policy.

3.1 THE IMPORTANCE OF GLOBAL HEALTH RESEARCH

Health research at its broadest encompasses everything from molecular and cellular biology to clinical research to population health. Most global health research focuses on the public health end of the spectrum. The goals of public health research include identifying and classifying new health problems, determining risk factors for disease, developing and testing new interventions for preventing or treating illness, evaluating the impact of health policies on health outcomes, and synthesizing existing knowledge.

Epidemiology is the study of the distribution and determinants of morbidity, mortality, and disability in populations. Epidemiologists and other public health researchers collect and disseminate data about the health-related conditions that occur in particular populations and the characteristics of the people who are most at risk for developing those conditions. This information helps clinicians to diagnose illnesses, prescribe appropriate therapies, and encourage healthy lifestyles for their patients. It also helps communities to set their own public health priorities and design and evaluate programs to address these issues, especially when a process called **community-based participatory research (CBPR)** is used. Research reports also inform the development of evidence-based policies and programs.

Several significant global health reports are released by major international organizations each month, and thousands of new global health-related academic and professional journal articles are published each month. A basic understanding of health research methods makes all of these resources— including the more than 500 references cited in this book—accessible to those seeking additional information about a particular health topic.

3.2 THE RESEARCH PROCESS

Health research follows a fixed set of steps (**Figure 3–1**).[1] Researchers start by identifying a focused study question and selecting an appropriate study design. They then work out the logistics of the study and collect data, which could take the form of interviewing people, running laboratory tests, acquiring documents for review, or other methods. After analyzing the collected data, the findings are disseminated through oral presentations and written publications.

The basic unit of population health research is the **primary study** that collects new data from individuals drawn from a well-defined population, such as the students at one school or a sample of residents of one suburban area. Most primary studies are observational and simply ask participants to complete a questionnaire. Some primary studies are experimental ones in which researchers assign at least some of the participants to do something new, perhaps to start taking a daily multivitamin or to take a new drug for their health condition. When the results of primary studies are published, they are said to add to the literature on a particular topic. (A **secondary study** also contributes to the body of knowledge on a topic by analyzing and reporting on existing data that someone else collected.) The summaries of these articles are often indexed in abstract databases such as PubMed that allow the contents of the manuscripts to be searched.

For global health, it is often important to have a worldwide perspective on disease incidence and prevalence rates, risk factors for disease, and other health information. A **tertiary study** seeks to identify all the primary (and secondary) studies that have been published on a particular topic and to summarize what those studies say. These systematic reviews and

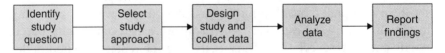

Figure 3–1 The research process.

Source: Reproduced from Jacobsen KH. *Introduction to health research methods: a practical guide*. Sudbury MA: Jones & Bartlett; 2012.

meta-analyses provide a comprehensive picture of what is known about a particular issue, and the findings and estimates from these studies can be used to predict health status in populations for which no data are currently available and to forecast future situations. Most of the global health reports published by the World Health Organization and other international agencies are based on primary studies (including country-level surveillance reports) and on meta-analyses that synthesize primary studies. These reports provide comparable data from around the world that can be used by policymakers, public health professionals, and others to foster improved health in their communities and countries.

3.3 OBSERVATIONAL STUDY DESIGNS

Most population-based public health research uses an observational study design. An **observational study** simply observes what people are doing or asks about what they have done in the past. No intervention is assigned to participants. The goal is to learn about a population as it is. **Descriptive studies** seek to describe the members of a population, the prevalence of risk factors within that population, or the rate of disease within that population. Descriptive studies often seek to answer questions about person (who?), place (where?), and time (when?). **Analytic studies** aim to understand the associations between risk factors and disease within a population and to answer "why?" questions.

3.3.A Prevalence Surveys

A **prevalence survey**, also called a **cross-sectional survey**, can be used to get a snapshot of a population's health status at one point in time. The research plan is fairly simple: recruit a representative sample of the population the researcher wants to know about, ask the participants a series of questions, and then analyze the collected data to see what proportion of the population reported various characteristics. The questionnaire can cover a wide variety of topics, including demographics (such as the age, sex, household income, and educational level of the participant), risk behaviors and other risky exposures, and illnesses and disabilities. The survey instrument can also include "KAP" questions about *k*nowledge, *a*ttitudes/beliefs, and *p*ractices/behaviors.

Prevalence surveys are one of the most common study designs used in public health research. They are often used as part of community needs assessments, and they are also used for conducting program evaluations. They are especially useful when there are time and budget constraints, because data can be collected quickly and inexpensively.

There are two key cautions about conducting and critically assessing cross-sectional surveys. First, it is very important for prevalence studies to recruit participants who are truly **representative** of the population the researchers say they want to examine. For example, a study about the health of women in a community should not be limited to including only women who are currently pregnant, because that recruiting strategy would systematically exclude older women who are of post-reproductive age. And a study about the health of college students should not recruit only students who are members of sports teams at the school, because those students are likely to be fitter than the general student body. Second, no conclusions about causality can be made from cross-sectional data, because all the questions about exposures and diseases are asked at the same time. For example, a cross-sectional survey of chewing tobacco use and dental cavities among a group of 1000 high school students might find a significantly higher prevalence of cavities among people who use chew, but that would not prove that chew caused cavities nor would it prove that cavities cause people to chew. This type of survey cannot show whether the chew or the cavities happened first.

3.3.B Case Series

A **case series** looks at the characteristics of a group of people who all have the same disease (or all had the same exposure). (A **case study** is a description of one patient. A case series describes two or more patients.) Most case series studies are written by and for clinicians, and most summarize the information in the medical records of people who were treated at a particular hospital for a particular condition. The goal of a case series may be to understand the demographic and other characteristics of people with a particular disease, to describe an unusual presentation of a disease, or to clarify the typical progression of a disease. Because a case series does not include a comparison group of healthy people, it is not possible to examine risk factors for the disease.

3.3.C Case-Control Studies

Case-control studies recruit people with a disease (**cases**) and similar people who do not have that disease (**controls**) so that their past exposures can be compared. After confirming that a participant has the disease of interest or does not have the disease, the participant is asked about his or her health behaviors (such as diet, physical activity, tobacco use, and alcohol use now and in the past), environmental exposures, and health history. After a sufficient number of cases and controls have completed the questionnaire, statistical analysis is used to identify the exposures that were reported more often by cases than by controls.

Case-control studies are ideal for learning about rare diseases. They can also be helpful for identifying past exposures that might increase the risk of disease, but the results of case-control studies must be interpreted cautiously because participants may have difficulty accurately recalling exposures that took place years or even decades before the study.

The most common way to look at the association between an exposure and a disease outcome is to create a **2 × 2 table** that has two rows for exposure status and two columns for disease status. Each individual in the study population is classified into one of the four groups created by the 2 × 2 table—exposed and diseased, exposed but not diseased, not exposed but diseased, and not exposed and not diseased. The count of the number of individuals in each of the four groups is filled into the cells of the 2 × 2 table, and various measures of association can then be calculated from those values.

The typical measure of association between an exposure and an outcome in a case-control study is the odds ratio. This is the same type of measurement used in betting (**Figure 3–2**). If someone thinks that a horse has a 25% chance of winning a race (and a 75% chance of losing), then the **odds** on the horse are 25:75, which can be simplified to 1:3 or 1/3 or 0.33—one chance of winning compared to 3 chances of losing. The **odds ratio (OR)** compares the odds of a case having a history of a particular exposure to the odds of a control having been exposed to the potential risk factor (**Figure 3–3**). An OR near 1 means that there was no association between the disease and the exposure in the study population, because cases and controls were equally likely to report the exposure. An OR greater than 1 indicates that people with the disease were more likely than people without disease to have a history of the exposure, which implies that the exposure was risky. An OR less than 1 indicates that cases were less likely than controls to have a history of the exposure, which implies that the exposure was protective.

Because a relatively small number of people sampled from a larger population cannot exactly describe the population as a whole, ORs and other statistical measures are often reported using confidence intervals. A **95% confidence interval** for an OR can be interpreted as saying "based on the sample of people the researchers took from the larger population, we can be 95% confident that the true OR in the

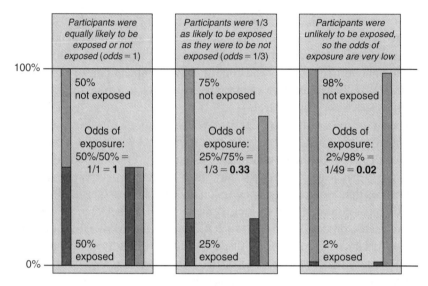

Figure 3–2 Odds.

Source: Reproduced from Jacobsen KH. *Introduction to health research methods: a practical guide.* Sudbury MA: Jones & Bartlett; 2012.

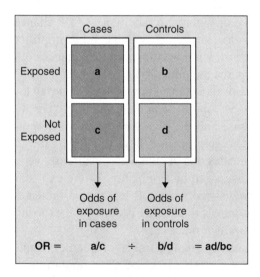

Figure 3–3 Case-control study analysis: odds ratio (OR).

Source: Reproduced from Jacobsen KH. *Introduction to health research methods: a practical guide.* Sudbury MA: Jones & Bartlett; 2012.

population as a whole is somewhere within this range of possible ORs" (**Figure 3–4**). If the entire confidence interval is greater than 1, the result is said to be statistically significant, and the conclusion is that the exposure appears to be risky. If the entire confidence interval is less than 1, the result is also statistically significant, and the conclusion is that the exposure appears to be protective. If the confidence interval overlaps 1, it means that there is not strong evidence that the exposure is risky or protective, and the conclusion is that there is no statistically significant association between the exposure and the outcome in the study population. In the example shown in **Figure 3–5**, the OR and 95% confidence interval is 0.56 (0.32, 0.93). Because the entire range is less than 1, the association between the exposure and disease is said to be statistically significant, and the conclusion is that cases were much less likely than controls to have had the exposure.

3.3.D Cohort Studies

A **cohort** is a group of similar people, and **cohort studies** recruit a group of similar people and follow them forward in time. At the start of the study, the researchers ask all of the participants about a variety of health behaviors and other exposures and characteristics, and they confirm that

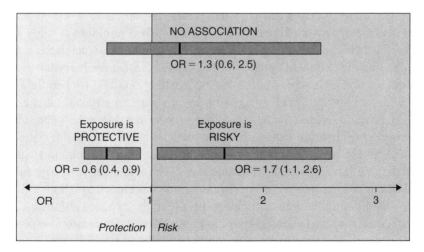

Figure 3–4 Case-control study analysis: 95% confidence interval for the OR.

Source: Adapted from Jacobsen KH. *Introduction to health research methods: a practical guide.* Sudbury MA: Jones & Bartlett; 2012.

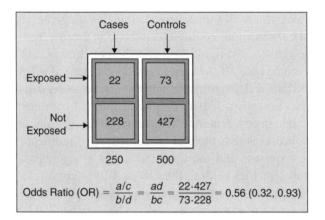

Figure 3–5 Example of a case-control study.

no one enrolled in the study already has the disease outcome of interest. The participants are then tracked for months or years, so that researchers can count the number of people who develop the disease or disability of interest. Statistical analysis is used to compare the rate of incident (new) disease among those with a particular exposure and those without that exposure.

Because the data collected at the start of the study can prove that an exposure existed before the onset of disease, cohort studies are very helpful for establishing whether an exposure causes a disease. Cohort studies are also useful for measuring the incidence of new disease in a population. The population studied can be a representative sample of a whole community or even a whole country. For example, the Framingham study has been following thousands of residents of one town in Massachusetts since 1948,[2] and the Whitehall studies have followed British civil servants from all occupational classes since the 1960s.[3] Another option is for people with an unusual exposure, such as an exposure to a particular industrial chemical, to be recruited and tracked for a long time so that researchers can study the impact of that rare exposure on the participants' future health status.

Two of the most common measures of association for a cohort study are the rate ratio and the attributable risk. The incidence **rate ratio** (also called the **risk ratio** or **relative risk**, or simply shortened to **RR**) is calculated by dividing the rate of incident disease in the exposed cohort by the rate in the unexposed cohort (**Figure 3–6**). An RR near 1 means that exposed and unexposed participants were equally likely to develop the disease during the study period. An RR greater than 1 indicates that the exposure was associated with increased risk of disease. An RR less than 1 indicates that the exposure was protective. Confidence intervals can be used

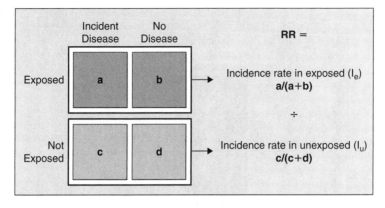

Figure 3–6 Cohort study analysis: rate ratio (RR).

Source: Reproduced from Jacobsen KH. *Introduction to health research methods: a practical guide*. Sudbury MA: Jones & Bartlett; 2012.

to show the level of certainty about the RR in the larger population from which participants were drawn (**Figure 3–7**). The **rate difference** (also known as **excess risk** or **attributable risk**) subtracts the rate of disease in the unexposed from the rate of disease in the exposed. If the exposed and unexposed populations were similar except for their exposure status, then this difference in disease rates represents cases of disease among exposed people that would not have occurred if they had not been exposed (**Figure 3–8**). In the example shown in **Figure 3–9**, the RR and 95%

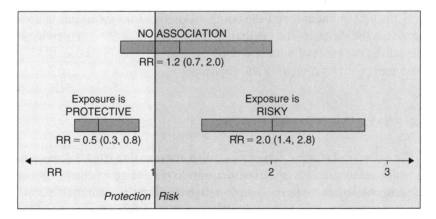

Figure 3–7 Case-control study analysis: 95% confidence interval for the RR.

Source: Reproduced from Jacobsen KH. *Introduction to health research methods: a practical guide*. Sudbury MA: Jones & Bartlett; 2012.

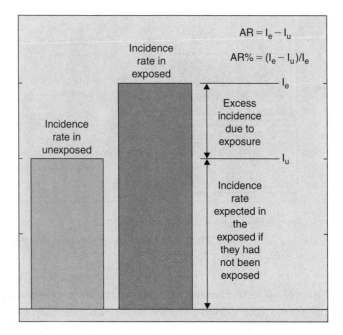

Figure 3–8 Cohort study analysis: attributable risk (excess risk).

Source: Reproduced from Jacobsen KH. *Introduction to health research methods: a practical guide*. Sudbury MA: Jones & Bartlett; 2012.

confidence interval is 2.00 (1.46, 2.74). Because the entire range is greater than 1, the association between the exposure and disease is said to be statistically significant, and the conclusion is that the exposure is a risk factor for the disease. The attributable risk percent is 50%, which means that half of the cases of disease among the exposed participants could have been prevented by removing the exposure.

3.4 EXPERIMENTAL STUDIES

Experimental studies, sometimes called **intervention studies**, are studies in which the researchers assign participants to receive a particular exposure. Experimental trials are the best study design for assessing causation, because the researchers intentionally subject participants to an exposure and then see what happens afterward. But because the researchers may be placing participants at risk of unexpected and potentially serious adverse outcomes, there are some special ethical concerns associated with experimental studies.

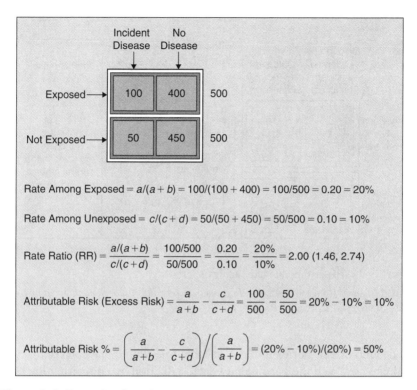

Figure 3–9 Example of a cohort study.

Some studies are deemed too risky to be conducted. Those that are approved are closely monitored by research ethics committees.

Some experimental studies are **clinical trials** of a new medication, a new vaccine, another new medical product, or some other intervention. Most clinical trials use a **randomized controlled trial (RCT)** design in which some people are assigned by chance to the active intervention and others are assigned by chance to a comparison group. The comparison may be a placebo, like a sugar pill or saline injection, or may be an active control such as the best drug already on the market or a lower dose of the new medication being tested. Most clinical trials are **double blind**, which means that neither the participants nor the people assessing the participants' health outcomes know whether a participant is receiving the trial drug or a placebo. That way neither the participants nor the examiners will be tempted, even subconsciously, to find a better outcome in a patient who they know is taking the new drug.

The most common outcome measure for an RCT is the **efficacy** of the intervention, which measures the ability of the intervention to produce

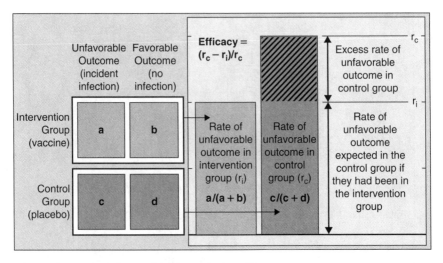

Figure 3–10 Experimental study analysis: efficacy.

Source: Adapted from Jacobsen KH. *Introduction to health research methods: a practical guide*. Sudbury MA: Jones & Bartlett; 2012.

the desired effect. For example, a vaccine trial with a placebo control will evaluate how well the vaccine prevented infection by comparing the rates of infection in the vaccine group and the placebo group (**Figure 3–10**).

Most new vaccines, medications, and other pharmaceutical agents undergo several rounds of testing before the product is released to the public. The first phases of the study test the safety of the product in small numbers of people. Later phases recruit hundreds or thousands of people to ensure the safety and effectiveness of the new product. Ongoing safety monitoring continues after the product is in wide use.

3.5 RESEARCH ETHICS

Nearly all health research projects that involve contact with people or access to identifiable personal information are supervised by ethics committees, commonly called **Institutional Review Boards (IRBs)** or **Research Ethics Committees (RECs)**. Review boards will not approve studies that do not meet the three main ethical considerations of health research: beneficence, respect for persons, and distributive justice.

Beneficence means that the study should be beneficial for the participants and for their communities. This call to do good is often paired with

nonmaleficence, from the root words for nonbadness, which call for the study to do no harm.

Respect for persons demands that all potential participants have the **autonomy** to choose whether they want to volunteer to participate in a study and that all potential participants are given all the information they need to be able to make an informed decision about whether to participate. Candidates for a research study should be told about the goals of the study, the potential risks and benefits of participation, the study procedures, the time requirements of participation, and the process for withdrawing from the study if they change their mind about participating. The process of sharing information and agreeing to participate is called **informed consent**. No one should feel pressured to participate in a research study. Respect for persons also requires researchers to keep the safety of participants as their top priority and to protect the privacy of participants and the confidentiality of the information participants choose to disclose.

Distributive justice aims to ensure that the populations that bear the risks of research participation have access to the benefits of that research. For example, this means that a community that took on the risk of volunteering to test a new medication or a new vaccine should also have the benefit of having access to that product after it is approved and marketed.

Adherence to these standards prevents the types of research misconduct that occurred in the mid-20th century when medical experiments were often conducted without participant consent. One of the most widely known examples from the United States is the Tuskegee Syphilis Experiment, which was conducted by the U.S. Public Health Service in Alabama for 40 years beginning in 1932.[4] Nearly 400 African-American men with late-stage syphilis were offered free medical care by doctors who were conducting a study on the progression of the disease. The men were not told that they had syphilis and many were not treated with antibiotics even after penicillin became the standard cure for the infection in 1947. Treatment was provided only after a major newspaper reported on the study in 1972. By that time many of the men had died of syphilis and many of their wives had been infected.

In order to protect the "human subjects" of research, new and ongoing research projects must be approved by an independent IRB in each country where study data will be collected. Research ethics committees will not approve studies that they deem to be unreasonably dangerous, poorly planned, or unnecessarily targeting members of a vulnerable population. After approval, the IRBs monitor ongoing studies. Researchers must seek prior approval for any changes they want to make to their research protocols, and they must immediately report any adverse event to the IRBs that are overseeing the project. These rules help researchers to design and implement high-quality research plans, and they help to ensure the protection and safety of all research participants.

3.6 SYNTHESIS STUDIES

Some research investigations synthesize the results of dozens or hundreds of previous primary studies. By combining and analyzing the results of multiple similar research studies from different parts of the world or various points in time, these tertiary analysis studies provide a comprehensive summary of the scientific literature on a particular topic, a foundation for projections about health problems and needs, and new insight about risk factors for particular diseases.

3.6.A Correlational Studies

A **correlational study**, sometimes called an **ecological study**, uses numeric data about a particular exposure and a particular health outcome from several populations to look for trends. The results of correlational studies are often displayed using a scatterplot. For each population, a point is placed on the graph by using the value for the exposure in that population as the x-coordinate and the value for the health outcome in that population as the y-coordinate. After all the points are plotted, a line that represents the best fit to the points is added to the graph.

The value of the **correlation** coefficient, r (which is often reported as r^2), measures how well the line predicts the location of the points (**Figure 3–11**). An r near 1 means that all of the points fall almost exactly on a line, so if the exposure level in a population is known, the outcome can be predicted with a high level of certainty. An r near 0 is extremely weak and means that the line has no predictive value. In other words, when r is close to 0, the exposure is not associated with the disease outcome. An r near 0.5 indicates a moderately strong correlation.

The slope of the line shows the direction of association. A positive value for r indicates a positive slope (one that goes up from left to right) and signifies that an increase in the rate of the exposure is associated with an increase in the rate of the outcome. For example, a study of 37 countries found that countries with greater income inequalities also had greater rates of bullying among middle school students ($r = 0.62$).[5] A negative value for

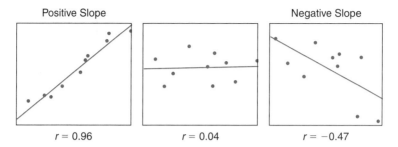

Figure 3–11 Analysis for a correlational study: correlation.

r indicates a negative slope and shows that an increase in the exposure rate is associated with a decrease in the outcome rate. For example, a study of 43 African countries found that countries with a higher proportion of adults who could read had a significantly lower proportion of women who died in childbirth ($r = -0.52$).[6]

These two examples highlight a key aspect of ecological study design: most ecological studies are designed to examine population-level exposures and outcomes, like income inequality, literacy rates, air quality, and maternal mortality rates. Ecological studies are not used to test individual-level correlations. Thus, the results of ecological studies that use population-level data can be applied to populations but cannot necessarily be applied to individuals. For example, if an ecological survey using data from dozens of cities shows a strong positive correlation between the number of tanning beds per 1000 adults and the number of new skin cancer diagnoses each year per 10,000 adults, this finding would not prove that the individuals who used tanning beds were the ones who were diagnosed with skin cancer. It is possible (though unlikely) that none of the individuals who use tanning beds developed skin cancer. The **ecological fallacy** describes when population-level correlations are incorrectly interpreted to be measures of individual risk. However, even with this limitation, ecological surveys can be a very helpful first step in testing a hypothesis about a possible risk factor for disease.

3.6.B Systematic Reviews and Meta-Analyses

Systematic reviews identify as many articles and reports about a particular topic as can be found, then check each one to see if it meets the predefined criteria for inclusion in the analysis. Information from each eligible article is extracted and compared with the other studies in order to paint a comprehensive picture of what is known (and what is not known) about the topic.

For example, a systematic review might show strong agreement in the literature about a particular exposure being a risk factor for a specific disease. Or the review might suggest that a particular exposure does not appear to increase the prevalence of a disease. Or a review might determine that the previous studies have mixed results and no consensus can be reached about the association based on the current scientific literature. (To ensure a fair conclusion, systematic reviews usually consider the potential effects of publication bias on their findings. **Publication bias** occurs when studies that find a statistically significant result are more likely than "null result" studies to published.)

When the study designs and the statistics used for each of the included studies in a systematic review are quite similar, it is sometimes possible to pool the results from the independent studies to create one summary statistical measure. This combined statistical analysis is called a **meta-analysis**.

3.6.C Forecasting and Modeling

Mathematical models can be used to estimate disease rates in populations lacking good data and to predict future health trends. For example, global burden of disease studies generally start with a systematic review of the disease of interest, and usually find incomplete data for many countries in the world. A mathematical model that incorporates the information that is available for a country (such as the distribution of the population by age) and estimates of morbidity and mortality from other countries with similar geographic and socioeconomic profiles can provide a good foundation for understanding the likely health profile of the understudied country. Similarly, if health and demographic data from several points in time in one country or world region are added to a model, researchers can create projections about the likely health situation in that area in 10, 25, or even 50 years. Models can also be modified to simulate the short-term and long-term effects of public health interventions and other population-level changes.

3.7 INTERPRETING STATISTICS

The only way to have a 100% accurate measure of health in a population is to collect data from every individual in that population. However, this is rarely done for large populations because of time and money constraints. Instead, a small proportion of the population is recruited for the study, and statistical tests are used to provide estimates of the health status in the whole population based on measures taken from the sample population.

Figure 3–12 shows an example of sampling. Of the 100 people in the population from which participants will be sampled, 32 are obese. If 10 individuals are sampled at random from that population, it is likely that the prevalence of obesity in the sample population will be 20% or 30% or 40%, something relatively close to 32%. However, some samples will, by chance, have a prevalence of 80% or 90% or even 100%. So a sample of 10 will not allow a high level of precision about the prevalence rate in the total population, even though it can provide a reasonable rough estimate.

The uncertainty about what the sample measure says about health in the larger population from which participants were drawn can be captured in a 95% confidence interval (95% CI) similar to the ones used for ORs and RRs. For example, the obesity prevalence estimate and its 95% CI for a sample of 10 individuals may be 30% (8%, 62%). This means that based on one sample of 10 people, we are 95% confident that the true prevalence in the larger population is somewhere between 8% and 62%. That range does indeed capture the 32% that is the true prevalence. (There is a 5% chance that this sample happened to be extreme, and that the 95% CI does not include the true value of the prevalence.) If a narrower CI is desired, then a larger sample population must be used. For example, if 50 individuals participate in the study instead of 10, then the estimate of the prevalence might be 34% (22%, 48%). That would mean that based on one sample of 50 people we are 95% confident that the true prevalence is somewhere between 22% and 48%. If more people are sampled, the 95% CI would become even narrower and closer to the true value of 32%.

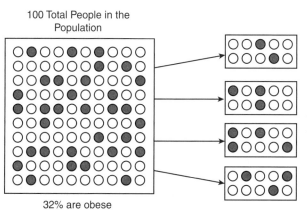

Figure 3–12 Sampling from a population.

A **p-value** (or probability value) is another measure of uncertainty. P-values are usually used with statistical tests of difference to indicate how likely it is that a difference exists between two or more populations. For example, a **t-test** can be used to see if there is a difference in the mean age of men and women who participated in a cross-sectional study, and a **Chi-squared test** can be used to see if there is a difference in the proportion of adults with diabetes in four different neighborhoods in one city. The p-value for these tests gives the estimated probability that, given the number of people in the sample, an even bigger difference between the groups than the one found for the sample might occur by chance even if there really was no difference between the groups being compared. Just as a larger sample size results in a narrower confidence interval, a larger sample size makes it easier to have a small p-value. A larger sample gives the test greater statistical **power**, a better ability to detect a difference between two or more groups when the groups really are different.

A small p-value (usually less than 0.05, or 5%) means that the statistical test found that it is unlikely that a larger difference between groups would occur by chance. Tests that produce p-values less than 0.05 are said to have statistically significant results and are deemed to show a difference between the groups being compared. For example, if a t-test comparing the mean ages of men and women has a p-value of 0.02, there is only a 2% likelihood that such an extreme difference in mean age would be observed by chance if there was really no difference between the populations. Because it is so unlikely that the apparent difference in mean ages of men and women was due to chance, the conclusion for this test is that the mean ages for men and women in that population are different. If the t-test has a p-value of 0.68, there is a 68% likelihood that an even bigger difference could be observed by chance if samples were drawn from populations with the same mean age. In this situation, the conclusion is that the means are not different. Other examples of p-value interpretation are shown in **Table 3–1**.

Knowing the meaning of CIs and p-values allows a reader to interpret almost all statistical results. A p-value of less than 0.05 means that a difference exists. A larger p-value means that no difference has been observed. A CI provides a range of likely values for a measure in a population, and that range gets narrower as the sample size increases. The CIs for ratios (like ORs and RRs) are centered around 1; if the CI does not include 1, then there is a difference between the two populations being compared by the ratio.

Table 3–1 Examples of p-value interpretation.

Goal of Test	*p-value*	*Is the p-value "extreme" (p < 0.05)?*	*Conclusion*
To compare mean ages of men and women	0.13	No	The mean age of the populations is **not different**.
To compare mean scores on a test for children in grades 1, 3, and 5	0.002	Yes	The mean test scores by grade are significantly **different**.
To compare the proportion of employees in different divisions of a company who walk or bike to work each day	0.43	No	The distribution of responses by the various groups is **not different**.
To compare the prevalence of diabetes in two cities	0.03	Yes	The proportions of people with diabetes in the two cities are significantly **different**.

3.8 CRITICAL READING

Several characteristics of good public health and medical research reports are listed in **Table 3–2**. Beyond these factors, there are several other important considerations for readers who are assessing and applying the results of published studies. These cautions include bias, measurement validity, and target populations.

Bias is a systematic error in study design, data collection, or data analysis that might create a difference between what the study intended to measure and what it actually measured. Bias of any type can lead to an overestimation or an underestimation of the association between an exposure and an outcome. **Selection bias** occurs when the people who participate in a study are not representative of the intended sample population. One example of selection bias is **volunteer bias**, which occurs when people who volunteer to be part of a research study turn out to be different from the desired sample population, perhaps because they are systematically healthier or less healthy than the population as a whole.

Table 3–2 Characteristics of good public health and medical research reports.

- The article has been peer-reviewed and published in a respected journal or by a trusted organization.
- The population studied is clearly defined and the number of participants in the study was reasonably large.
- An appropriate epidemiological study design was used (with a control group, if required).
- The methods used to measure exposures/interventions and health outcomes are explained in detail.
- The results of statistical tests are presented using easy-to-read charts, graphs, and tables.
- The relationship of the new study to previous studies is discussed, and many other articles are cited.
- The strengths and limitations/biases of the study are acknowledged and discussed.
- The conclusions seem reasonable and are based on the new results.
- The article is well written and follows a logical outline (usually Introduction/ Background, Methods, Results, Discussion/Conclusion).
- The article states that the study was approved and overseen by an ethics review committee, and there are no obvious conflicts of interest that may have influenced the findings.

Information bias occurs when incorrect information is given to researchers. For example, **recall bias** may happen when participants do not accurately recall past events. When there is differential recall—say, when people with cancer strain to recall any potentially harmful past exposure but people in the control group of a case-control study are not similarly motivated to remember past exposures—the results of a study may be inaccurate. Bias can be avoided or minimized when a study is carefully designed, conducted, and analyzed. The discussion sections of articles usually include an explanation of the limitations of the study and the possible sources of bias (as well as potential issues related to confounding, effect modification, or other scenarios that could affect the results). Readers can also make their own evaluations about whether bias in a study may have influenced the findings.

   Validity asks how well a test measures what it is supposed to measure (internal validity) and how well a study measures the true situation in a population (external validity or **generalizability**). A test should be **accurate** (valid), which means that it gives the actual values of height, blood pressure, or some other measure. A test should also be **precise (reliable)**, which means that when the test is given several times to the same person the results are consistent. Most global health research articles provide details in their methods sections about their survey instruments (questionnaires), clinical and laboratory tests, and other assessments. Readers should check to be sure that the questions used for a survey appear to accurately capture the exposure of interest. Self-reported measures (like "how many calories did you eat today?" and "how many miles did you walk today?") may not be as accurate as observed measures (such as having a researcher quantify the actual portions of various foods eaten during the day and using a pedometer to record the number of steps taken). Additionally, different types of questions may yield different responses (such as "how many servings of vegetables did you eat today?" versus "how many servings of vegetables do you eat in a typical day?").

A third consideration relates to the populations to which the results of a study can be applied. The conclusions of a study that included only male participants between 20 and 24 years of age should not be applied to women ages 80 to 89. The conclusions of a study of women living in California probably do not apply to women living in Malawi. The conclusions of a study of nonsmokers should probably not be applied to smokers. Results from tests done in rats do not necessarily apply to humans. Caution should be used when applying the results of any study conducted in one place at one point in time to another population.

3.9 EVIDENCE-BASED GLOBAL HEALTH

Clinicians often use a process called **evidence-based medicine (EBM)** to guide them as they seek to make the best decisions about how to care for their patients. The goal of EBM is to use facts rather than anecdotes or ideology to make clinical decisions. Like EBM, evidence-based public health and evidence-based global health require a careful and critical review of the literature prior to implementing any intervention (**Figure 3–13**).[7] The goal of this review process is to learn what has worked for others and what has not worked. There is no need to "reinvent the wheel" when the global health literature is full of examples of successful public health programs and policies. There is also a substantial benefit to learning from the mistakes others have made and not repeating them. Ideally, evidence-based global health promotes the cost-efficient and effective use of limited health resources to solve public health problems. The tools in this chapter

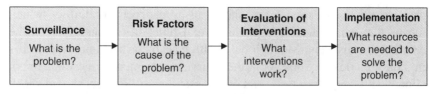

Figure 3–13 The public health approach.

Source: Adapted from Holder Y, Peden M, Krug E, Lund J, Gururaj G, Kobusingye O, editors. *Injury surveillance guidelines*. Geneva: WHO; 2001.

provide the foundation for conducting a valuable analysis of any global health concern or intervention. It is not an overstatement to say that health research saves lives.

3.10 DISCUSSION QUESTIONS

1. Look at the health webpage for a popular Internet news site. What topics are covered? How many of the stories present the results of a research project?
2. Would you participate in a health research study? Why or why not? Would your answer be different for an observational study and an experimental study?
3. Use PubMed or another abstract database to find an academic journal article on a health topic of interest to you. Read the article to find the answers to these questions: (a) What was the main study question?, (b) Who participated in the study, where did it take place, and when was it conducted?, (c) What study design was used?, and (d) What was the answer to the main study question?
4. Look up the most recent issue of the *State of the World's Children* or another United Nations report and examine the statistical annex. What sources of data contributed to these tables?
5. Find a recent news story from the popular press about a newly released health research report. Look up and read the scientific article on which the news report was based. Was the news story accurate? Did it leave out any critical information?
6. How have the results of health research studies contributed to improving your quality of life?
7. How do the results of health research studies contribute to improving global health?

REFERENCES

1. Jacobsen KH. *Introduction to health research methods: a practical guide*. Sudbury MA: Jones & Bartlett; 2012.
2. Splansky GL, Corey D, Yang Q, et al. The Third Generation Cohort of the National Heart, Lung, and Blood Institute's Framingham Heart Study: design, recruitment, and initial examination. *Am J Epidemiol*. 2007;165:1328–1335.
3. Marmot M, Brunner E. Cohort profile: the Whitehall II study. *Int J Epidemiol*. 2005;34:251–256.
4. White RM. Unraveling the Tuskegee Study of Untreated Syphilis. *Arch Intern Med*. 2000;160:585–598.
5. Elgar FJ, Craig W, Boyce W, Morgan A, Vella-Zarb R. Income inequality and school bullying: multilevel study of adolescents in 37 countries. *J Adolesc Health*. 2009;45:351–359.
6. Alvarez JL, Gil R, Hernández, Gil A. Factors associated with maternal mortality in sub-Saharan Africa: an ecological study. *BMC Public Health*. 2009;9:462.
7. Buekens P, Keusch G, Belizan J, Bhutta ZA. Evidence-based global health. *JAMA*. 2004;291:2639–2641.
8. Holder Y, Peden M, Krug E, Lund J, Gururaj G, Kobusingye O, editors. *Injury surveillance guidelines*. Geneva: WHO; 2001.

CHAPTER 4

Socioeconomic Determinants of Health

Income, education, occupation, and other determinants of socioeconomic position have a significant impact on health status and the ability to access healthcare services. Culture influences health beliefs and behaviors and shapes decisions about when and where to seek health care.

4.1 SOCIAL DETERMINANTS OF HEALTH

Socioeconomic status (SES), or **socioeconomic position (SEP)**, indicates an individual's (or family's) standing in a society based on social, economic, and educational characteristics. There is no one measure of SES, but proxies such as ownership of various assets (like a house, car, bicycle, television, radio, or livestock), occupation, amount and type of education, residential area, and other social and economic characteristics can be used to evaluate a person's relative position in a community or larger population group.

Three of the key components that contribute to the socioeconomic status of an individual or household—economic status, occupational status, and educational status—are inextricably linked to each other and to health status (**Figure 4–1**). Any intervention aimed at one of these three categories will likely impact the others. New reading skills may lead to a better job. Increased job skills may lead to a higher hourly wage. Extra income may be used to pay for additional training. And any one of these improvements can lead to increased health.

Income, employment, education, social class, sex, race, ethnicity, and other living conditions that influence health status and access to health services are collectively called the **social determinants of health**. These factors can be summarized using the acronym **PROGRESS**, as shown in **Table 4–1**.[1]

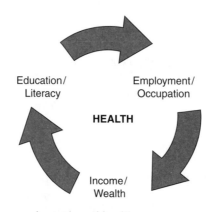

Figure 4–1 Socioeconomic status and health.

Table 4–1 PROGRESS-Plus list of the social determinants of health.

P	Place of residence (rural/urban; particular state or province; housing characteristics)
R	Ethnicity
O	Occupation (and employment status)
G	Gender (male/female/other)
R	Religion
E	Education
S	Social capital (neighborhood, community, and family support)
S	Socioeconomic position (income, wealth, and other measures)
Plus	Age
	Disability (physical or mental disability)
	Sexual orientation
	Other vulnerable groups

Source: Adapted from Kavanagh J, Oliver S, Lorenc T. Reflections on developing and using PROGRESS-Plus. *Equity Update*. 2008;2:1–3.

Children and adults who have low socioeconomic status (either in terms of absolute poverty or relative poverty compared to neighbors) tend to have significantly reduced health status compared to those from wealthier socioeconomic groups.[2] These differences in health status between population groups are called **health disparities**, and one of the key goals of global public health is to reduce health disparities by increasing the health status of disadvantaged populations.

4.1.A Income, Wealth, and Health

The two most common ways of measuring the economic status of a household are income and wealth. **Income** is the amount of take-home pay earned by household members in a given time period. **Wealth** is the accumulated worth of the household's resources and can include a house, car, television or radio, livestock, and other consumer goods. Low-income households generally have very little wealth, so they have few resources to draw on when someone in the household develops a severe illness or disability.

About 1.4 billion people worldwide—1 in 5 people—survive on less than the international poverty line of $1.25 per person per day (**Figure 4–2**).[3] Many of the poorest households try to grow enough as subsistence farmers with a small plot of land to feed all the household members. Others are the urban poor, who often live in informal settlements with no amenities. Poverty impacts the type of dwelling a household lives in (which can be unstable, unventilated, and/or built with harmful materials), how crowded the home is (which can facilitate spread of infectious diseases like tuberculosis),

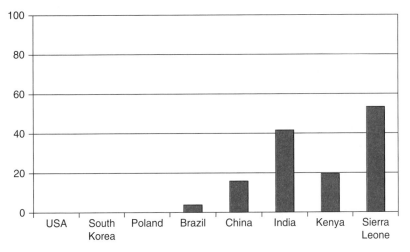

Figure 4–2 Percentage of the population living on less than $1.25 per day, the international poverty line, between 2000 and 2009.

Source: Data from *Human development report 2011*. New York: UNDP; 2011.

and whether it is in proximity to schools, healthcare facilities, public transportation, waste dumps, and clean water sources.

Poverty is often linked to an unhealthy living environment. Many poor communities do not have a source of consistently safe drinking water, properly installed latrines, or enough water to practice good hygiene, so the risk of contracting an infection is greatly increased. In some places, dwindling availability of wood for fuel limits the ability of households to boil water and cook food. And without electricity for refrigeration it is difficult to store food safely. In rural areas, the lack of infrastructure for communication (such as telephones and radios) and transportation makes it difficult to access health education and health care. Furthermore, poor households may not have money for disease prevention, such as the purchase of insecticide-treated bednets for malaria, because they must dedicate all income to immediate survival needs like food, housing, clothing, and emergency medical care.

Poverty affects the health of people of all ages. For example, **Figure 4–3** shows that children of relatively poor families have a much lower chance of survival than children of relatively wealthy families.[4–6] Low-resource

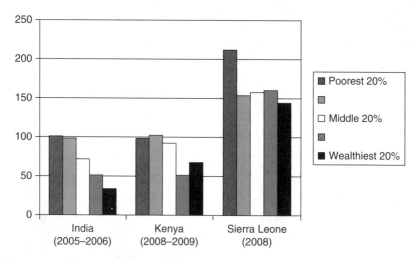

Figure 4–3 Comparison of mortality rates of children less than 5 years old per 1000 live births, by wealth quintile.

Source: Data from *India: DHS, 2005–06—final report*. Calverton MD: International Institute for Population Sciences and Macro International Inc.; 2007 Sep.; and *Kenya: DHS, 2008–09—final report*. Nairobi and Calverton MD: Kenya National Bureau of Statistics and ICF Macro; 2010 Jun.; and *Sierra Leone: DHS, 2008—final report*. Freetown and Calverton MD: Statistics Sierra Leone, Ministry of Health and Sanitation, and ICF Macro; 2009 Jul.

households must make healthcare decisions very carefully and consider all the costs of health care, including transportation to a healthcare facility, food for the patients and caregivers (as many hospitals do not provide food for inpatients), fees for seeing clinicians, the price of medications and supplies like bandages, and lost wages for the patient and caregiver. When people from poor households decide to seek medical attention they may receive substandard care because they have to seek care at an underfunded, understocked, and understaffed clinic. Hospitals that primarily serve the poor rarely have highly trained specialists on staff and may not have the support staff and technology to offer advanced care.

Wealthier people generally have better access to advanced health care when they are sick. They can afford the best diagnostic tests and the best therapies, and they have the resources to seek care for relatively mild conditions that if untreated could develop into severe problems. And because wealthier people have better access to good nutrition, work jobs that are less dangerous, and have usually had previous injuries and infections treated, they are usually in better overall health than poorer people. Thus, income and wealth directly contribute to enhanced health status.

4.1.B Employment and Occupational Status

Employment of at least one wage earner is generally critical for keeping a household out of poverty. In addition to income, employment often provides health insurance, compensation for on-the-job injuries, and sometimes also housing, food allowances, and schooling for children of employees. These benefits can have a significant and positive impact on the health of workers and their families.

However, not all jobs are equally beneficial to health. People with limited job skills often have the most dangerous jobs, receive little compensation for their labor, and have little or no job security. Injured or ill workers may not receive adequate treatment for their conditions because they cannot afford to take time off to see a doctor or to recuperate at home, and because they cannot afford to pay for health care. Manual laborers have higher all-cause mortality rates than skilled nonmanual workers, and much higher mortality rates than professionals.[7] Men who do manual labor are more likely than nonmanual workers to die from injuries, some of which are job related, and are also more likely to die of heart disease, stroke, lung diseases, gastrointestinal diseases, and cancer.[8]

Being unemployed or underemployed is also associated with reduced health status. Unemployed women and men who are healthy enough to be actively seeking work have higher rates of physical and mental illness than working people of the same age.[9,10] Unemployed working-age adults also have significantly higher suicide rates and all-cause mortality rates than employed men and women.[11]

4.1.C Literacy and Educational Level

Formal education and the ability to read are both correlated with a variety of measures of health. **Literacy** is usually defined as functional literacy, the ability to understand written words well enough to complete normal daily tasks. Educational level is usually measured in terms of years of education completed and diplomas, certificates, or degrees earned.

Literacy allows readers to acquire health information and navigate health systems. Readers can learn about food preparation and exercise programs in newspapers and magazines, comprehend health and safety warnings on consumer products, access air and water quality reports, read posters advertising immunization and screening campaigns, follow directions on medication bottles and hospital discharge orders, understand the health benefits packages offered by employers and the government, apply for aid and benefits, read brochures about their health conditions, use signs to navigate hospitals, and seek out additional information online or at libraries. People who cannot read will have difficulty with all of these health-related activities. They may delay seeking a diagnosis or treatment for a health problem because they worry about being unable to complete paperwork at the doctor's office or being ridiculed for not knowing how to read or write. They may have difficulty taking their prescribed medications properly if their healthcare providers have not fully explained dosage and timing and they cannot read the instructions on the label. They may not be able to read the safety information provided by a pharmacist or know when to return for a follow-up examination.

Female literacy and education are particularly important for family and child health. Women who can read and have at least several years of formal education are able to learn about improved home-health practices and can more easily gain the knowledge and skills they need to reduce their children's risk of malnutrition, illness, and death.[12] Women with more education also tend to report fewer problems accessing health care

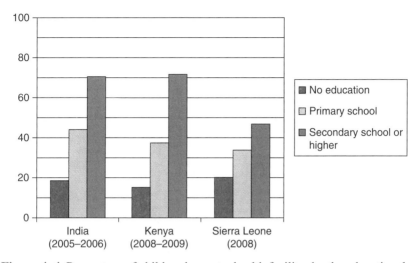

Figure 4–4 Percentage of children born at a health facility, by the educational level of the mother.

Source: Data from *India: DHS, 2005–06—final report*. Calverton MD: International Institute for Population Sciences and Macro International Inc.; 2007 Sep.; and *Kenya: DHS, 2008–09—final report*. Nairobi and Calverton MD: Kenya National Bureau of Statistics and ICF Macro; 2010 Jun.; and *Sierra Leone: DHS, 2008—final report*. Freetown and Calverton MD: Statistics Sierra Leone, Ministry of Health and Sanitation, and ICF Macro; 2009 Jul.

than other women do.[4,6] As a result, women with more formal schooling are more likely to give birth at a healthcare facility (**Figure 4–4**), which means that both mothers and newborns are more likely to survive if there are complications during or after delivery. The children of women with more education are also more likely to receive appropriate preventive and therapeutic medical services (**Figure 4–5**).[4–6]

Unfortunately, even though the economic and health benefits of education are well established, in most world regions fewer girls than boys are enrolled in primary school (elementary school) and secondary school (middle school and high school), and fewer women than men can read.[13] Some health intervention programs focus on helping girls to enroll in primary school and complete their basic education, which is usually considered to be about seven years of classroom learning. Other health-related education programs focus on female adult literacy and sponsor reading classes for mothers and other adult women. General education has health benefits for women and their families and communities.

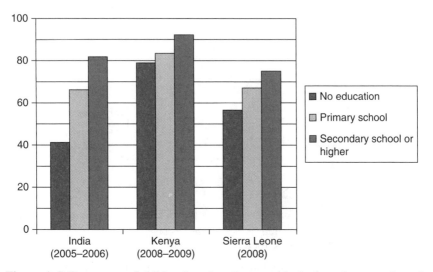

Figure 4–5 Percentage of children less than 5 years old who have been vaccinated against measles, by the educational level of the mother.

Source: Data from *India: DHS, 2005–06—final report*. Calverton MD: International Institute for Population Sciences and Macro International Inc.; 2007 Sep.; and *Kenya: DHS, 2008–09—final report*. Nairobi and Calverton MD: Kenya National Bureau of Statistics and ICF Macro; 2010 Jun.; and *Sierra Leone: DHS, 2008—final report*. Freetown and Calverton MD: Statistics Sierra Leone, Ministry of Health and Sanitation, and ICF Macro; 2009 Jul.

4.2 SOCIOECONOMIC INDICATORS

Just as the health status of individuals and families is related to their socioeconomic position, the health status of communities and nations is linked to their economic status. High-income countries have different health profiles than low-income countries, with higher-income countries typically having lower fertility rates, lower mortality rates, longer life expectancies, a higher proportion of deaths and disability from noncommunicable diseases (NCDs), and a lower proportion of deaths from infectious diseases.

Health economists use a variety of macroeconomic indicators to measure the amount of economic activity in a country. The GDP, GNI, and GNP are three of the most common measures. To make the distinction between these measures clear, consider the way the GDP, GNI, and GNP of Canada would be calculated. The **gross domestic product (GDP)** is the total amount of goods and services produced in Canada by both Canadian corporations and foreign corporations. It includes consumer spending, investment, government spending, and exports. The **gross national income (GNI)** is similar to the GDP, but puts the focus on the total income from the selling of goods and services produced in the country. The **gross national product (GNP)** is the total amount of goods and services produced by Canadian companies in Canada and by Canadian corporations working in other countries.

Because the amount of goods and services that can be purchased with a given amount of money varies from place to place, these values are often recorded in terms of **purchasing power parity (PPP)**, which measures how many goods, services, and other products can be purchased in each country with a fixed amount of money (like $1000 U.S. dollars). A popular example of PPP is the "Big Mac Index" that determines the relative price of a McDonald's burger in two different countries and uses that exchange rate to determine the relative value of other items.[14] If a Big Mac costs $2 in one country and $3.50 in another, it is likely that the costs of living are much higher in the $3.50-per-hamburger country, and workers in the higher-priced country will have to earn a much higher salary to stay above the local poverty line than workers in the $2-per-burger country.

GDP, GNI, and GNP can also be recorded in per capita (per person) terms by dividing the total monetary value by the population of the country. The GNI per capita of a country is about equal to the average income of an individual. Although these numbers are only a rough guide to the economic profile of a country, they do allow for comparisons between countries. **Figure 4–6** shows where the richest and poorest countries are located. High-income countries generally have high life expectancies and low-income countries generally have low life expectancies (**Figure 4–7**).[15,16]

Summary values like the GDP and GNI have some major limitations if they are being used to estimate health and development. They do not count unpaid labor like work caring for children and growing food to feed a family. They ignore issues of sustainability, environmental damage, and the distribution of wealth and quality of life (standard of living) in a country. These values show the economic experience of the "average" person living in each country, but the "average" economic measure may be misleading if most people in a given country are very poor and some are extremely rich and there is almost no middle class. Even when a large proportion of the population experiences something near the average reported for the country, there will still be variability in the experiences of individuals. There are millionaires in every country, even the countries with the poorest "average" person. And there are people in every country, even the wealthiest ones, who live on almost nothing.

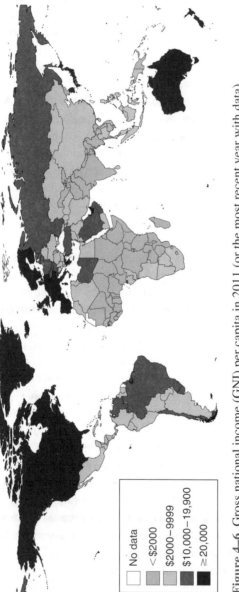

Figure 4–6 Gross national income (GNI) per capita in 2011 (or the most recent year with data).

Source: Data from *World development indicators database.* Washington DC: World Bank.

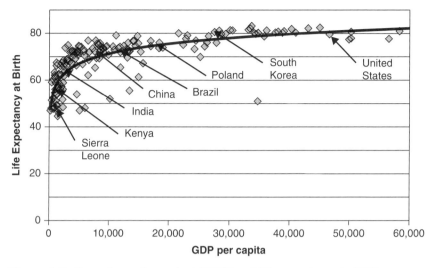

Figure 4–7 Gross domestic product (GDP) and life expectancy in 2010.
Source: Data from *Human development report 2010*. New York: UNDP; 2010.

The **Gini Index** is a measure of the inequality in the distribution of incomes within a particular country. A country in which everyone has exactly the same income has an index of 0 (perfect equality) and a country in which one person has all the income and everyone else has zero income has an index of 100 (perfect inequality). For example, Namibia has a Gini Index of 74.3 and a very unequal distribution of income,[16] with the richest 10% of the population making about 107 times more than the poorest 10%.[17] In contrast, Denmark has a Gini Index of 24.7 and a relatively equal income distribution, with the richest 10% making 8 times more than the poorest 10%. The United States has a Gini Index of 40.8, and the richest 10% make about 16 times more than the poorest 10%. In general, European countries have the greatest income equality and countries in Africa and the Americas have the greatest income inequalities. Income inequalities are associated with higher mortality rates, especially among younger adults.[18,19]

Some measures of socioeconomic status combine economic data with other markers of development, including health status. For example, the **Human Development Index (HDI)**, developed by the World Bank, is an estimate of national development based on composite data on longevity (life expectancy at birth), knowledge (school enrollment and adult literacy rate), and income (GDP per capita in purchasing power parity dollars). Some of these measures are highlighted in **Table 4–2**. There is a connection between

Table 4-2 Socioeconomic indicators by country in 2011.

Country	USA	South Korea	Poland	Brazil	China	India	Kenya	Sierra Leone
GDP per capita ($) (2009)	45,989	27,100	18,905	10,367	6828	3296	1573	808
GNI per capita (PPP$)	43,017	28,230	17,451	10,162	7476	3468	1492	737
Mean years of schooling (for ages ≥25)	12.4	11.6	10.0	7.2	7.5	4.4	7.0	2.9
HDI value	0.910	0.897	0.813	0.718	0.687	0.547	0.509	0.336
Inequality-adjusted HDI	0.771	0.749	0.734	0.519	0.534	0.392	0.338	0.196
Quintile income ratio, richest 20% to poorest 20% (2000–2011)	8.5	4.7	5.6	17.6	8.4	5.6	11.3	8.1
Gini Index for income (2000–2011)	40.8	31.6	34.2	53.9	41.5	36.8	47.7	42.5
Overall life satisfaction (on a scale from 0 to 10, with 10 representing high satisfaction)	7.2	6.1	5.8	6.8	4.7	5.0	4.3	4.1

Source: Data from *Human development report 2011*. New York: UNDP; 2011.

these indicators and health status, with more economically developed countries experiencing a high burden from NCDs and less developed countries continuing to have a high burden from infectious diseases even as NCDs are a growing concern.

4.3 HEALTH OF VULNERABLE POPULATIONS

Access to health care and other services is associated with wealth, employment, and education, but it is also related to power. Power can be conferred by political position and socioeconomic position. Government officials may have the authority to demand certain services, and business leaders may have the money and connections to access care that is denied to others. Power can also be conferred by cultural systems. A tribal or religious leader may have the power to mobilize people and resources at will. A husband may have power to control his wife's movements and activities.

Powerful people can choose to limit or grant access to goods and resources like property, technology, social networks, and health care. In many populations, some people have the power to secure health for themselves and their families while others without power have limited or no access to the resources they need to be safe and healthy. Members of potentially vulnerable groups—such as ethnic, racial, religious, and tribal minorities; immigrants, refugees, and internally displaced people; prisoners; people with mental illnesses or physical impairments; and older persons—may not have the power to demand access to an equitable level of healthcare. The resulting **inequalities** in health, differences in health experience and health status, exist at many levels. These differences are largely a function of social, political, and economic environments, and not innate biological differences. Some of these differences are avoidable, unfair, and unjust, and are referred to as **inequities**.[20]

4.3.A Race, Ethnicity, and Health

Ethnicity is based on many dimensions of cultural heritage, tribal affiliation, nationality, race, religion, and language. **Race** refers to superficial categories that group individuals based primarily on physical attributes like skin color. Significant cultural and genetic diversity is present within most "racial" groups. For example, in the United States government surveys include only five racial categories: American Indian or Alaskan Native, Asian, Black or African American, Native Hawaiian or other Pacific Islander, and White.[21] The "White" category includes most people whose ancestors were Europeans, North Africans, Middle Easterners, or Latin Americans; the "Asian" category includes people with ancestors from countries as diverse as China, India, the Philippines, and Thailand. (These surveys also include only one measure of "ethnicity": whether a person self-identifies as having "Hispanic or Latino" origin.)

Significant differences in health status often exist between different racial and ethnic groups. An assortment of explanations each partly explains the reasons for these health disparities.[22] Racial and ethnic categories may capture some genetic differences between population groups, and genes may predispose people to particular diseases and conditions. For example, Tay-Sachs disease, a fatal neurological disease of young children, is mostly found among people whose ancestors were Jews from Eastern Europe, and sickle cell anemia, also a genetic disorder, is more common in people of African and Mediterranean heritage. Race and ethnicity may also be markers for health behaviors. If members of a particular ethnic group tend to have the same dietary preferences and favorite foods, alcohol and tobacco use habits, and physical activity routines, these practices may account for some of the health differences observed between populations. Race and ethnicity may also be associated with socioeconomic position. Members of marginalized population groups may have lower socioeconomic status than other people in their town or city, and poverty is known to be associated with reduced health status. Additionally, discrimination on the basis of race or ethnicity may cause chronic psychosocial stress that leads to poor health outcomes.

Celebrations of the various cultural traditions that exist within a nation or community can bring people with diverse backgrounds together. However, race and ethnicity can also be used to divide people. At worst, these divisions can lead to abuse, violence, hate crimes, war, and genocide. On a day-to-day basis, people who belong to minority racial, ethnic, tribal, or religious groups may encounter discrimination along with language, cultural, and belief barriers. These obstacles may exist in the workplace and marketplace, and also within the healthcare system. Medical practitioners may be unfamiliar with the special health needs of patients from other backgrounds (in part because many population groups remain understudied by health researchers), and patients may be uncomfortable discussing health concerns and being examined by a doctor who is not a member of their group.

For example, women from traditional cultural and religious sects may be uncomfortable being examined by a male doctor. And in some cases barriers to healthcare access are legally sanctioned, such as when proof of legal residency is required before health care can be offered. Because of these obstacles to accessing health care, the health status of minority populations tends to be worse than that of the majority populations.

Indigenous populations tend to have especially low health status compared to other residents of their countries. More than 350 million people worldwide are members of indigenous population groups that have maintained unique cultural traditions (and often also languages) for many generations after the colonization or domination of their traditional homeland by another group. These populations include the Cherokee (and many other groups) of the United States, the Sami of Scandinavia, the Torres Strait Islanders of Australia, the Tangata Whenua (Māori) of New Zealand, the Quichua of Ecuador, the Maasai of Kenya, and the Hmong of Southeast Asia.[23] Members of indigenous people groups are more likely to be poor than their nonindigenous neighbors, and usually have higher rates of morbidity and premature mortality.[24]

4.3.B Immigrants

People move from one community or country to another for a variety of reasons. Some move voluntarily to be closer to family, to start a new job, or to pursue educational opportunities, while others are forced to move because of violence, persecution, or natural disasters. Some migrants intend to settle permanently in their new host country, while others are temporary guest workers. Some immigrants may experience an increase in access to health care when they move from a country with a poor health infrastructure to a country with an easily accessible healthcare system, but many immigrants experience reduced access to health care in their new communities. Thus, it is impossible to speak generically about the health effects of migration.[25]

However, many migrants do face heightened health risks during their journeys and as they settle in to their new places of residence.[26] For example, smuggled migrants, victims of trafficking, asylum seekers, and refugees may experience violence and deprivation as well as other traumas during their travels. And after arriving, many voluntary and involuntary migrants face obstacles to accessing health care and staying healthy because of poverty, language barriers, and risky jobs.

4.3.C Prisoners

On any given day, nearly 10 million people across the globe are incarcerated (**Figure 4–8**).[27] (That 10 million includes more than 2 million adults in the United States, the country with the highest proportion of incarcerated people in the world.[27]) Prisons, jails, and detention centers house convicted criminals and may also accommodate suspects waiting for trial, juvenile offenders, and illegal immigrants. Many people entering prison already have health problems related to mental illness, drug abuse, malnutrition, and poverty. Severe overcrowding, poor ventilation, poor nutrition, unhygienic conditions, lack of access to medical care, abuse by guards, and prisoner-on-prisoner violence, including beatings and sexual assault, may all facilitate the spread of disease within prisons. However, contracting potentially life-threatening infections is not part of any prisoner's sentence, and it is considered unjust not to provide incarcerated people with medical and dental care, adequate nutrition, protection from infectious diseases, and safe conditions.[28] Prisoners are entitled to all fundamental human rights, and need to be protected from medical neglect, starvation, abuse, forced medical experimentation, and other civil rights violations.

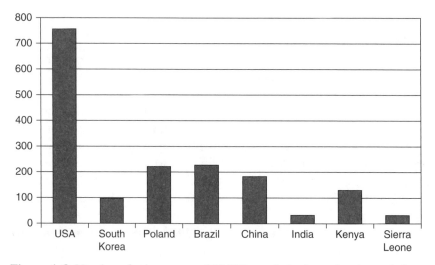

Figure 4–8 Number of prisoners per 100,000 people in the national population in 2008.

Source: Data from Walmsley R. *World prison population list*, 8th edition. London: International Centre for Prison Studies; 2008.

Tuberculosis (TB) is one of the diseases that has become a major health crisis in prisons, especially in the former Soviet Union and in parts of the world with relatively high TB rates in the general population.[29] Tuberculosis spreads easily in crowded prison blocks, and late diagnosis and inadequate treatment may allow prisoners with TB to have a contagious form of the disease for lengthy periods of time. The prevalence of TB in prisons in some places has been reported to be up to 100 times higher than in the general population (**Figure 4–9**).[29] Over time, an increase in TB in prisons will increase the amount of TB in the general population too, because once persons infected with TB are released from prison they may spread TB to their family and friends. Furthermore, each prisoner may become infected with several different strains of TB, contributing to the emergence of multidrug-resistant TB (MDR-TB) strains that are not able to be cured by the standard antibiotics used to treat TB. To prevent further increases in the prevalence of TB in prisons, it is important for every case of TB in prisoners to be detected early and treated consistently with no interruptions in antibiotic therapy.

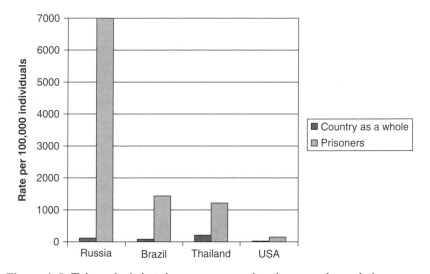

Figure 4–9 Tuberculosis in prisoners compared to the general population.
Source: Data from Dara M, Grzemska M, Kimerling ME, Reyes H, Zagorskiy A. *Guidelines for control of tuberculosis in prisons.* Washington DC: USAID and Tuberculosis Coalition for Technical Assistance; 2009.

4.4 CULTURE AND HEALTH

Culture is a way of living, believing, behaving, communicating, and understanding the world that is shared by members of a social unit. Culture includes a group's norms, values, morals, rules, and customs. Culture also often defines the foods people eat, the clothes they wear, the language they use, the ways they interact with those inside and outside the cultural group, and how they describe and experience **illness** (feeling unhealthy) and **sickness** (how a person with poor physical or mental health relates to and is regarded by the community).[30] Thus, people with a shared culture may engage in similar health-related behaviors, have similar health beliefs, and have similar preferences about when and where to seek health care.

Different cultures may have distinct explanations about what causes disease. A mechanistic approach sees disease as a dysfunction or breakdown of the human body, which is supposed to function like a well-oiled machine. A moralistic perspective considers health to be the result of clean living and disease to be a type of punishment for wrongdoing. A supernatural viewpoint blames illness on demonic possession, evil eye, or the anger of God or the gods or ancestors. A disequilibrium approach considers disease to be caused by imbalance within the body, such as an imbalance between hot and cold, yin and yang, or the four humors of blood, phlegm, yellow bile, and black bile. Disease may also be attributed to energy or qi imbalances; to emotions like fright or grief or jealously; or to stress, weather, food, germs, sex, genes, or age.

These beliefs about health and illness may influence the way people interpret symptoms and diagnoses, the timeline for seeking treatment, and the type of therapy that will be effective. Those with a mechanistic viewpoint may prefer to be treated by an allopathic practitioner like a physician or a nurse; those with a spiritual perspective may visit a religious advisor; those who see illness as the result of disequilibrium may seek the services of an acupuncturist, a chiropractor, or a massage therapist.

A growing number of people around the world now blend Western medicine and traditional medicine (TM), mixing prescription medications with herbal remedies, manual techniques, and spiritual therapies. **Complementary/alternative medicine (CAM)** refers to the use of healthcare practices outside of a person's own tradition or that are not part of conventional medical practice. The distinction between TM/CAM and Western medicine is blurring. Many pharmaceutical formulations are made from plants first used in traditional treatments, and CAM therapies are increasingly being integrated into allopathic medical practice. In some countries, allopathic and traditional practitioners work alongside one another in the healthcare system so that patients can receive both conventional and complementary care.[31,32]

Culture plays a role in how health and disease are experienced across the lifespan, everything from the way childbirth is approached to decisions about end-of-life care. An understanding of the global diversity of perspectives on health, disease, illness, sickness, medicine, and healing is necessary for those working in medicine and in the global public health arena. Public health initiatives and medical interventions must be culturally acceptable as well as socioeconomically affordable and accessible.

4.5 DISCUSSION QUESTIONS

1. Describe yourself using the PROGRESS-Plus list of the social determinants of health shown in Table 4–1. How do these characteristics affect your health status?
2. How would you survive if you earned only $1.25 per day?
3. If you had a very small income and limited wealth, how would you prioritize spending on food, housing, utilities, clothing, education, health care, and entertainment?
4. What are some of the conditions related to poverty that increase the risk of infectious diseases? Noncommunicable diseases (NCDs)? Neuropsychiatric disorders? Injuries?
5. What health disparities are present within your own community?
6. Do you identify with a particular ethnic group? Do you know of any health conditions that you are at special risk for because of your ethnic background? Are these conditions genetic? Are they related to health behaviors?
7. How do your beliefs about the causes of disease influence your approach to health, well-being, and healing?
8. What complementary and alternative medical (CAM) therapies have you tried? Do you use CAM to complement or replace conventional medical treatment?

REFERENCES

1. Kavanagh J, Oliver S, Lorenc T. Reflections on developing and using PROGRESS-Plus. *Equity Update*. 2008;2:1–3.
2. Wilkinson R, Marmot M. *Social determinants of health: the solid facts.* Copenhagen: WHO; 2003.

3. *Human development report 2011.* New York: UNDP; 2011.

4. *India: DHS, 2005–06—final report.* Calverton MD: International Institute for Population Sciences and Macro International Inc.; 2007.

5. *Kenya: DHS, 2008–09—final report.* Nairobi and Calverton MD: Kenya National Bureau of Statistics and ICF Macro; 2010.

6. *Sierra Leone: DHS, 2008—final report.* Freetown and Calverton MD: Statistics Sierra Leone, Ministry of Health and Sanitation, and ICF Macro; 2009.

7. Geyer S, Peter R. Occupational status and all-cause mortality: a study with health insurance data from Nordrhein-Westfalen, Germany. *Eur J Public Health.* 1999;9:114–118.

8. Kunst AE, Groenhof F, Mackenbach JP; EU Working Group on Socioeconomic Inequalities in Health. Occupational class and cause specific mortality in middle aged men in 11 European countries: comparison of population based studies. *BMJ.* 1998;316:1636–1642.

9. Jin RL, Shah CP, Svoboda TJ. The impact of unemployment on health: a review of the evidence. *CMAJ.* 1995;153:529–540.

10. Paul KI, Moser K. Unemployment impairs mental health: meta-analysis. *J Vocational Behav.* 2009;74:264–282.

11. Roelfs DJ, Shor E, Davidson KW, Schwartz JE. Losing life and livelihood: a systematic review and meta-analysis of unemployment and all-cause mortality. *Soc Sci Med.* 2011;72:840–854.

12. King EH, Hill MA. *Women's education in developing countries: barriers, benefits, and policies.* Baltimore MD: Johns Hopkins University Press; 1993.

13. *State of the world's children 2012.* New York: UNICEF; 2012.

14. Ong LL. Burgernomics: the economics of the Big Mac standard. *J Int Money Finance.* 1997;16:865–878.

15. *World development indicators database.* Washington DC: World Bank.

16. *Human development report 2010.* New York: UNDP; 2010.

17. *Human development report 2009.* New York: UNDP; 2009.

18. Dorling D, Mitchell R, Pearce J. The global impact of income inequality on health by age: an observational study. *BMJ.* 2007;335:873.

19. Wilkinson RG, Pickett KE. Income inequality and population health: a review and explanation of the evidence. *Soc Sci Med.* 2006;62:1768–1784.

20. Gwatkin DR. Health inequalities and the health of the poor: What do we know? What can we do? *Bull World Health Organ.* 2000;78:3–18.

21. *Revisions to the standards for the classification of federal data on race and ethnicity.* Washington DC: Office of Management and Budget (OMB); 1997.

22. Dressler WW, Oths KS, Gravlee CC. Race and ethnicity in public health research: models to explain health disparities. *Ann Rev Anthropol.* 2005;34:231–252.

23. Bartlett JG, Madariaga-Vignudo L, O'Neil JD, Kuhnlein HV. Identifying indigenous peoples for health research in a global context: a review of perspectives and challenges. *Int J Circumpolar Health.* 2007;66:287–307.

24. Gracey M, King M. Indigenous health part 1: determinants and disease patterns. *Lancet.* 2009;374:65–75.

25. *International migration, health & human rights.* Geneva: WHO; 2003.

26. Gushulak BD, MacPherson DW. The basic principles of migration health: population mobility and gaps in disease prevalence. *Emerg Themes Epidemiol.* 2006;3:3.

27. Walmsley R. *World prison population list*, 8th edition. London: International Centre for Prison Studies; 2008.

28. *Standard minimum rules for the treatment of prisoners.* Geneva: Office of the United Nations High Commissioner for Human Rights; 1977.

29. Dara M, Grzemska M, Kimerling ME, Reyes H, Zagorskiy A. *Guidelines for control of tuberculosis in prisons.* Washington DC: USAID and Tuberculosis Coalition for Technical Assistance; 2009.

30. Boyd KM. Disease, illness, sickness, health, healing and wholeness: exploring some elusive concepts. *Med Humanities.* 2000;26:9–17.

31. *Legal status of traditional medicine and complementary/alternative medicine: a worldwide review.* Geneva: WHO; 2001.

32. *Traditional medicine strategy 2002–2005 (WHO/EDM/TRM/2002.1).* Geneva: WHO; 2002.

CHAPTER 5

Child Health

Nearly all child mortality occurs in low-income countries, where the lack of medical care for newborns, infections like diarrhea and pneumonia, and undernutrition cause millions of deaths each year. Most of these deaths could be prevented by low-cost interventions and health education, and many local and global initiatives are succeeding in their efforts to improve child health and survival.

5.1 INEQUALITIES IN CHILD DEATH

In 2010, about 8 million children died.[1] About half of these deaths happened in sub-Saharan Africa and about one-third in South Asia. Less than 1% occurred in high-income countries. About 1 in 5 newborns in central Africa and 1 in 13 newborns in South Asia do not survive to their fifth birthdays.[2] In contrast, about 1 in 167 newborns in North America and 1 in 270 newborns in Western Europe die during their first five years. Thus, although the child mortality rate is decreasing in nearly every region of the world (**Figure 5–1**), significant gaps remain (**Figure 5–2**).[1,3]

Most of the children who die this year will be in their first five years of life, the age group professionals working in the field of **maternal and child health** (often shortened to just "MCH") call "**under-5s.**" About one-third of under-5 deaths occur in **neonates** (newborns in their first 28 days after birth), about one-third in **infants** 29 days through 1 year old, and about one-third in children between their first and fifth birthdays. **Table 5–1** summarizes the leading causes of under-5 death: neonatal conditions, diarrhea, pneumonia, malaria, other infections, injuries, and undernutrition.[4]

Figure 5–3 shows the distribution of causes of death for under-5s who survived for at least one month after birth (to the postneonatal period).[4] The vast majority of these pediatric deaths are due to preventable or treatable conditions like diarrhea, pneumonia, malaria, measles, and other infections (such as HIV/AIDS, meningitis, and pertussis). If malnutrition, which contributes to at least one-third of child deaths,[5] is also considered, then

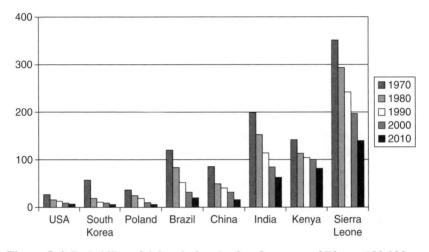

Figure 5–1 Probability of dying during the first five years of life per 100,000 live births between 1970 and 2010.

Source: Data from Rajaratnam JK, Marcus JR, Flaxman AD, et al. Neonatal, postneonatal, childhood, and under-5 mortality for 187 countries, 1970–2010: a systematic analysis of progress toward Millennium Development Goal 4. *Lancet*. 2010;375:1988–2008.

the proportion of preventable deaths is even higher. The majority of child deaths can be prevented with simple, low-cost interventions that have been proven to be effective. The following sections provide an overview of each of the most common causes of child death and the interventions for each condition that already save thousands of lives each year and could save thousands more if they were implemented more widely.

5.2 NEONATAL MORTALITY

Most deaths of newborns occur because the babies are born too early and are underdeveloped, because of complications during labor and delivery that may result in asphyxia or birth trauma that damages the brain or other organs (complications that are common when women do not have access to a healthcare professional when giving birth), and because of infections acquired around the time of birth.[6] About 3.5 million neonates die each year (**Table 5–2**),[4] with most deaths occurring in low-income countries (**Figure 5–4**).[7] (That number includes only live births; it does not include the approximately 3 million stillbirths that occur each year.[6])

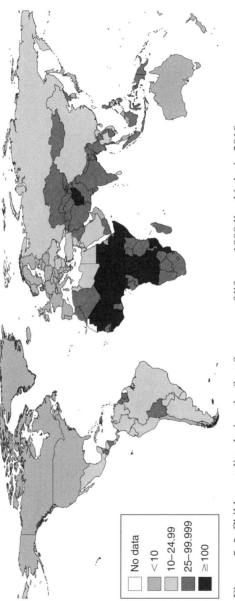
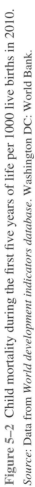

Figure 5–2 Child mortality during the first five years of life per 1000 live births in 2010. *Source:* Data from *World development indicators database.* Washington DC: World Bank.

Table 5–1 Causes of mortality in children during their first five years of life. Undernutrition is not listed separately but is a contributing factor to about one-third of these deaths.

Cause	Estimated Number of Deaths Worldwide in 2008	Estimated % of All Pediatric Deaths
Neonatal deaths, including preterm birth complications, birth asphyxia, sepsis, and other conditions	3,600,000	41%
Diarrheal diseases	1,300,000	14%
Acute respiratory infections (ARIs)	1,200,000	14%
Malaria	750,000	8%
Injuries	300,000	3%
HIV/AIDS	200,000	2%
Measles	100,000	1%
Other infections	1,100,000	13%
All other causes	350,000	4%

Note: These are estimates based on prediction models, rather than actual counts, because reporting systems in most countries are incomplete. Other research groups report slightly different estimates.

Source: Data from Black RE, Cousens S, Johnson HL, et al.; Child Health Epidemiology Research Group (CHERG) of WHO and UNICEF. Global, regional, and national causes of child mortality in 2008: a systematic analysis. Lancet. 2010;375:1969–1987.

The implementation of several proven interventions before birth, during delivery, and in the minutes, hours, and days after birth significantly improves the likelihood of survival of newborns (**Table 5–3**).[8]

5.3 DIARRHEA

Diarrhea is an increase in the volume of stool and the frequency of defecation, and it can quickly cause dehydration and death in young children. Diarrhea causes the loss of excessive amounts of water and

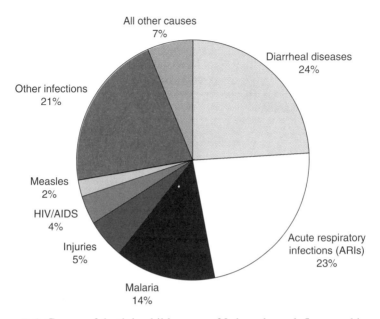

Figure 5–3 Causes of death in children ages 29 days through 5 years old.

Source: Data from Black RE, Cousens S, Johnson HL, et al.; Child Health Epidemiology Research Group (CHERG) of WHO and UNICEF. Global, regional, and national causes of child mortality in 2008: a systematic analysis. *Lancet*. 2010;375:1969–1987.

the loss of electrolytes like sodium, potassium, and bicarbonate. Severe dehydration can cause low blood pressure (because fluid loss decreases blood volume), a fast and weak pulse, rapid breathing (but insufficient oxygen intake), sunken dry eyes, loss of skin elasticity, muscle contractions and convulsions, and delirium. Electrolyte imbalances can lead to kidney and heart failure, and eventually to death.

Diarrhea is usually caused by an infection like rotavirus (which is vaccine-preventable) or bacteria such as *E. coli*, *Shigella*, *Campylobacter*, or *Salmonella*. (It can also be caused by conditions like lactose intolerance that cause poor absorption of water, and by food allergies, some antibiotics and other medications, and some chemicals, such as caffeine and toxins.) The infectious agents that cause diarrhea are transmitted through contaminated food and water, by physical contact with people who have an infection that causes diarrhea, and by contact with feces. Together, unsafe drinking water, inadequate availability of water for hygiene, and lack of access to sanitation (such as a toilet or latrine) are estimated to contribute to about 90% of deaths from diarrhea each year.[9] Prevention of diarrhea

Table 5–2 Causes of neonatal mortality.

Cause	Estimated Number of Neonatal Deaths Worldwide in 2008	Estimated % of All Neonatal Deaths
Preterm birth complications	1,000,000	29%
Birth asphyxia	800,000	23%
Sepsis	500,000	15%
Pneumonia	400,000	11%
Congenital abnormalities	300,000	8%
Diarrhea	80,000	2%
Tetanus	60,000	2%
Other	400,000	11%

Source: Data from Black RE, Cousens S, Johnson HL, et al.; Child Health Epidemiology Research Group (CHERG) of WHO and UNICEF. Global, regional, and national causes of child mortality in 2008: a systematic analysis. *Lancet*. 2010;375:1969–1987.

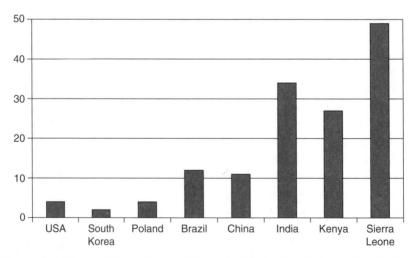

Figure 5–4 Neonatal mortality rate (death during the first 28 days after birth) per 100,000 live births in 2010.

Source: Data from *State of the world's children 2012*. New York: UNICEF; 2012.

Table 5–3 Examples of effective interventions for neonatal health.

Time	*Intervention*
Preconception	• Folic acid supplementation to prevent neural tube defects • Birth spacing
Antenatal/ prenatal (before birth)	• Tetanus toxoid immunization • Syphilis screening and treatment • Intermittent preventive treatment in pregnancy (IPTp) of malaria (in endemic areas) • Maternal supplementation with iron, iodine, zinc, and calcium • Maternal antihelminthic (deworming) treatment • Prevention of mother-to-child HIV transmission
Intranatal/ intraparturm (during delivery)	• Clean delivery • Detection and management of breech births (by Caesarian section, if required) • Antibiotics for preterm premature rupture of membranes • Corticosteroids for preterm labor • Early diagnosis of complications during labor
Postnatal (after birth)	• Newborn resuscitation • Delayed umbilical cord clamping • Breastfeeding • Kangaroo mother care (keeping low birthweight babies in an upright position on a parent's bare chest so they have skin-to-skin contact and the baby's ear is near the parent's heart) • Prevention and management of hypothermia • Nevirapine and replacement feeding for babies born to mothers with HIV infection • Pneumonia case management • Neonatal vitamin A supplementation • Insecticide-treated bednets for malaria prevention

Source: Information from Darmstadt GL, Bhutta ZA, Cousens S, Adam T, Walker N, Bernis L; Lancet Neonatal Survival Steering Team. Evidence-based, cost-effective interventions: how many newborn babies can we save? *Lancet*. 2005;365:977–985.

requires access to clean water for drinking, food preparation, handwashing, and bathing, and the safe disposal of feces.

About 2.5 billion cases of diarrhea occur in under-5 children each year,[10] and more than 1 million children die from diarrhea each year.[11] Once a child has diarrhea, the most important method for preventing death is the administration of **oral rehydration therapy (ORT)**. Sometimes called oral rehydration solution or salts (ORS), ORT is a solution of sugar, salt, and clean drinking water that replaces lost fluids and restores the balance of electrolytes in the blood. Oral rehydration salts are sometimes distributed in packets at clinics, usually in a relatively new "low osmolarity" formula. Parents can also make their own ORS solution by mixing 8 teaspoons of sugar and one half teaspoon of salt into one liter of boiled water. Potassium can be added to the solution through fruit juice, coconut water, or mashed bananas. Children with diarrhea need to drink ORT every time they pass watery stool for a total of at least one liter each day. If they also have vomiting they need to drink more ORT in order to replace those lost fluids. Zinc supplementation also helps prevent diarrhea deaths.[12]

Adequate nutrition is also important because malnutrition increases the risk of death from diarrhea. Children with diarrhea should be encouraged to eat the same foods that they normally consume (as long as they are not vomiting too much to keep food down), and breastfed children should continue to breastfeed during their illness. After children recover from diarrhea they should be encouraged to eat more food than normal to regain lost weight and lost nutrients.

ORT combined with **continued feeding** leads to the best health outcomes for children with diarrhea, but in developing countries fewer than half of children with diarrhea receive this care.[7] Additional health education for parents and communities is needed in order to increase the use of ORT, to promote continued feeding for sick children, and to facilitate water and sanitation development and other actions that prevent diarrhea (**Table 5–4**).

5.4 PNEUMONIA

The main function of the body's respiratory system is the exchange of gases, which mostly means taking in oxygen and getting rid of carbon dioxide (**Figure 5–5**). When a person takes a breath, the air enters the lungs and fills little air sacs called alveoli. Each alveolus is wrapped in tiny blood vessels called capillaries and has a very thin surface so that gas exchange

Table 5–4 Key methods for preventing and treating diarrhea.

Prevention (primary prevention to reduce new infections)	*Treatment* (secondary prevention to reduce disease severity and death once a child is ill)
• Rotavirus and measles immunization	• Fluid replacement to prevent dehydration
• Early and exclusive breastfeeding of infants, followed by complementary feeding	○ Oral rehydration therapy (ORT)
	○ Breastfeeding
• Vitamin A supplementation	○ Continued feeding during illness
• Hand washing with soap	• Zinc supplementation
• Improved water supply quantity and quality	
• Community-wide sanitation (safe disposal of stool, latrine use instead of open defecation)	

Information from *Diarrhoea: why children are dying and what can be done*. New York/Geneva: WHO/UNICEF; 2009.

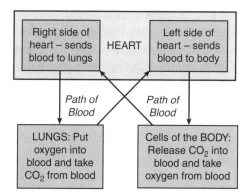

Figure 5–5 Path of blood through the heart, lungs, and body.

can take place. When a person inhales, oxygen is absorbed into the blood in those capillaries. This oxygenated blood is pumped into the heart and then to the rest of the body so that all of the cells can receive the oxygen they need to function properly. When the cells take in oxygen from nearby capillaries, they can also get rid of carbon dioxide and other waste products by dumping them into the blood. Carbon dioxide and other waste products can then be released from the blood into the alveoli. When a person exhales, these wastes are expelled from the body.

Pneumonia occurs when part of a lung fills with fluid. If the alveoli are filled with fluid, they cannot efficiently exchange oxygen and carbon dioxide. The symptoms of an **acute respiratory illness (ARI)** of the lower respiratory tract usually include a cough accompanied by difficult rapid breathing. People with pneumonia can feel like they are drowning as fluid fills their lungs and they develop **hypoxia** (lack of oxygen). A child with severe infection may even turn bluish in color due to hypoxia.

Approximately 150 million cases of pneumonia occur in under-5 children worldwide each year.[13] Acute lower respiratory infections can be caused by a variety of pathogens, but most often are caused by bacteria. The most common bacterial causes of pneumonia are pneumococcus (*Streptococcus pneumoniae*) and *Haemophilus influenzae* type b (Hib). Both of these infections are vaccine-preventable. Other common agents include *Staphylococcus aureus* and *Klebsiella pneumoniae*.[13]

Bacterial infections can often be cured by inexpensive oral antibiotics if treatment is sought soon after the onset of symptoms. However, only about 60% of the world's children with suspected pneumonia are taken to a healthcare provider and only about one-third are treated with antibiotics.[7] Thus, one component of improving child survival is educating caregivers about the importance of seeking medical care as soon as the symptoms of pneumonia appear, so that a course of antibiotics can be started. (Antibiotics will not speed recovery from colds and other upper respiratory infections like bronchitis that are usually caused by viruses, but they are usually effective against early-stage bacterial pneumonia.)

5.5 MALARIA

Malaria is a parasitic infection spread by the bites of infected mosquitoes. Malaria usually presents with a fever and flu-like symptoms, but children with malaria can deteriorate quickly and enter into a coma (cerebral malaria). In many cases, children with malaria can be successfully treated with inexpensive antimalarial tablets, but malaria can cause weeks or even months of illness due to relapses and severe anemia (too few red blood cells). Reinfection with malaria is common, and in many tropical areas the average child may have several bouts of malaria each year. Furthermore, babies born to women with malaria have an increased risk of low birth weight, birth complications, and stillbirths. One of the most effective ways to prevent infection is the use of insecticide-treated bednets (ITNs) that shield sleeping people from the bites of mosquitoes, yet many households in regions where malaria is common do not have ITNs or fail to use them consistently.

5.6 VACCINE-PREVENTABLE DISEASES

Hundreds of thousands of children die each year from vaccine-preventable diseases. Measles remains one of the most common causes of vaccine-preventable mortality, even though the rates of measles mortality have dropped significantly in recent years.[14,15] Measles is a highly contagious viral infection that is spread from one person to another through the air or by contact with secretions from the nose or throat of people with the infection. The common symptoms are a fever, runny nose, cough, and sore eyes, followed by a rash that starts on the face and spreads down the body. But measles may also cause diarrhea, ear infections, pneumonia, and encephalitis (brain swelling), and these severe complications can lead to permanent disabilities, especially in children who are undernourished. There is no treatment available for measles, so prevention through immunization is crucial. Other vaccine-preventable infections that cause many deaths of children each year include *Haemophilus influenzae* type b (Hib), pneumococcus, and rotavirus, among others. **Table 5–5** lists all childhood vaccinations currently recommended by the World Health Organization (WHO) and by the U.S. Centers for Disease Control and Prevention (CDC).[16,17]

5.7 UNDERNUTRITION AND BREASTFEEDING

Undernutrition occurs when children do not consume enough calories or do not take in adequate amounts of specific nutrients like proteins, fats, vitamins, and minerals. In addition to deaths directly caused by undernutrition, being malnourished increases the risk of death from infectious diseases. Many cases of undernutrition could be prevented by a simple set of nutritional interventions that include having infants consume only breastmilk during their first six months of life, continuing to provide breastmilk after introducing solid foods into the infant's diet, and providing vitamin A and zinc supplementation when necessary.[5]

New mothers should be encouraged to breastfeed their babies so that they can pass both nutrients and disease-fighting antibodies to their children.

Table 5–5 Recommended childhood immunizations. The WHO schedule is for most children worldwide. The CDC schedule is for children in the United States.

Agent	Agent Type	WHO Schedule	CDC Schedule
Chickenpox (varicella)	Virus		●
Cholera	Bacterium	○	
Diphtheria	Bacterium	●	●
Hepatitis A virus	Virus	○	●
Hepatitis B virus	Virus	●	●
Haemophilus influenzae type b (Hib)	Bacterium	●	●
Human papillomavirus	Virus	●	●
Influenza	Virus	○	●
Japanese encephalitis	Virus	○	
Measles	Virus	●	●
Meningococcal	Bacterium	○	●
Mumps	Virus	○	●
Pertussis (whooping cough)	Bacterium	●	●
Pneumococcal	Bacterium	●	●
Polio (poliovirus)	Virus	●	●
Rabies	Virus	○	
Rotavirus	Virus	●	●
Rubella (German measles)	Virus	○	●
Tetanus	Bacterium	●	●
Tuberculosis	Bacterium	●	
Typhoid	Bacterium	○	
Yellow fever	Virus	○	

● Recommended for all children
○ Recommended for children in some countries or some high-risk areas and population groups

Source: Data from *Recommended routine immunization: summary of WHO position papers*. Geneva: WHO; 2010 Oct 21; and *2011 childhood & adolescent immunization schedules*. Atlanta GA: CDC; 2011.

Breastmilk contains all of the nutrients and water babies need, and it also includes digestive enzymes and antibodies and other immune factors that protect against harmful infections and promote health. For example, bifidus factor encourages the multiplication of helpful bacteria called *Lactobacillus bifidus* in the baby's intestines. Colostrum, the milk produced in the first days after giving birth, is especially beneficial because it contains large quantities of an antibody called secretory immunoglobulin A (IgA).[18] **Early breastfeeding**, breastfeeding within the first hour after giving birth, also increases the neonatal survival rate.

In ideal circumstances, infants should be exclusively breastfed for the first 6 months of life. **Exclusive breastfeeding** means that breastmilk is the only substance the baby consumes, and that no supplemental water, juice, cow or goat milk, porridge, rice water, or any other foods are fed to the baby. However, only about one in three children worldwide is exclusively breastfed for the first six months of life.[7] This low percentage contributes to illness and death from undernutrition and diarrhea.

After six months of exclusive breastfeeding, **complementary foods** should be introduced into the infant's diet while continuing breastfeeding for up to 2 years or more (**Figure 5–6**).[19] "Complementary" means that the foods accompany breastmilk and do not immediately replace it.

Not all women are able to exclusively breastfeed. Some mothers do not produce adequate milk for their babies and have to supplement with formula at an early age, some have HIV infection and do not want to risk passing the virus to their babies through breastmilk, and some have work schedules that do not allow them to feed their babies every few hours. Newborns whose mothers have died in childbirth are also not able to be breastfed by their mothers. Breastmilk substitutes for infants must provide hydration plus all of the essential nutrients. Commercial infant formula is usually the best substitute for breastmilk, because cow's milk, tea, rice water, and other substitutes do not provide all the nutrients of breastmilk or infant formula.

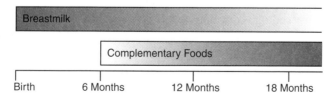

Figure 5–6 Breastfeeding timeline. Babies should have only breastmilk for the first 6 months of life, and complementary foods should be added as the baby is weaned.

However, using infant formula can be a challenge for mothers and families with a lack of access to clean water, difficulties reading and following the mixing instructions, or limited incomes to pay for commercial products.

Additional concerns about the use of formula in lower-income countries stem from the marketing strategies used by Nestlé and other infant formula companies in the 1970s.[20] Hospital maternity wards in developing countries were sponsored by formula companies, and new mothers would be sent home with formula samples and no breastfeeding education. New mothers who do not breastfeed quickly lose the ability to produce milk and must then rely on breastmilk substitutes, so providing a limited amount of free formula may create a dependency on the product. Worse, some companies hired "milk nurses" to go into communities in nursing uniforms to advertise formula, implying that formula was better than breastmilk. In 1981 the World Health Assembly addressed these problematic marketing practices with their adoption of the International Code of Marketing of Breast-milk Substitutes.[21] The Code recognizes that "when mothers do not breastfeed, or only do so partially, there is a legitimate market for infant formula." But it stresses that breastmilk is the best option, and says that new mothers who are given information about the use of infant formula must be informed about the "social and financial implications of its use, the health hazards of inappropriate foods or feeding methods, and, in particular, the health hazards of unnecessary or improper use of infant formula and other breast-milk substitutes."[21] The Code stipulates that marketing personnel (even if they are healthcare professionals) should not directly contact pregnant women or new mothers, health facilities should not promote formula use, and samples of formula should not be distributed at hospitals or by retailers. Nestlé and other major formula producers have adopted the International Code of Marketing of Breast-milk Substitutes and no longer directly market to pregnant women or new mothers in developing countries.

Mothers do need to be provided with the information to make an informed choice about whether to breastfeed and how long to breastfeed. Attitudes toward breastfeeding also need to be addressed, as in many cultures breastfeeding is discouraged. Employers rarely have a private room available for mothers who would like to use a breast pump. Women are not always free to breastfeed in public areas, even the "public" areas of their own homes. And new grandmothers who bottlefed their own babies may discourage their daughters from choosing breastfeeding. It is particularly important to promote breastfeeding as an option for new mothers in places where breastfeeding is not the cultural norm. The phrase "breast is best" needs to be accompanied by conditions that support breastfeeding.

Older infants and young children need access to a variety of nutrient-rich, age-appropriate foods. While most child hunger stems from a lack of food at the household level, it may be possible in some cases to improve the nutritional status of children by changing social eating practices. In cultures where food is traditionally served to men first and to children last, children may not get an adequate amount of high-quality proteins. In cultures where everyone at the meal eats from a common pot, small children may not eat quickly enough to secure adequate calories. New serving practices, such as giving children their own plate or bowl of food, may help children to consume the food they need to be healthier.

5.8 GLOBAL CHILD HEALTH INITIATIVES

Several multinational initiatives have sought to standardize efforts to improve global child health (**Table 5–6**).[22,23] One of the first efforts supported primary health care (PHC), a system of community-based health that employs community health workers and focuses as much on prevention as on cures. PHC became the focus of most international health work following the Alma-Ata Conference of 1978, which developed the goal of "Health for All by 2000" through the reduction of barriers to healthcare access, especially in poor and rural areas. PHC prioritizes prevention of locally common infectious diseases, promotion of nutrition, provision of essential drugs and treatments for common diseases and injuries, coordination of health services with traditional health practitioners, and programming for maternal and child health (including immunization and family planning). PHC is a "horizontal" approach to health care that emphasizes routine

Table 5–6 Acronyms for global child health programs.

Acronym	Program
PHC	Primary Health Care
EPI	Expanded Program on Immunization
GOBI	Growth monitoring, Oral rehydration therapy, Breastfeeding, and Immunization
GOBI/FFF	Growth monitoring, Oral rehydration therapy, Breastfeeding, and Immunization + Family planning, Food production, and Female education
IMCI	Integrated Management of Childhood Illness

access to comprehensive primary care, rather than a "vertical" approach that targets selected diseases with specific interventions (like special vaccination days) that are managed outside the public healthcare system.[24]

A hallmark of PHC is regularly scheduled health clinics for children under 5 years of age that monitor child growth and provide necessary immunizations for children from birth through their fifth birthdays. Because all children, whether sick or healthy, are encouraged to have frequent interactions with the healthcare system through these under-5 health clinics, warning signs for potentially life-threatening conditions in relatively healthy children can be detected early and treated. For example, growth monitoring tracks child weight so that caregivers will know if a child has lost weight or is failing to gain weight. Weight loss or stagnation can be a sign of serious illness, and early detection means that a nutritional intervention can be implemented before a health crisis occurs.

The Expanded Program on Immunization (EPI) was started in the mid-1970s by the World Health Organization and expanded the number and types of vaccines typically given to children. EPI succeeded in significantly increasing the percentage of children receiving essential immunizations.

GOBI, an initiative started in the 1980s by UNICEF, focused on increasing child survival through promotion of four simple interventions: growth monitoring, oral rehydration therapy for diarrhea, breastfeeding, and immunization. Later, a partnership between UNICEF, WHO, and the World Bank added three community-focused components to the mix—family planning, food production, and female education—creating a program called GOBI/FFF.

Integrated Management of Childhood Illness (IMCI) is a package of simple, affordable, and effective interventions for major childhood illnesses and undernutrition that was first developed in the 1990s by UNICEF and WHO.[25] The term "integrated" has several layers of meaning. One aspect of integration is the emphasis on the interrelatedness of children's health conditions. A child with malaria is more vulnerable to diarrhea. A child with vitamin A deficiency is more vulnerable to death from measles. Clinicians working under an IMCI framework complete a series of medical assessments on each sick child that allow for diagnosis of underlying conditions in addition to the primary illness. Integration also emphasizes families and communities working together with the staff of various levels of healthcare facilities to care for sick children, and the staff of outpatient clinics knowing when to refer sick children to inpatient hospital departments or specialty clinics.

The aim of IMCI is to improve family and community health practices and to improve case management skills of healthcare staff. To further this goal, IMCI provides home healthcare guidelines for families with young children (**Table 5–7**)[26] and evidence-based decision charts for

Table 5–7 Key family practices under IMCI.

	#	*Practice*
Physical and Mental Growth	1	Breastfeed infants exclusively for at least six months (if the mother does not have HIV infection)
	2	From 6 months of age, feed children good-quality complementary foods while continuing to breastfeed up to two years (or longer)
	3	Ensure that children receive adequate amounts of micronutrients (especially vitamin A, iron, and zinc) either in their diet or through supplementation
	4	Promote mental and social development by responding to a child's needs for care and by talking, playing, and providing a stimulating environment
Disease Prevention	5	Dispose of feces safely and wash hands after defecation or contact with children's feces, before preparing meals, and before feeding children
	6	Protect children in malaria-endemic areas from mosquito bites by ensuring that they sleep under insecticide-treated bednets
	7	Provide appropriate care for HIV-infected people and those affected by HIV (especially children orphaned by HIV/AIDS), and take action to prevent further HIV infections
Appropriate Home Care	8	Continue to feed and offer more fluids, including breastmilk, to children when they are sick
	9	Give sick children appropriate home treatment for infections (such as ORT for diarrhea and first aid for injuries)
	10	Protect children from injuries and accidents, and provide treatment when necessary
	11	Prevent child abuse and neglect, and take action when it does occur
	12	Involve fathers in the care of their children and in the reproductive health of their families
Care Seeking and Compliance	13	Recognize when sick children need treatment outside the home and seek care from appropriate providers
	14	Take children to complete a full course of recommended immunizations before their first birthday
	15	Follow the health provider's advice on treatment, follow-up, and referral
	16	Ensure that every pregnant woman has adequate antenatal care, and seeks care at the time of delivery and afterward

Source: Information from *Child health in the community—"community IMCI" briefing package for facilitators*. Geneva: WHO; 2004.

clinicians to use when assessing children and treating common illnesses. For example, consider the ideal integrated response to a child who has diarrhea. The family of the child should know how to prepare ORT correctly and know what symptoms require the child to be taken to the local clinic or hospital. The clinic should support community health education programs and be prepared to provide care for advanced cases of dehydration and to make referrals for hospital-based treatment if necessary. Or perhaps a family is concerned about its children contracting malaria. In an integrated response, the parents would be instructed to install and consistently use ITNs to prevent mosquito bites and to monitor their children for fevers and other symptoms of malaria. The local clinic should support community health education efforts, be prepared to effectively treat cases of malaria that do occur, and make referrals for advanced treatment if needed.

Each of these global programs had contributed to significant improvements in global child health, but infant and child health statistics show that there is still a great deal of work to be done. In order to ensure that as many children as possible have a healthy start in life, it is important to further increase access to essential drugs and immunizations, to educate parents about the use of ORT and ITNs, to promote breastfeeding, to improve access to safe drinking water and nutritional foods, and to implement other important public health measures.

5.9 THE RIGHTS OF CHILDREN

In addition to infectious disease and malnutrition, children may be at risk for injury and abuse. Both boys and girls may be subjected to physical, emotional, and sexual abuse by family members or other adults or children. In 1989, the General Assembly of the United Nations adopted the Convention on the Rights of the Child. Several of the articles of the Convention are related to child health and survival. The rights of the child include an adequate standard of living, freedom from all forms of exploitation, protection from all forms of violence, access to education and appropriate information, the right to be heard, and the right to rest, leisure, and play. Acknowledging the right of every child in the world to these basic protections is a start, but this recognition must be acted on to be meaningful. The sad reality is that millions of children are denied these protections.

Many children are sent to work at an early age. Some types of work, such as when rural children work alongside their parents on the family farm, can be a positive experience. But some children develop lasting physical and psychological scars from long hours doing domestic labor, agricultural work, or factory work. The International Labor Organization (ILO) makes a distinction between children participating in economic activity—working (whether for pay or not) for a few hours or full time doing activities other than household chores or schooling—and children who are involved in "child labor." It is permissible for children 12 years old and older to spend a few hours a week doing light work that is not hazardous. But it is a child labor violation when a child has an excessive workload, unsafe work conditions, or extreme work intensity, because any of these conditions may harm a child's physical health, mental health, or moral development. At worst, a child may be sold by his or her family into bonded labor, forced into sex work, or forced into armed conflict. The ILO estimates that more than 300 million children between the ages of 5 and 17 were engaged in labor in 2008, of whom about 115 million conducted hazardous work.[27]

Girls are especially vulnerable to abuse and neglect. In some parts of the world, they are subject to infanticide, heavy domestic responsibilities at a very early age, female genital mutilation (FGM), violence, and sexual abuse. When a family has limited resources, girls may face discrimination in food allocation, may not be allowed to attend school, and may be forced into early marriage, sometimes even before reaching puberty. In 1995, the United Nations adopted the Beijing Declaration that affirms several strategic objectives for promoting the rights of the "girl-child," including eliminating educational discrimination, the exploitation of child laborers, and violence against children.[28] Although some improvements have been achieved, such as increasing school enrollment, significant inequalities between boys and girls remain in many regions of the world.

Children with special needs are also vulnerable, especially those who require early medical intervention in order to live life to the fullest. Babies with a cleft lip or cleft palate, which is when the upper lip or the roof of the mouth is separated, may require surgery to be able to suck properly and receive adequate nutrition. Children born with cerebral palsy or spina bifida can develop their motor skills to their highest potential only if they have physical therapy and the use of braces, crutches, and walkers at an early age. Language and communication skills are learned best in the early years (until about age 7), so children who are deaf or hearing impaired do best when they start speech and language therapy as early as possible. Children with other sensory impairments, such as blindness, or with developmental disorders also benefit from early therapy that focuses on skills such as mobility, orientation (the ability to locate oneself in space), and communication. Unfortunately, many parents do not have the resources or ability to have their children start therapy at an early age, do not know what therapy to provide at home for their children, and are not able to help their disabled children access education.[29]

Several groups are dedicated to protecting children. The most prominent is UNICEF. UNICEF (initially called the United Nations International Children's Emergency Fund but now shortened to the United Nations Children's Fund) has a mandate to advocate for the protection of children's rights, to help meet their basic needs, and to expand opportunities for children to reach their full potential. UNICEF advocates for children by promoting prenatal health care, girls' education, childhood immunizations and nutrition, HIV/AIDS prevention among young people, and protective environments free of violence, abuse, and exploitation. UNICEF also responds to emergencies in order to protect the rights of children and to relieve the suffering of children and their caregivers. About two-thirds of the UNICEF budget comes from governments, but the rest must be obtained from nongovernmental organizations, partnerships, and private donations. Additionally, a wide variety of other public and private organizations promote child health, nutrition, and education, both locally and internationally.

5.10 DISCUSSION QUESTIONS

1. Do you know any parents who have experienced the death of a child? How did they respond to their loss? How do you think you would react if you had a son or daughter die at a young age?
2. In some regions of the world, more than 1 in 5 children die at a young age. How do you think the loss of so many children impacts families and communities?
3. Do you know any children who have died from pneumonia, diarrhea, malaria, measles, or undernutrition? What does your answer indicate about global health inequalities?
4. What do you notice about the differences between the WHO childhood immunization recommendations and the CDC schedule?
5. If you had an infant, would you plan to breastfeed (or encourage your partner to breastfeed)? Why or why not? Would you feel comfortable breastfeeding (or having your partner breastfeed) outside the privacy of your home?

6. Have you seen advertisements or public service announcements promoting vaccination, nutrition, or other child health practices? What
organizations sponsor these ads? What do these ads suggest are key
child health issues in your community?
7. What educational and other resources are available for children in your
community who have special needs?

REFERENCES

1. Rajaratnam JK, Marcus JR, Flaxman AD, et al. Neonatal, postneonatal, childhood, and under-5 mortality for 187 countries, 1970–2010: a systematic analysis of progress toward Millennium Development Goal 4. *Lancet*. 2010;375:1988–2008.
2. Murray CJL, Laakso T, Shibuya K, Hill K, Lopez AD. Can we achieve Millennium Development Goal 4? New analysis of country trends and forecasts of under-5 mortality to 2015. *Lancet*. 2007;370:1040–1054.
3. *World development indicators database*. Washington DC: World Bank.
4. Black RE, Cousens S, Johnson HL, et al.; Child Health Epidemiology Research Group (CHERG) of WHO and UNICEF. Global, regional, and national causes of child mortality in 2008: a systematic analysis. *Lancet*. 2010;375:1969–1987.
5. Black RE, Allen LH, Bhutta ZA, et al.; Maternal and Child Undernutrition Study Group. Maternal and child undernutrition: global and regional exposures and health consequences. *Lancet*. 2008;371:243–260.
6. *Neonatal and perinatal mortality: country, regional and global estimates*. Geneva: WHO; 2006.
7. *State of the world's children 2012*. New York: UNICEF; 2012.
8. Darmstadt GL, Bhutta ZA, Cousens S, Adam T, Walker N, Bernis L; Lancet Neonatal Survival Steering Team. Evidence-based, cost-effective interventions: how many new-born babies can we save? *Lancet*. 2005;365:977–985.
9. Prüss-Üstün A, Corvalán C. How much disease burden can be prevented by environmental interventions? *Epidemiology*. 2007;18:167–178.
10. *Diarrhoea: why children are dying and what can be done*. New York/Geneva: WHO/UNICEF; 2009.
11. Boschi-Pinto C, Velebit L, Shibuya K. Estimating child mortality due to diarrhoea in developing countries. *Bull World Health Organ*. 2008;86:710–717.
12. Fischer Waler CL, Black RE. Zinc for the treatment of diarrhoea: effect on diarrhoea morbidity, mortality and incidence of future episodes. *Int J Epidemiol*. 2010;39 (suppl 1):i63–i69.
13. Rudan I, Boschi-Pinto C, Biloglav Z, Mulholland K, Campbell H. Epidemiology and etiology of childhood pneumonia. *Bull World Health Organ*. 2008;86:408–416.
14. Wolfson LJ, Strebel PM, Gacic-Dobo M, Hoekstra EJ, McFarland JW, Hersh BS; Measles Initiative. Has the 2005 measles mortality reduction goal been achieved? A natural history modelling study. *Lancet*. 2005;369:191–200.
15. van den Ent MMVX, Brown DW, Hoekstra EJ, Christie A, Cochi SL. Measles mortality reduction contributes substantially to reduction of all cause mortality among children less than five years of age, 1990–2008. *J Infect Dis*. 2011;104(suppl 1):S18–S23.

16. *Recommended routine immunization: summary of WHO position papers.* Geneva: WHO; 2010.

17. *2011 childhood & adolescent immunization schedules.* Atlanta GA: CDC; 2011.

18. Hanson LA. Feeding and infant development: breast-feeding and immune function. *Proc Nutr Soc.* 2007;66:384–396.

19. *Complementary feeding: report of the global consultation, and summary of guiding principles for complementary feeding of the breastfed child.* Geneva: WHO; 2002.

20. Brady JP. Marketing breast milk substitutes: problems and perils throughout the world. *Arch Dis Child.* 2012;97:529–532.

21. *International Code of Marketing of Breast-milk Substitutes.* Geneva: World Health Organization; 1981. Retrieved from http://www.who.int/nutrition/publications/code_english.pdf

22. Cueto M. The origins of primary health care and selective primary health care. *Am J Public Health.* 2004;94:1864–1874.

23. Claeson M, Waldman RJ. The evolution of child health programmes in developing countries: from targeting diseases to targeting people. *Bull World Health Organ.* 2000;78:1234–1245.

24. Msuya J. *Horizontal and vertical delivery of health services: what are the trade offs?* Washington DC: World Bank; 2004.

25. Lambrechts T, Bryce J, Orinda V. Integrated management of childhood illness: a summary of first experiences. *Bull World Health Organ.* 1999;77:582–594.

26. *Child health in the community—"community IMCI" briefing package for facilitators.* Geneva: WHO; 2004.

27. International Programme on the Elimination of Child Labour (IPEC). *Children in hazardous work: what we know, what we need to do.* Geneva: ILO; 2011.

28. *The Platform for Action, UN Fourth World Conference on Women*; 1995.

29. *World report on disability 2011.* Geneva: WHO; 2011.

CHAPTER 6

Health of Younger Adults

Mental health disorders, infections, and injuries cause a large proportion of the illnesses and disabilities experienced by young adults around the world. Reproductive health issues like safe sex, family planning, and the risk of maternal mortality are also significant concerns for both young men and women.

6.1 HEALTH IN EARLY ADULTHOOD

It is fairly easy to summarize the main causes of disease, disability, and death for children (poverty) and older adults (chronic diseases), but the health risk profile for young adults varies considerably by sex and in different parts of the world. For example, HIV/AIDS is the leading cause of death of reproductive-age adults in Africa, while cardiovascular disease is the most common cause of mortality among younger adults in Europe.[1] Even so, there are several common issues that young adults face across the globe. The leading causes of morbidity, mortality, and disability of young adults worldwide include mental health disorders, injuries (primarily due to road-traffic accidents), infectious diseases, and pregnancy-related conditions (**Table 6–1**).[2,3] As adults age, the primary causes of death shift from injuries, HIV/AIDS, and suicide to heart disease and stroke (**Table 6–2**).[1]

6.2 MENTAL HEALTH

Neuropsychiatric conditions such as depression, bipolar disorder, and schizophrenia are the leading cause of disability in young adults in every region of the world, accounting for about half of all lost disability-adjusted life years (DALYs).[2] Some mental health disorders cause only occasional interference with normal activities, but others are severe and cause extreme disability. For example, people with schizophrenia may have distorted

Table 6–1 Top five causes of morbidity and mortality in adolescents and young adults worldwide, by sex and age, in 2004, with mental health and injury-related conditions shaded in grey.

		Females		Males	
		15–19 years	20–24 years	15–19 years	20–24 years
Leading Causes of Illness and Disability	1	Unipolar depressive disorders	Unipolar depressive disorders	Unipolar depressive disorders	Road-traffic accidents
	2	Schizophrenia	HIV/AIDS	Road-traffic accidents	Violence
	3	Bipolar disorder	Abortion	Alcohol use	Unipolar depressive disorders
	4	Abortion	Schizophrenia	Schizophrenia	Alcohol use
	5	Panic disorder	Bipolar disorder	Bipolar disorder	Self-inflicted injuries
Leading Causes of Death	1	Self-inflicted injuries	HIV/AIDS	Road-traffic accidents	Road-traffic accidents
	2	Road-traffic accidents	Tuberculosis	Violence	Violence
	3	Pneumonia	Self-inflicted injuries	Self-inflicted injuries	Self-inflicted injuries
	4	Tuberculosis	Fire-related death	Drownings	HIV/AIDS
	5	Fire-related death	Maternal hemorrhage	Pneumonia	Tuberculosis

Source: Data from Gore FM, Bloem PJ, Patton GC, et al. Global burden of disease in young people aged 10–24 years: a systematic analysis. Lancet. 2011;377: 2093–2102; and Patton GC, Coffey C, Sawyer SM, et al. Global patterns of mortality in young people: a systematic analysis of population health data. Lancet. 2009;374:881–892.

perceptions of reality (including hallucinations and delusions) that cause them to be socially excluded or to isolate themselves from others. People with severe depression may not have the energy to get out of bed, eat, go to work, meet with friends, or conduct other normal daily activities.

Table 6–2 Major causes of death for young and middle-aged adults, by age and sex in 2004.

Females			*Males*		
15–29 years	30–44 years	45–59 years	15–29 years	30–44 years	45–59 years
HIV/AIDS	HIV/AIDS	Ischemic heart disease	Road-traffic accidents	HIV/AIDS	Ischemic heart disease
TB	TB	Stroke	Violence	Road-traffic accidents	Stroke
Self-inflicted injuries	Self-inflicted injuries	HIV/AIDS	HIV/AIDS	TB	HIV/AIDS
Road-traffic accidents	Ischemic heart disease	Breast cancer	Self-inflicted injuries	Ischemic heart disease	COPD
Fires	Road-traffic accidents	COPD	TB	Violence	Lung cancer
Maternal hemorrhage		Diabetes		Self-inflicted injuries	TB

COPD: Chronic obstructive pulmonary disease; TB: tuberculosis

Source: Data from *The global burden of disease: 2004 update.* Geneva: WHO; 2008.

A survey of mental health conducted in more than a dozen diverse countries estimated that between 1% and 4% of the populations of most countries had serious mental illnesses, and approximately 9% to 17% of those surveyed reported having at least one episode of a mental illness in the 12 months before the survey.[4] Worldwide, more than 450 million people have a psychiatric disorder, including about 120 million with depression, 70 million with alcohol dependence, 40 million with dementia, and 25 million with schizophrenia.[5] Mental and behavioral health disorders account for at least 12% of the global burden of disease and cause as many days of lost work as physical illnesses.[5] Nearly 1 million people commit suicide each year, and 10 million to 20 million make a suicide attempt.[5]

In many communities, people with mental illness are treated badly.[6] They may be imprisoned or involuntarily detained in hospitals for long periods of time without any legal recourse, or they may be denied access to hospitalization when it is needed. Some people with mental illness are subjected to forced labor and some are physically or sexually abused. And because of poverty and discrimination, many people with mental illnesses do not have access to the health care that could improve their mental and physical health status.

Many mental illnesses are treatable. Medications can relieve symptoms and prevent relapses, therapy can help those with mental illnesses to understand and change their thoughts and behaviors, and social rehabilitation that focuses on practical skills can help people with mental illnesses return to normal living activities. Unfortunately, mental health therapies are extremely underused. Considerably fewer than half of adults with severe mental illnesses receive any mental healthcare services, and an even lower proportion of those with mild or moderate mental illness receive medical care.[7] Many people do not know that help is available and so they do not seek clinical help. For others, the stigma of being diagnosed with a mental illness prevents them from seeking treatment. And many people who would like mental health assistance do not have access to a mental health specialist. In most African and Asian countries there are more than 100,000 people for every one psychiatrist (**Figure 6–1**).[8] The risk factors for mental illness include living in poverty, experiencing a conflict or disaster, and having a major physical disease, so the populations that have the greatest need for mental health services often have the least access to them.

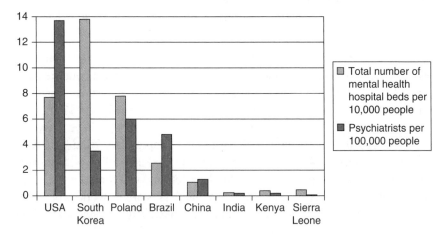

Figure 6–1 Healthcare resources for severe mental illnesses in 2005.

Source: Data from Jacob KS, Sharan P, Mirza I, et al. Mental health systems in countries: where are we now? *Lancet*. 2007;370:1061–1077.

The public health actions for improving mental health care include educating the public about mental illness, providing mental health treatment as part of primary health care, and involving communities and families in caring for people with mental illnesses. When a support system is in place and the public sector (including the healthcare, education, and justice systems) as well as private employers are prepared to work with persons with mental health conditions, an environment can be created in which most people with mental illnesses can participate in the economy, be included in social events, and be protected from discrimination and violence.[9]

6.3 INJURIES

The all-cause mortality rates for both young men and young women have decreased in recent decades (**Figure 6–2**),[10] but young men continue to have a higher likelihood of death than young women. Much of this difference is due to the higher rate of injuries in males.[1] Males are significantly more likely than females to die from all major types of injuries other than burns (**Figure 6–3**).[11] This disparity is due to men being more likely than women to work in hazardous occupations, to participate in dangerous recreational

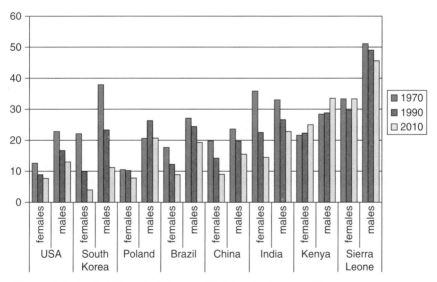

Figure 6–2 Probability of a 15 year old dying before age 60.

Source: Data from Rajaratnam JK, Marcus JR, Levin-Rector A, et al. Worldwide mortality in men and women aged 15–59 years from 1970 to 2010: a systematic analysis. *Lancet.* 2010;375:1704–1720.

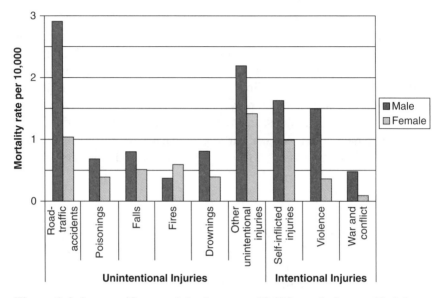

Figure 6–3 Sex-specific annual death rate per 10,000 people for specific injury-related causes worldwide in 2008.

Source: Data from *The global burden of disease: 2004 update (May 2011 update)*. Geneva: WHO; 2011.

activities, to spend time on the road, to use alcohol, and to be involved armed conflict. (Women spend more time cooking than men do, so women are more likely to fall into fires or scald themselves by dropping a pot of boiling liquid.)

However, females are more likely than males to be the victims of domestic violence (violence by intimate partners and family members) and other acts of physical aggression, including rape, and the rate of injuries due to physical and sexual violence is probably significantly under-reported. In a multi-country study of violence against women, 15% to 71% of women of reproductive age (15 to 49 years old) at each study site reported having been physically or sexually abused by an intimate partner.[12] In that same study, a large number of women indicated that they believed that a man has good reason to beat his wife if she does not complete housework, disobeys her husband, is unfaithful, or if the husband suspects infidelity.[13] Many women reported that they did not think it was acceptable for a woman to refuse sex with her husband even if she did not want to have sex, her partner was drunk or mistreating her, or she was sick.

Females may have little power over their own bodies both because of gender norms that give men authority over women and because women

Table 6–3 Examples of violence against women throughout the life cycle.

Phase	Type of Violence
Prebirth and Infancy	• Sex-selective abortion • Effects of battering during pregnancy on birth outcomes • Female infanticide
Girlhood	• Physical, sexual, and psychological abuse by family members and acquaintances (child abuse) • Female genital mutilation (FGM) • Forced sexual initiation (including child marriage) • Child prostitution and pornography
Adolescence and Adulthood	• Physical, sexual, and psychological abuse by family members • Dating and courtship violence (including acid throwing and date rape) • Intimate partner abuse (including dowry abuse, honor killings, marital rape, and forced pregnancy) • Forced prostitution (including trafficking) • Nonpartner coerced sex, including rape

Source: Information from Watts C, Zimmerman C. Violence against women: global scope and magnitude. *Lancet*. 2002;359:1232–1237.

tend to be smaller and physically weaker than men. The immediate health consequences of violence against women include serious injuries, death, damage caused to fetuses when pregnant women are attacked, and psychological trauma. Sexually abused women may also have an unwanted pregnancy or contract sexually transmitted infections (STIs), including HIV. Violence against females may occur at any stage of their lives (**Table 6–3**).[14]

6.4 SEX, GENDER, AND HEALTH

Men and women face different health challenges because of both biological characteristics related to sex and social structures related to gender.[15] Sex refers to the biological classification of people as male or female based on genetics (the presence of XX or XY sex chromosomes) and reproductive anatomy. Males and females also have somewhat different body chemistry, hormones, physiology, and brain function. These differences mean that men and women sometimes have different symptoms for the same disease and different prognoses and pathways to recovery. For example, men are more likely to have "dramatic" heart attacks with crushing chest pain, while women often have subtle symptoms like feeling more tired than normal, and this difference is a key reason why heart disease in women has traditionally been under diagnosed.[16] There are many other significant differences in health risks between the sexes (**Table 6–4**),[17] and these differences must be considered when planning for and implementing health education and preventive, diagnostic, and therapeutic health services.

Gender refers to social, cultural, and psychological aspects of being male or female, and is shaped by the sociocultural environment and experience in addition to biology. There is tremendous variability in the

Table 6–4 Comparison of the burden of disease for women and men. Although all of these conditions occur in both females and males, the risk of developing these conditions varies by sex.

Women Are More Likely Than Men To . . .	Men Are More Likely Than Women To . . .
. . . have cancers of the reproductive system	. . . have lung, bladder, mouth, esophageal, and stomach cancer
. . . have complications from sexually transmitted infections like chlamydia and gonorrhea	. . . become infected with trypanosomiasis, schistosomiasis, leishmaniasis, lymphatic filariasis, and other tropical infections
. . . die from burns	
. . . have depressive disorder, posttraumatic stress disorder, panic disorder, and migraines	. . . die from traffic accidents, poisonings, falls, drowning, violence, and war
. . . develop vision problems related to glaucoma, cataracts, and trachoma	. . . commit suicide and have drug-use disorders
. . . have Alzheimer's and other dementias	. . . develop liver disorders such as cirrhosis, hepatitis B, and hepatitis C
. . . die from diabetes	. . . have lung diseases like TB and COPD (chronic obstructive pulmonary disease)
. . . develop musculoskeletal disorders like rheumatoid arthritis and osteoarthritis	
. . . develop autoimmune disease like Lupus	
. . . develop iron-deficiency anemia	
. . . live to very old age	

Source: Data from World health report 2004. Geneva: WHO; 2004.

way individual women and individual men express their gender and in the ways cultures define gender roles. **Gender roles** describe how a culture believes men and women should behave. For example, gender roles may indicate what tasks women are expected to do, such as cooking, cleaning, and taking care of children. They may also define what tasks women cannot do, which might include working with heavy machinery, being in religious leadership, or driving cars. Traditional cultures often consider women to be under the authority of their fathers (or other male relatives) until marriage and of their husbands after marriage, and they may limit the ability of a woman to own property or manage her own finances. Some cultures have strict rules about what women can wear in public and whether they can be in public spaces unaccompanied by a male. This can limit the ability of women to participate in the marketplace and government, to attend school and religious meetings, and to acquire medical attention and information. Gender roles also define the social and behavioral norms for men. For example, young men may feel pressure to engage in risky behaviors like reckless driving or tobacco use in order to demonstrate their masculinity.

6.5 REPRODUCTIVE HEALTH AND MATERNAL MORTALITY

Reproductive health encompasses issues of safe sex, prevention and treatment of sexually transmitted infections, contraception, fertility and infertility, sexual health, pregnancy, and childbirth. Reproductive health is a critical issue for both men and women who are young adults. Both men and women need to have access to reproductive health care and the tools to maintain their reproductive health. And both men and women need to be aware of the risks associated with childbearing.

For many pregnant women, the hours of labor and delivery are precarious ones. Pregnancy and childbirth are still among the leading causes of death among women of reproductive age in low-income countries. About 350,000 women worldwide die each year as a result of pregnancy or childbirth, which translates to nearly 40 deaths every hour.[18] The most common cause of **maternal mortality**—death during pregnancy, childbirth, or soon after—is severe postpartum bleeding (**hemorrhage**) (**Figure 6–4**). Other common causes of maternal death include **eclampsia** (which starts as pre-eclampsia, characterized by high blood pressure and protein in the urine, and can develop into convulsions and possible organ failure), unsafe abortions, infections (like sepsis, an infection of the blood), and obstructed labor.[19,20]

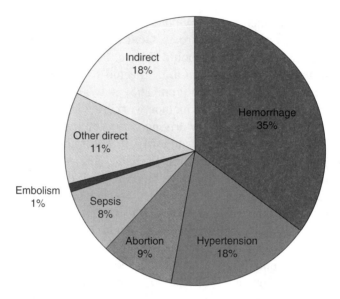

Figure 6–4 Causes of maternal death in 2005.

Source: Data from *Countdown to 2015 decade report (2000–2010): taking stock of maternal, newborn and child survival*. Geneva: WHO/UNICEF; 2010; and Khan KS, Wojdyla D, Say L, Gülmezoglu AM, Van Look PFA. WHO analysis of causes of maternal death: a systematic review. *Lancet.* 2006;367:1066–1074.

Each pregnancy carries risks, but pregnancy is especially risky when a woman has existing health problems, has had a high-risk pregnancy in the past, is having twins or higher numbers of children, or will not have access to a trained birth attendant.

The difference in risk of maternal death between high-income and low-income regions is huge. In Sierra Leone, one of the poorer countries in sub-Saharan Africa, more than 900 women die for every 100,000 births, compared to about 20 maternal deaths for every 100,000 births in the United States (**Figure 6–5**).[21] Most women in Sierra Leone have several pregnancies, so the lifetime risk of maternal death is about 1 in 23. In the United States, where women tend to have fewer pregnancies and a lower risk of death for each pregnancy, the lifetime risk of maternal death is about 1 in 2400.[22] On average, women in sub-Saharan Africa are about 140 times more likely to die while giving birth than women in the United States, Canada, or Europe (**Figure 6–6**).[23] There are also significant variations in the maternal mortality rate within most countries, with higher-income women experiencing a much lower mortality rate than lower-income women.[24]

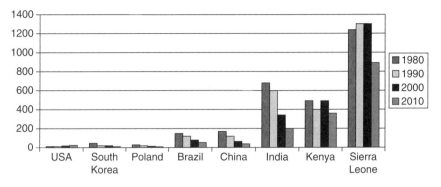

Figure 6–5 Number of deaths of women from pregnancy-related causes per 100,000 live births between 1980 and 2010.

Source: Data from Hogan MC, Foreman KJ, Naghavi M, et al. Maternal mortality for 181 countries, 1980–2008: a systematic analysis of progress towards Millennium Development Goal 5. *Lancet.* 2010;375:1609–1623; and *Trends in maternal mortality: 1990 to 2010.* Geneva: WHO, UNICEF, UNFPA, World Bank; 2012.

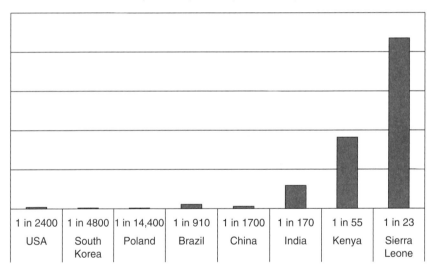

Figure 6–6 Lifetime risk of death due to pregnancy-related causes for women as of 2010.

Source: Data from *Trends in maternal mortality: 1990 to 2010.* Geneva: WHO, UNICEF, UNFPA, World Bank; 2012.

Many of these deaths could have been prevented if the women had access to advanced medical care. However, about one-third of women worldwide—including half of women in sub-Saharan Africa and South Asia—give birth without the assistance of a skilled birth attendant (sometimes called a trained birth attendant, or TBA), such as a nurse or midwife, who is trained to manage complications (**Figure 6–7**).[21] Maternal healthcare workers also facilitate the reproductive health of women more generally by educating women and men about contraceptives and child spacing, increasing access to prenatal care and delivery assistance, and fostering conditions in which women can make informed health decisions for themselves.

Women who survive pregnancy and delivery complications may be left with permanent disabilities. For example, some women who are small, as is often the case with girls who become pregnant in their early teenage years, develop a condition called obstructed labor, which is when the unborn baby is wedged so tightly into the birth canal that blood flow to surrounding tissues is cut off and the tissue starts to die. Women who are able to get to a hospital can have surgery (a Cesarean section) to deliver the baby before too much damage is done. Women who do not have access to a surgeon may be in labor for several days. The outcome, if the woman survives, is often the formation of an **obstetric fistula**, a hole between the rectum or bladder and the vagina that constantly leaks urine or feces. Because of the odor, most women with an obstetric fistula are ostracized by their communities. Some women are left paralyzed because of nerve damage and many are left infertile. In nearly all of these cases the baby is stillborn. About 3 million women worldwide are estimated to be living with an obstetric fistula, and

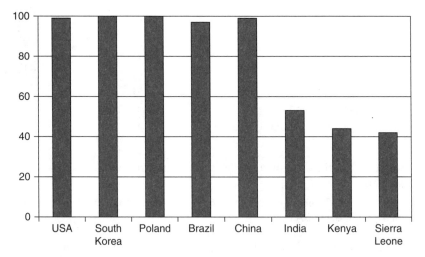

Figure 6–7 Percentage of births attended by skilled personnel (doctors, nurses, or midwives) between 2006 and 2010.

Source: Data from *State of the world's children 2012*. New York: UNICEF; 2012.

more than 50,000 new cases occur every year.[25] Fistulas can be surgically corrected, but the better option is preventing obstructed labor by delaying pregnancy until women are fully grown and by ensuring access to medical professionals during delivery if help is needed.

Women who have been circumcised (also called female genital cutting, female genital mutilation, or FGM), a common practice in some parts of Africa and the Middle East, have particularly high risks of adverse reproductive health outcomes, including a greater risk of infection, tearing during delivery, and postpartum hemorrhage, and a greater need for Caesarean sections.[26]

Safe motherhood programs need to address issues from prior to conception through the time after delivery (**Table 6–5**).[27,28] All women and men of reproductive age need to have access to information about reproduction and contraception so they are better prepared to make decisions about sex and are able to prevent unwanted pregnancies, unsafe abortions, and sexually transmitted infections. During pregnancy, women need information about how to stay healthy, eat well, and recognize potential complications so they can be addressed as soon as possible.

Table 6–5 Preventive and treatment interventions for maternal mortality.

Preventive Interventions (promoting healthy pregnancies)	Treatment Interventions (addressing birth complications)
• Family planning/birth spacing • Diagnosis and treatment of medical conditions that could complicate a healthy pregnancy, such as anemia, asthma, diabetes, heart disease, hypertension, or infections • Iron and folic acid supplements, deworming treatment, and malaria treatment to prevent or treat anemia • Antiretroviral drugs for women with HIV infection • Calcium supplements for women at high risk of pre-eclampsia • Tetanus toxoid immunization	• Detection and management of pregnancy complications such as pre-eclampsia • Antibiotics for premature rupture of membranes to prevent sepsis • Skilled attendants during labor, delivery, and the postpartum stage • Early detection of postpartum maternal complications such as hemorrhage • Early referral to professional obstetric care for women experiencing maternal complications during pregnancy, labor, delivery, or after delivery

Source: Data from Campbell OMR, Graham WJ; The Lancet Maternal Survival Series steering group. Strategies for reducing maternal mortality: getting on with what works. *Lancet*. 2006;368:1284–1299.

All deliveries should be attended by a trained healthcare provider, the woman and her baby should be observed after delivery, and both should be examined several weeks later to be sure that they are recovering and healthy.

6.6 FAMILY PLANNING

Family planning is an important decision for both young men and young women. Women and their babies are usually healthier when women have fewer pregnancies. Mothers, babies, and children also benefit from **birth spacing**. When the time between the birth of one baby and the next one is short, the older baby is at risk for malnutrition because of being weaned from breastmilk at a young age and having fewer household resources per child, and the younger baby has an increased risk of low birthweight and preterm birth.[29,30] **Family planning** helps women and men to make decisions about how many children they want to have and how many years apart they want those pregnancies to be.

Contraception is the intentional prevention of pregnancy. Contraceptive methods include abstinence, barriers, medications, and surgery.[31] Complete sexual abstinence is the only guaranteed way to prevent pregnancy. Some couples practice periodic abstinence and avoid intercourse during the days after a woman ovulates (when an egg is released from an ovary), the time when a woman is most fertile, but this is an imperfect method.

Condoms and diaphragms are used as a physical barrier during sexual intercourse to prevent sperm from coming into contact with an egg.

Oral contraceptives (birth control pills) prevent ovulation when taken as prescribed, so no eggs are released from the ovaries and a pregnancy cannot occur. In many parts of the world, oral contraceptives are called the "family planning pill" in recognition of their importance for birth spacing. Oral contraceptive pills must be taken at the same time every day, without skipping any doses, for this method to be effective. Some women prefer a longer-term method of pregnancy prevention and choose hormonal contraceptives that are delivered through a weekly patch, monthly injections, or vials placed under the skin of the upper arm that release medication for up to 5 years.

IUDs (intrauterine devices) prevent fertilization of eggs by creating a uterine environment that is unfavorable to sperm (which must pass through the uterus to reach unfertilized eggs). IUDs may also inhibit the implantation of fertilized eggs in the endometrium that lines the uterus. For permanent sterilization, women can opt to have tubal ligation surgery and men may choose to have vasectomies. The relative effectiveness of a variety of contraceptive methods is shown in **Table 6–6**.

Table 6–6 Contraceptive methods.

Type	Approach	Approximate Pregnancy Rate in 1st Year of Typical (not perfect) Use	Protection Against Sexually Transmitted Infections?	Notes
Complete abstinence	Abstinence	0%	Yes	No intercourse
Male sterilization (vasectomy)	surgery	~0%	No	Permanent
Subdermal implant contraceptives	Hormones	~0%	No	Effective for about 3 to 5 years after implantation
Female sterilization (tubal ligation)	Surgery	<1%	No	Permanent
Intrauterine device (IUD)	IUD	<1–2%	No	Effective for 5 or more years after insertion
Injection contraceptives	Hormones	<1–3%	No	One injection every 1 to 3 months
Oral contraceptives	Hormones	8%	No	Pill must be taken daily to be effective
Transdermal (patch) contraceptives	Hormones	8%	No	The patch must be replaced weekly
Intravaginal (ring) contraceptives	Hormones	8%	No	The vaginal ring must be replaced monthly
Male condom	Barrier	15%	Yes	Must be used during every act of intercourse
Diaphragm or cervical cap with spermicide	Barrier + spermicide	20%	No	Must be used during every act of intercourse
Female condom	Barrier	21%	Some	Must be used during every act of intercourse
Spermicide alone	Spermicide	29%	No	Must be used during every act of intercourse
Periodic abstinence (fertility-awareness–based methods)	Behavior	12–25%	No	Requires daily monitoring of body functions and periods of abstinence
Withdrawal method	Behavior	27%	No	Must be used during every act of intercourse
No contraceptive method used	None	85%	No	

Source: Data from Black KI, Gupta S, Rassi A, Kubba A. Why do women experience untimed pregnancies? A review of contraceptive failure rates. *Best Pract Res Clin Obstet Gynaecol.* 2010;24:443–455.

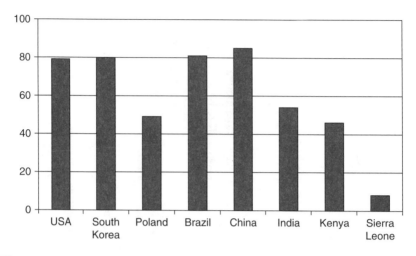

Figure 6–8 Proportion of sexually active women ages 15 to 49 using contraceptives between 2006 and 2010.

Source: Data from *State of the world's children 2012*. New York: UNICEF; 2012.

Abortion is the termination or loss of a pregnancy. (Miscarriages are called spontaneous abortions by medical professionals.) Induced abortions are chemically or surgically terminated pregnancies. Abortions are not a form of contraception because they end a pregnancy rather than prevent it. Increased access to contraception reduces the number of induced abortions by preventing unplanned pregnancies.

Many sexually active reproductive-age women and men around the world do not use any contraceptive method (**Figure 6–8**).[21] Because only abstinence and condoms help to prevent the spread of sexually transmitted infections (STIs), all sexually active people of all ages—even women who are not able to become pregnant and men who are infertile—are encouraged to consider what methods they will use to prevent STIs.

6.7 FERTILITY

There are a number of different ways to report a woman's reproductive history. **Gravidity** refers to the total number of times a woman has been pregnant, and includes miscarriages, abortions, stillbirths, and live births. **Fertility** is the total number of births, whether the result was a stillbirth or a live birth. **Parity** refers to the total number of live births. Because very few miscarriages and abortions are reported to healthcare professionals, most global health reports use fertility to measure pregnancies in a population. The goal of family planning is to minimize unplanned pregnancies (to reduce gravidity) and to maximize the health of babies from pregnancies that do occur (so that parity is as close as possible to gravidity).

The **fertility rate** is the average number of children a woman gives birth to during her childbearing years. In most countries the fertility rate has decreased significantly in recent decades (**Figure 6–9**).[21,23] Still, in general, lower-income countries have much higher fertility rates than higher-income countries (**Figure 6–10**).[32] One of the best predictors of decreased fertility is increased female education (**Figure 6–11**).[32] Educated women have smaller families for many reasons.[33] One is that the work outside the home that is made possible by literacy may delay marriage and a first pregnancy. Another reason is that educated women can make better decisions about contraception and childbearing with their partners because they have the ability to read and act on information about good health practices, nutrition, disease prevention, and child-rearing strategies.

The fertility rate has an impact on population health, not just the health of individual women, babies, and families. If each woman has, on average, about 2 children (and those children live to adulthood), then each couple will produce only a **replacement population** (2 parents producing

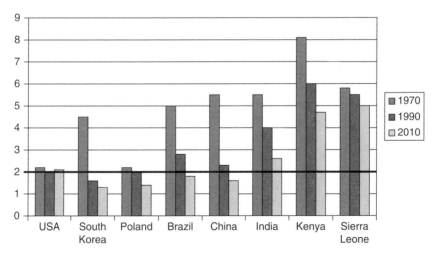

Figure 6–9 Total fertility rates between 1970 and 2010. A fertility rate less than 2 is below replacement levels.

Source: Data from *State of the world's children 2012*. New York: UNICEF; 2012; and *State of the world's children 2011*. New York: UNICEF; 2011.

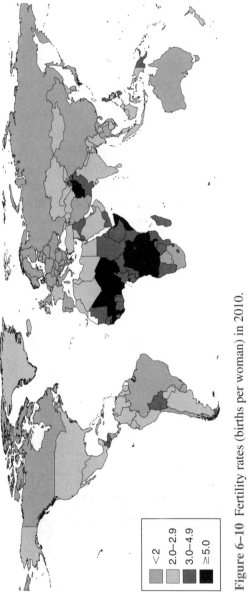

Figure 6–10 Fertility rates (births per woman) in 2010.
Source: Data from *World development indicators database.* Washington DC: World Bank.

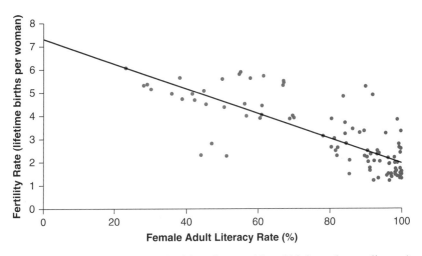

Figure 6–11 Female literacy (% of females age 15 and higher who are literate) and fertility (total births per woman) in 2009.

Source: Data from *World development indicators database*. Washington DC: World Bank.

2 offspring), and over the generations the population size will remain about the same. If the total fertility rate is greater than 2, then the size of the population will increase over time. If the fertility rate is less than 2, then the average age of the population will increase and the number of people in the total population will begin to decrease. (These stages are part of the demographic transition associated with economic development.) The high fertility rates in some parts of the world, and the low rates in others, have created concerns about global population growth and about appropriate policies for promoting healthy fertility rates.

Reproductive rights have been a controversial topic on the global health agenda. For example, when the Cairo Conference on Population and Development in 1994 focused on women's empowerment and reproductive rights—and, more specifically, on the ability of a woman or couple to decide how many children they want without interference from governments or other organizations—it sparked the concern of religious groups. The Roman Catholic Church was particularly vocal about the use of contraceptives and possible increases in the number of induced abortions.

Even so, most communities now recognize the importance of all adults and adolescents, both males and females, understanding their options for contraception and family spacing. Population planning programs target both women and men because household reproductive decisions involve both partners, and because a woman whose partner does not want her to use contraception will often follow her partner's wishes. Although millions of people who would like to use contraception do not have access to family planning services, thousands of healthcare providers, governments, partners of the United Nations Population Fund (UNFPA, formerly the United Nations Fund for Population Activities), Planned Parenthood affiliates, and other organizations seek to bring information and supplies to men and women worldwide who want to make informed reproductive decisions.

6.8 POPULATION GROWTH

Picture a small island in the middle of an ocean. It is arable (can grow food) and has a variety of plant and animal species. Say that at first 10 people settle on the island. They build homes, develop a system for collecting freshwater (because ocean water is too salty to drink or to use for irrigation), and begin to farm the land. They also begin to have children, and eventually those children have children. Soon the population has reached 100, and then it grows to 1000. The amount of land available for farming decreases as more homes are built, yet the need for food is greater because there are more people to feed. Getting rid of waste products and finding energy sources are growing problems. The limited amount of freshwater available is becoming a source of stress as the demand for water increases, but water quality becomes poorer as waste pollutes water sources. Some plants and animals are threatened and at risk of extinction. Crime is increasing as resources become scarce. What would happen if the population increased to 10,000, or to a million? Is there a limit to the number of people a small island could support?

Many people have similar concerns about the growth of the global human population. For a long time the size of the Earth's population was relatively steady, but recent population growth has been exponential. **Figure 6–12** is a plot of the size of the world's human population over time, and it shows a "J-shaped" growth pattern. After many years of relatively limited population growth, there has been a very steep increase in the total world population in recent centuries. The doubling time, the number of years it takes for the world's population to double, is getting shorter. It took only 40 years—from 1950 until 1990—for the number of humans to double from 2.5 billion to 5 billion. The current world population is approximately 7 billion, and it is expected to level off at about 9 billion by 2100.[34]

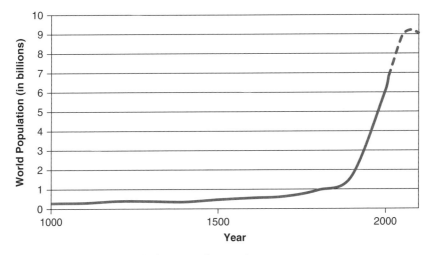

Figure 6–12 World population growth over time.

Source: Data from United Nations Department of Economic and Social Affairs. *World population to 2300.* New York: UN; 2004.

Carrying capacity is the maximum human population the Earth can sustain. There is no easy way to calculate carrying capacity because it depends on the standard of living and cultural factors in addition to population density (measured as land area per person or as arable land area per person), climate, and the land and natural resources that are available. Carrying capacity can be approximated with **ecological footprint** estimates based on the per capita area of land needed to meet a population's consumption patterns (**Figure 6–13**).[35] Earth could likely not support the current world population if everyone had the current ecological footprint of the United States, but most countries aspire to higher standards of living that come with larger ecological footprints.

So what will happen if the world population continues to grow? One famous scenario was proposed in 1798 by Thomas Malthus, who predicted that at some point the population would exceed food supply, and the result would be mass famine, epidemics, and war.[36] These **Malthusian catastrophes** have not occurred, and at present global food production is growing faster than the population. However, food and other resources are not distributed equally, and fertility rates and population growth are highest in the poorest parts of the world where food production is often low. There are valid reasons to be concerned about the unequal distribution of

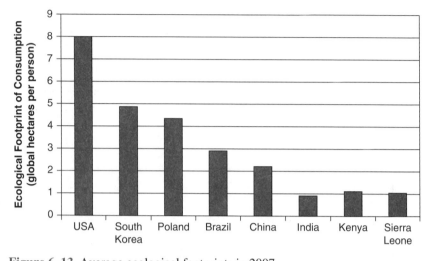

Figure 6–13 Average ecological footprints in 2007.

Source: Data from Ewing B, Moore D, Goldfinger S, Oursler A, Reed A, Wackernagel M. *The Ecological Footprint Atlas 2010*. Oakland, CA: Global Footprint Network; 2010.

food and natural resources, the risks of increased pollution and congestion that will occur with continued population growth, and the possibility of increased crime and war as resources in some regions of the world become scarce. One check on exponential growth is that fertility rates generally decrease when economic conditions in a region improve. Another check is the increased use of modern family planning methods.

6.9 POPULATION PLANNING POLICIES

The goal of population planning policies at the regional, national, and international levels is to promote a population growth rate in line with desired demographic and socioeconomic profiles. In most lower-income countries, population policies focus on encouraging reduced fertility rates (**Table 6–7**).[37] Middle-income countries generally view their growth rates as satisfactory. And in some high-income countries where fertility rates are below replacement level and population aging is a concern, the goal of population policies is to provide incentives for increased fertility. Effective population planning policies often aim to increase the ability of women and men to choose how many children they want and how they want to space their children's births.

Table 6–7 Population policies.

Country	USA	South Korea	Poland	Brazil	China	India	Kenya	Sierra Leone
Annual Growth Rate (1990–2010)	1.0%	0.6%	0.0%	1.3%	0.8%	1.7%	2.7%	1.9%
Expected Annual Growth Rate (2010–2030)	0.8%	0.2%	–0.1%	0.6%	0.2%	1.1%	2.4%	1.9%
Total Fertility Rate (2010)	2.1	1.3	1.4	1.8	1.6	2.6	4.7	5.0
View on Population Growth/Fertility Level	Satisfactory	Too low	Too low	Satisfactory	Satisfactory	Too high	Too high	Too high
Policy on Population Growth/Fertility	No intervention	Raise	Raise	No intervention	Maintain	Lower	Lower	Lower

Source: Data from United Nations Department of Economic and Social Affairs. *World population policies 2009*. New York: UN; 2010.

Nearly all low-income countries have relatively high fertility rates. To promote reduced fertility, most low-income countries provide direct government support for the distribution of family planning information and contraceptives,[37] but their specific policies vary. For example, Kenya has had a government population policy since 1967, and since 2005 has allocated government funds directly for contraceptives in order to improve infant and maternal survival.[38] Many of Kenya's population policies stem from the Kilimanjaro Programme of Action adopted at the Second African Population Conference, which met in Arusha, Tanzania, in 1984, and provided a framework for population policies on the African continent. The recommendations of the Arusha Conference stated that governments should acknowledge that family planning and child spacing strengthen families, that family planning services should be incorporated into maternal healthcare services, that governments should ensure access to family planning for all individuals seeking it and should offer services at free or subsidized prices, and that a variety of family planning methods should be made available to users. As a comparison, India has had government-sponsored family planning programs since 1951, and has shifted from an original focus on the distribution of barrier contraceptives to an emphasis on sterilization, especially sterilization of relatively young women, along with a focus on birth spacing.[39]

China has been one of the most aggressive countries in limiting population growth. The "late, long, few" policy of the 1970s encouraged delayed childbearing, longer spacing between children, and fewer children, and cut the total fertility rate in half. The goal of China's one-child policy, which was adopted in 1979, is to use economic and educational incentives to promote one-child families, especially in urban areas. Because there are exemptions to the policy for rural residents, for highly educated or wealthy parents, for parents who are both only children, and for some minority groups, the actual fertility rate in China is currently about 1.8 children per couple, not 1 child per couple.[40] The program has been controversial since its inception because of reports that, despite official policy, there have been instances of forced abortions and sterilizations, infanticide (especially of females in rural areas), and other human rights abuses. Another concern is that the preference for male children may have made sex-selective abortions common enough to skew male-female birth ratios (even though the Chinese government expresses a commitment to equalizing its sex ratio).[41,42] Within China, the main concern is that there are now many families with a "one-two-four" structure—only one grandchild to support two parents and four grandparents.[43] Still, as a result of those policies and programs, China now has what it deems to be a satisfactory population growth and fertility rate.

As a comparison with another middle-income country, Brazil's fertility rate has also decreased significantly in recent decades even though few formal government policies have promoted contraceptive use. The first agencies in Brazil that provided reproductive health services were nongovernmental organizations founded in the 1960s to address some of the demands for family planning. In the 1980s, the Ministry of Health initiated several maternal health programs that focused on comprehensive health care rather than emphasizing fertility control. Only in the 2000s did the federal government expand its commitment to supplying free or low-cost contraceptives to reproductive-age men and women and to increasing access to both sterilization surgery and infertility treatment.[44]

Higher-income countries have a different emphasis: most want to promote higher fertility rates. South Korea has one of the lowest fertility rates in the world, which prompted the government of the Republic of Korea to drop policies promoting low fertility rates in 1996. In 2006, the government introduced a new plan to promote childbearing that aims to help women balance work and family responsibilities. The government covers many of the costs associated with health care for pregnant women, provides tax breaks to cover childcare costs, pays for 90 days of maternity leave, and provides a subsidy for stay-at-home parents.[45]

Thus, population planning policies are designed to address country-specific needs and are responsive to changing socioeconomic and demographic trends. Ideally, these policies help increase the health status of infants and children, reproductive-age adults, their families, and their communities.

6.10 DISCUSSION QUESTIONS

1. What psychiatric and psychological health services are available in your community? Do you know where you could go to access mental health care? Do you know where you could refer a friend who was having suicidal thoughts?
2. What types of injuries are you most likely to have? What steps can you take to prevent injuries and injury-related disability?
3. What are some examples of gender roles in your community? How do these relate to health?
4. Before reading this chapter, did you consider pregnancy to be a risky time for a woman? What are the factors that account for the huge

difference in the risk of maternal mortality in low-income countries and high-income countries?

5. A growing number of American women want to give birth at home instead of at a hospital. What do you think about this practice? What environment would you prefer if you were giving birth or your partner was giving birth?

6. How many children do you want to have? What influences your ideas about your ideal number of offspring?

7. Do you think that there is a limit to the number of humans who can live on Earth? What factors contribute to the ability of the Earth to sustain (or fail to sustain) a large number of humans?

REFERENCES

1. *The global burden of disease: 2004 update*. Geneva: WHO; 2008.
2. Gore FM, Bloem PJ, Patton GC, et al. Global burden of disease in young people aged 10–24 years: a systematic analysis. *Lancet*. 2011;377:2093–2102.
3. Patton GC, Coffey C, Sawyer SM, et al. Global patterns of mortality in young people: a systematic analysis of population health data. *Lancet*. 2009;374:881–892.
4. Demyttenaere K, Bruffaerts R, Posada-Villa J, et al.; WHO World Mental Health Survey Consortium. Prevalence, severity, and unmet need for treatment of mental disorders in the World Health Organization World Mental Health Surveys. *JAMA*. 2004;291:2581–2590.
5. *World health report 2001*. Geneva: WHO; 2001.
6. *WHO resource book on mental health, human rights and legislation*. Geneva: WHO; 2005.
7. Wang PS, Aguilar-Gaxiola S, Alonsa J, et al. Use of mental health services for anxiety, mood, and substance disorders in 17 countries in the WHO world mental health surveys. *Lancet*. 2007;370:841–850.
8. Jacob KS, Sharan P, Mirza I, et al. Mental health systems in countries: where are we now? *Lancet*. 2007;370:1061–1077.
9. Herrman H, Saxena S, Moddie R, editors. *Promoting mental health: concepts, emerging evidence, practice: summary report*. Geneva: WHO; 2004.
10. Rajaratnam JK, Marcus JR, Levin-Rector A, et al. Worldwide mortality in men and women aged 15–59 years from 1970 to 2010: a systematic analysis. *Lancet*. 2010;375:1704–1720.
11. *The global burden of disease: 2004 update (May 2011 update)*. Geneva: WHO; 2011.
12. García-Moreno C, Jansen HAFM, Ellsberg M, Heise L, Watts CH; WHO Multi-country Study on Women's Health and Domestic Violence against Women Study Team. Prevalence of intimate partner violence: findings from the WHO multi-country study on women's health and domestic violence. *Lancet*. 2006;368:1260–1269.
13. García-Moreno C, Jansen HAFM, Ellsberg M, Heise L, Watts C. *WHO Multi-country Study on Women's Health and Domestic Violence against Women: Initial results on prevalence, health outcomes and women's responses*. Geneva: WHO; 2005.

14. Watts C, Zimmerman C. Violence against women: global scope and magnitude. *Lancet.* 2002;359:1232–1237.

15. Johnson JL, Greaves L, Repta R. Better science with sex and gender: facilitating the use of a sex and gender-based analysis in health research. *Int J Equity Health.* 2009;8:14.

16. Arslanian-Engoren C, Engoren M. Physiological and anatomical bases for sex differences in pain and nausea as presenting symptoms of acute coronary syndromes. *Heart Lung.* 2010;39:386–393.

17. *World health report 2004.* Geneva: WHO; 2004.

18. Hogan MC, Foreman KJ, Naghavi M, et al. Maternal mortality for 181 countries, 1980–2008: a systematic analysis of progress towards Millennium Development Goal 5. *Lancet.* 2010;375:1609–1623.

19. *Countdown to 2015 decade report (2000–2010): taking stock of maternal, newborn and child survival.* Geneva: WHO/UNICEF; 2010.

20. Khan KS, Wojdyla D, Say Lm, Gülmezoglu AM, Van Look PFA. WHO analysis of causes of maternal death: a systematic review. *Lancet.* 2006;367:1066–1074.

21. *State of the world's children 2012.* New York: UNICEF; 2012.

22. *Trends in maternal mortality: 1990 to 2010.* Geneva: WHO, UNICEF, UNFPA, World Bank; 2012.

23. *State of the world's children 2011.* New York: UNICEF; 2011.

24. Ronsmans C, Graham WJ; The Lancet Maternal Survival Series steering group. Maternal mortality: who, when, where, and why. *Lancet.* 2008;368:1189–1200.

25. Wall LL. Obstetric vesicovaginal fistula as an international public-health problem. *Lancet.* 2006;368:1201–1209.

26. Adam T, Bathija H, Bishai D, Bonnenfant YT, et al.; FGM Cost Study Group of WHO. Estimating the obstetric costs of female genital mutilation in six African countries. *Bull Wold Health Organ.* 2010;88:281–288.

27. AbouZahr C. Safe motherhood: a brief history of the global movement 1947–2002. *Br Med Bull.* 2003;67:13–25.

28. Campbell OMR, Graham WJ; The Lancet Maternal Survival Series steering group. Strategies for reducing maternal mortality: getting on with what works. *Lancet.* 2006;368:1284–1299.

29. Rutstein SO. Effects of preceding birth intervals on neonatal, infant and under-five years mortality and nutritional status in developing countries: evidence from the demographic and health surveys. *Int J Gynaecol Obstet.* 2005;89 (suppl 1):S7–S24.

30. Conde-Agudelo A, Rosas-Bermúdez A, Kafury-Goeta AC. Birth spacing and risk of adverse perinatal outcomes: a meta-analysis. *JAMA.* 2006;295:1809–1823.

31. Black KI, Gupta S, Rassi A, Kubba A. Why do women experience untimed pregnancies? A review of contraceptive failure rates. *Best Pract Res Clin Obstet Gynaecol.* 2010;24:443–455.

32. *World development indicators database.* Washington DC: World Bank.

33. Skirbekk V. Fertility trends by social status. *Demographic Res.* 2008;18:145–180.

34. United Nations Department of Economic and Social Affairs. *World population to 2300.* New York: UN; 2004.

35. Ewing B, Moore D, Goldfinger S, Oursler A, Reed A, Wackernagel M. *The Ecological Footprint Atlas 2010.* Oakland, CA: Global Footprint Network; 2010.

36. Malthus M. *An essay on the principle of population.* London: J. Johnson; 1798.

37. United Nations Department of Economic and Social Affairs. *World population policies 2009*. New York: UN; 2010.

38. Crichton J. Changing fortunes: analysis of fluctuating policy space for family planning in Kenya. *Health Policy Plan*. 2008;23:339–350.

39. Matthews Z, Padmadas SS, Hutter I, McEachran J, Brown JJ. Does early childbearing and a sterilization-focused family planning programme in India fuel population growth? *Demographic Res*. 2009;28:693–720.

40. Hesketh T, Lu L, Xing ZW. The effect of China's one-child family policy after 25 years. *N Engl J Med*. 2005;353:1171–1177.

41. Ding QJ, Hesketh T. Family size, fertility preferences, and sex ratio in China in the era of the one child family policy: results from national family planning and reproductive health survey. *BMJ*. 2006;333:371–373.

42. Zhu WX, Lu L, Hesketh T. China's excess males, sex selective abortion, and one child policy: analysis of data from 2005 national intercensus survey. *BMJ*. 2009;338:b1211.

43. Hvistendahl M. Has China outgrown the one-child policy? *Science*. 201;329:1458–1461.

44. Diniz Alves JE. The context of family planning in Brazil. *Demographic transformations and inequalities in Latin America: historical trends and recent patterns*. Rio de Janeiro: UNFPA; 2009: 297–302.

45. Westley SB, Choe MK, Retherford RD. Very low fertility in Asia: Is there a problem? Can it be solved? *Asia Pacific Issues*. 2010;94:1–12.

CHAPTER 7

Noncommunicable Diseases and Aging

The vast majority of adults worldwide die of heart disease, cancer, strokes, COPD, diabetes, or other chronic diseases. Many older adults live with sensory impairments, dementia, mobility issues, or other conditions that may limit their independence. As fertility rates decrease and life expectancies increase in many parts of the world, all countries must prepare to support a growing population of older adults.

7.1 GLOBAL AGING

Declining fertility rates and increasing life expectancy have significantly increased the percentage of the world population that is 65 years of age and older (**Figure 7–1**),[1] and that proportion is expected to continue to increase in the coming decades in every part of the world (**Figure 7–2**).[2] The number of people aged 60 and older worldwide is expected to increase from about 700 million in 2010 to 2 billion in 2050, and the number of adults aged 80 and older is expected to increase from about 100 million in 2010 to 400 million in 2050.[3] About two-thirds of all older adults currently live in less developed countries, and that proportion will increase in the coming years.[3]

Many older adults live active and independent lives. However, most will at some point develop hypertension or another cardiovascular disease, diabetes, cancer, a chronic lung disease, a musculoskeletal condition such as arthritis or osteoporosis, a neuropsychiatric condition such as dementia or depression, a sensory impairment like hearing or vision loss, or several of these chronic conditions at the same time.[4] Noncommunicable diseases (NCDs) are the most common causes of death of older adults in every region of the world (**Figure 7–3**), even though the rates of particular NCDs vary somewhat between regions (**Figure 7–4**).[4]

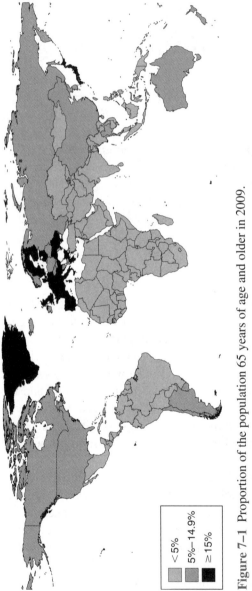

Figure 7–1 Proportion of the population 65 years of age and older in 2009.
Source: Data from *World development indicators database.* Washington DC: World Bank.

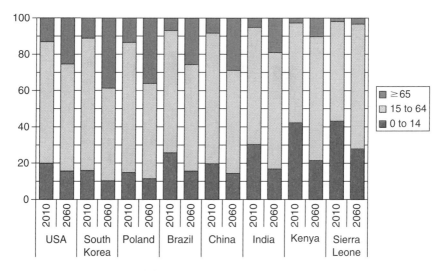

Figure 7–2 Proportion of the population by age in 2010 and projected for 2060.

Source: Data from Hughes BB, Kuhn R, Peterson CM, Rothman DS, Solórzano JR. *Improving global health forecasting the next 50 years*. Patterns of Potential Human Progress Series, Volume 3. Boulder CO: Paradigm Publishers; 2011.

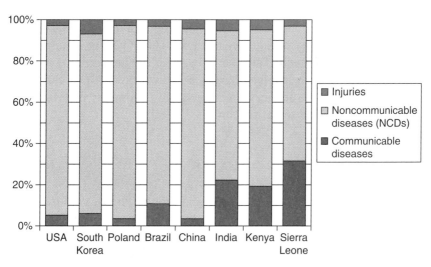

Figure 7–3 Percent of deaths in adults ages 60 and older due to communicable diseases, noncommunicable diseases, and injury in 2008.

Source: Data from *The global burden of disease: 2004 update (April 2011 update)*. Geneva: WHO; 2011.

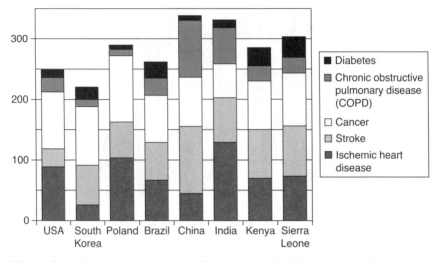

Figure 7–4 Estimated annual mortality rates per 10,000 adults ages 60 and older in 2008.

Source: Data from *The global burden of disease: 2004 update (April 2011 update)*. Geneva: WHO; 2011.

The number of years an individual adult lives without disability is a function of a lifetime of behaviors such as diet, physical activity, tobacco and alcohol use, and adherence to prescribed medical regimens, in addition to being influenced by personal characteristics like genetics and psychosocial factors.[5] Older adults also have a greater likelihood of maintaining a high quality of life when they have access to affordable preventive and therapeutic healthcare services, safe home and community environments, and strong family and social support.[5]

7.2 CARDIOVASCULAR DISEASES

More than one-third of older men and women die of cardiovascular disease, most often from a heart attack or a stroke or complications related to these events. The relative proportion of heart disease and stroke varies somewhat between countries, but within countries this ratio tends to be similar for females and males (**Figure 7–5**).[4]

Just like every other organ in the body, the tissues that make up the heart require a constant supply of oxygenated blood. **Atherosclerosis** occurs when the walls of the arteries that carry oxygen-rich blood from the heart to

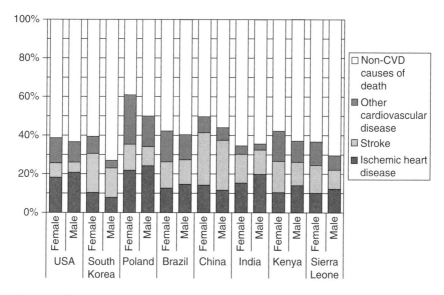

Figure 7–5 Proportion of deaths from cardiovascular disease (CVD) and other causes among adults ages 60 and older in 2008.

Source: Data from *The global burden of disease: 2004 update (April 2011 update)*. Geneva: WHO; 2011.

the rest of the body, including to the heart muscle itself, thicken and harden. The diameter of those vessels consequently narrows, limiting the blood supply to the tissues fed by those arteries. When atherosclerosis occurs in the arteries that provide blood to the heart, a condition known as **coronary artery disease**, the blood flow to the heart may be reduced. Reduced blood supply (**ischemia**) can present as chest pain (**angina**), and more serious blockage of the arteries may lead to a heart attack (more formally called a **myocardial infarction**), which causes a portion of the heart muscle to die due to a lack of oxygen.

A stroke (also called a **cerebrovascular accident**, or CVA) may occur when a blockage of a blood vessel, often due to a blood clot, causes ischemia in the brain. (Strokes can also be caused by bleeding in the brain, but hemorrhagic strokes are less common than ischemic strokes.) Common symptoms of a stroke include weakness on one or both sides of the body, confusion, trouble speaking or understanding, vision disturbances, a loss of balance, and a severe headache. Untreated hypertension (usually defined as a blood pressure higher than 140/90 mm Hg) is a major contributor to the risk of stroke, and also increases the likelihood of heart failure, kidney failure, aneurysms (bulges in blood vessels, which may rupture), and blindness.

The most significant predictor of cardiovascular disease is increasing age. However, there are also many modifiable risk factors, including tobacco use, physical inactivity, obesity, an unhealthy diet, consumption of excessive amounts of alcohol, unmanaged diabetes, and an unhealthy blood lipid profile (such as having elevated cholesterol and triglycerides), in addition to hypertension.[6] Lower socioeconomic status is also associated with an increased risk for cardiovascular disease, in part because people with lower incomes have fewer resources for addressing modifiable risk factors.[6]

7.3 CANCER

About one in six older adults worldwide dies of cancer.[7] Cancers (sometimes called **neoplasms**) occur when abnormal cells begin to reproduce uncontrollably, often invading nearby tissues and spreading to other parts of the body. Normal cells are genetically stable, and if mutations or other types of damage cannot be repaired the cell will undergo a process called **apoptosis** or programmed cell death. Cancer cells, in contrast, are genetically unstable and undergo unlimited reproductive cycles. Additionally, cancer cells can stimulate **angiogenesis**, the formation of new blood vessels to nourish a tumor, and the cells can **metastasize**, breaking away from the primary site and forming new tumors in other parts of the body. (Benign, noncancerous tumors usually remain encapsulated at their original site.)

It is a bit misleading to refer to cancer as though it is one disease because there are several hundred different types of cancer. Cancers are named for the part of the body where they originate and for the specific type of cell that has become cancerous. For example, carcinomas form in epithelial tissues, which usually line the inside or outside of the body, and sarcomas arise from connective tissues like bones or muscles. Cancers are also classified based on whether the cancer cells remain noninvasive and local, if they have spread to regional lymph nodes, or if they have spread to distant parts of the body.

The risk factors for cancer are specific to the type of cancer. For example, human papillomavirus (HPV) is an infection that specifically increases the risk of cervical cancer in women, occupational benzene exposure is associated with a significantly increased risk of leukemia, and sun exposure increases the likelihood of developing skin cancer. Advanced age is the most important risk factor for most types of cancer. Tobacco use, excessive alcohol consumption, physical inactivity, and an unhealthy diet are also risk factors for many types of cancer, and these are modifiable exposures. Inherited mutations are responsible for relatively few cases of cancer; most people diagnosed with cancer do not have a family history of that type of cancer. For many types of cancer, no major risk factors—modifiable or otherwise—have been identified.

Worldwide, the most commonly diagnosed cancers in men, from most common to less common, are cancers of the lung, prostate, colon/rectum (large intestine), stomach, and liver. The most common causes of cancer death for men are cancers of the lung, liver, stomach, colon/rectum, and esophagus.[8] For women worldwide, the most commonly diagnosed cancers are cancers of the breast, uterine cervix, colon/rectum, lung, and stomach. The most common causes of cancer death for women are cancers of the breast, lung, cervix, colon/rectum, and stomach.[8] However, there are important differences between countries and regions (Table 7–1).[8] For example, cervical cancer remains a leading cause of cancer death among women in low-income countries but is now fairly rare in high-income countries due to routine use of Pap smears for early detection of cancerous and precancerous lesions and also the use of the HPV vaccine, which prevents recipients from becoming infected with several of the most common strains of HPV that are associated with an increased risk of cervical cancer.

The proportion of people who live in high-income countries who develop cancer is much higher than the proportion in low- and middle-income countries (Figure 7–6),[9] partly because cancer is more common in older adults and more people in high-income countries reach older ages. However, the population mortality rates from cancer are only a little higher in high-income countries (Figure 7–7),[10] and because so many more people live in developing countries than in industrialized ones, the number of cancer deaths in low- and middle-income countries is considerably higher than the number of deaths in high-income countries (Figure 7–8).[9] This means, for example, that although a person who lives in a more developed country is more likely to be diagnosed with lung cancer or breast cancer than a person who lives in a less developed country, the total number of deaths each from these cancers is higher in less developed regions.[11]

Survival rates for those diagnosed with cancer also vary significantly between countries, with survival rates significantly lower in developing countries than in developed countries (Figure 7–9).[12] People living in low-income countries are often not diagnosed until the cancer is at an advanced stage and the available treatment options are limited. If access to screening and diagnostic tests, which allow for detection of cancer at an earlier, more treatable stage, and access to advanced therapies like chemotherapeutic

Table 7–1 Most common cancer diagnoses and causes of cancer mortality.

	USA	South Korea	Poland	Brazil	China	India	Kenya	Sierra Leone
Most Commonly Diagnosed Cancers in Men	Prostate	Stomach	Lung	Prostate	Lung	Lung	Esophagus	Prostate
	Lung	Colorectum	Prostate	Lung	Stomach	Mouth	Prostate	Liver
	Colorectum	Lung	Colorectum	Stomach	Liver	Throat	Stomach	Lung
Most Common Causes of Cancer Death in Men	Lung	Lung	Lung	Lung	Lung	Lung	Esophagus	Prostate
	Colorectum	Liver	Colorectum	Prostate	Liver	Throat	Prostate	Liver
	Prostate	Stomach	Stomach	Stomach	Stomach	Mouth	Stomach	Lung
Most Commonly Diagnosed Cancers in Women	Breast	Thyroid	Breast	Breast	Breast	Cervix	Breast	Cervix
	Lung	Breast	Lung	Cervix	Lung	Breast	Cervix	Breast
	Colorectum	Colorectum	Colorectum	Colorectum	Stomach	Ovary	Esophagus	Liver
Most Common Causes of Cancer Death in Women	Lung	Lung	Lung	Breast	Lung	Cervix	Cervix	Cervix
	Breast	Stomach	Breast	Cervix	Stomach	Breast	Breast	Breast
	Colorectum	Colorectum	Colorectum	Lung	Liver	Ovary	Esophagus	Liver

Source: Data from Ferlay J, Shin HR, Bray F, Forman D, Mathers C, Parkin DM. GLOBOCAN 2008 v1.2: Cancer Incidence and Mortality Worldwide. Lyon: IARC; 2010.

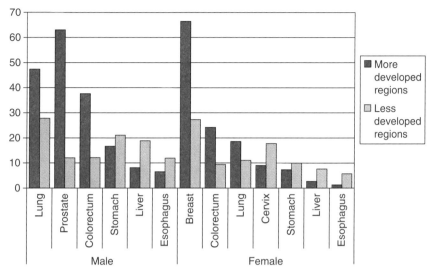

Figure 7–6 Estimated age-standardized annual number of new (incident) cases of cancer per 100,000 people in 2008.

Source: Data from Ferlay J, Shin HR, Bray F, Forman D, Mathers C, Parkin DM. Estimates of worldwide burden of cancer in 2008: GLOBOCAN 2008. *Int J Cancer.* 2010; 12:2893–2917.

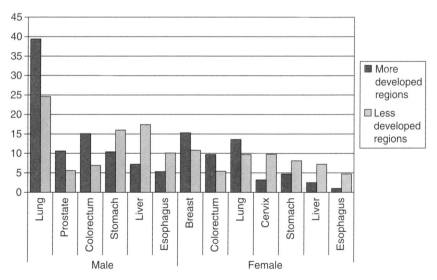

Figure 7–7 Estimated age-standardized number of cancer deaths per 100,000 people in 2008.

Source: Data from Ferlay J, Shin HR, Bray F, Forman D, Mathers C, Parkin DM. Estimates of worldwide burden of cancer in 2008: GLOBOCAN 2008. *Int J Cancer.* 2010; 12:2893–2917.

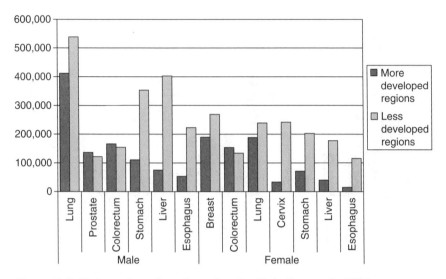

Figure 7-8 Estimated number of people who died of cancer in 2008.

Source: Data from Ferlay J, Shin HR, Bray F, Forman D, Mathers C, Parkin DM. Estimates of worldwide burden of cancer in 2008: GLOBOCAN 2008. *Int J Cancer.* 2010; 12:2893–2917.

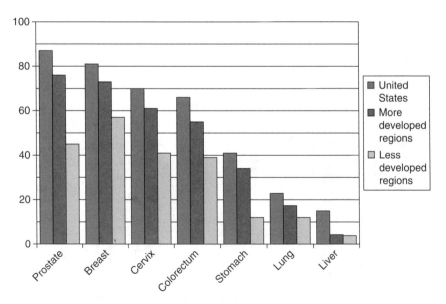

Figure 7-9 Estimated age-adjusted 5-year cancer survival rate for selected cancers in 2002.

Source: Data from Parkin DM, Bray F, Ferlay J, Pisani P. Global cancer statistics, 2002. *CA Cancer J Clin.* 2005; 55:74–108.

drugs, technology-enhanced surgical techniques, and radiology regimens were increased, many more people worldwide would survive their bouts with cancer.

7.4 CHRONIC LUNG DISEASE

Nearly 10% of older adults worldwide die of **chronic obstructive pulmonary disease (COPD) (Figure 7–10)**.[4,13] COPD is characterized by coughing, shortness of breath, wheezing, and tightness in the chest due to damage to airways (the bronchi and bronchioles) and the tiny air sacs (alveoli) in the lungs where gas exchange takes place. Progressive thickening and narrowing of the airways occurs because of inflammation and excess production of mucus that clogs breathing passages. This process causes **chronic bronchitis**. A reduction in gas exchange occurs as the alveoli lose elasticity and become distended or destroyed, which reduces the surface area available for intake of oxygen and release of carbon dioxide. This process is called **emphysema**. These symptoms are often accompanied by **asthma**, which makes the airways sensitive to exposures like air pollutants, cold air, and stress.

Although treatment can help manage some symptoms, the damage to the airways and lungs is not fully reversible with current therapies. Symptoms

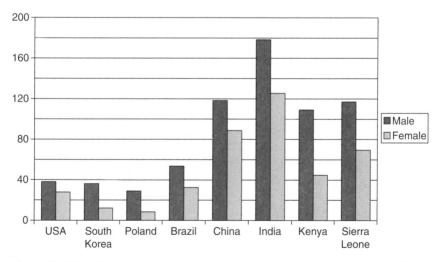

Figure 7–10 Estimated age-standardized chronic respiratory disease mortality rate per 100,000 people in 2008.

Source: Data from *Global status report on noncommunicable diseases 2010*. Geneva: WHO; 2011.

often worsen over time. Although not curable, COPD is often preventable. The most common risk factors besides age are exposure to tobacco smoke, indoor and outdoor air pollution, and industrial chemicals.[14]

7.5 DIABETES

Insulin is a hormone produced by the pancreas that helps the body to maintain a relatively constant level of glucose (sugar) in the bloodstream so that cells have a relatively constant supply of energy. **Type 1 diabetes** (previously called juvenile-onset diabetes or insulin-dependent diabetes) occurs when the body does not produce enough insulin. **Type 2 diabetes** (formerly known as adult-onset diabetes or non–insulin-dependent diabetes) is far more common and happens when the body stops responding appropriately to insulin even when the hormone is still being produced. The risk factors for type 2 diabetes include age plus obesity and related lifestyle characteristics, such as physical inactivity and an unhealthy diet. Signs of the initial onset of diabetes may include increased thirst and hunger, frequent urination, unexplained weight loss, fatigue, and frequent slow-healing infections.

The goal of diabetes management is to keep blood sugar levels from becoming too high (hyperglycemia) or too low (hypoglycemia). People with type 1 diabetes require frequent insulin injections to maintain a safe blood sugar level. For those with type 2 diabetes, the disease can often be managed with weight loss, a careful diet, and sometimes also oral medications. Failure to carefully maintain blood sugar levels can, over the years, cause complications like blindness (from diabetic retinopathy), kidney failure, nerve damage (diabetic neuropathy), and foot ulcers leading to amputation.

The prevalence of diabetes is increasing in both lower- and higher-income countries, and will continue to do so in the coming decades as the proportion of adults who are obese increases (**Figure 7–11**).[15] Diabetes and its complications, including an increased risk of cardiovascular death, are becoming major causes of premature death worldwide.[16]

7.6 SENSORY IMPAIRMENT

More than 300 million people worldwide are blind or have low vision.[17] Common causes of adult vision loss include **cataracts**, in which the lenses of the eyes become cloudy; **glaucoma**, which causes loss of peripheral vision due to elevated pressure within the eyeball; age-related macular degeneration, which causes loss of central vision; chronic diseases like

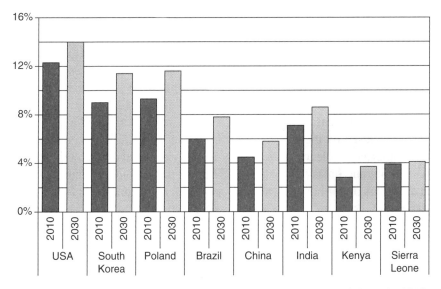

Figure 7–11 Estimated proportion of adults ages 20 to 79 with diabetes in 2010 and projected for 2030.

Source: Data from Shaw JE, Sicree RA, Zimmet PZ. Global estimates of the prevalence of diabetes for 2010 and 2030. *Diabetes Res Clin Pract.* 2010;87:4–14.

diabetes; and infections.[18] Many of these cases of blindness could be prevented with advanced medical care, and many individuals with low vision could regain at least some of their sight with glasses to correct refractive errors (like myopia and astigmatism) or surgery to replace lenses damaged by cataracts. Those with untreatable or untreated visual impairments may experience reduced quality of life, mobility, and independence.

More than 250 million people worldwide are deaf or hard of hearing.[19] Age-related hearing loss (presbycusis) often makes it difficult for older adults to hear high frequencies. Hearing loss is also often noise induced, as high-intensity sounds damage the special surfaces (stereocilia) of cells in the ears that receive noise signals and transmit them to the brain.

Vision and hearing disorders are responsible for more than 10% of the disability experienced by adults age 60 and older.[7]

7.7 DISABILITY

Skeletal diseases such as arthritis and osteoporosis, muscle weakness, nervous system disorders such as Parkinson's disease (which causes tremors), intellectual or cognitive impairments (perhaps resulting from a stroke or brain trauma), and sensory impairments that affect vision, hearing, and speech can all result in activity limitations and disability for older adults. A distinction is made between anatomical and physiological impairments and disabilities. Disability is both a health condition and a social context in which a person with impairment interacts with other people, institutions, and the environment (**Figure 7–12**).

One way of measuring disability is to ask how much functional impairment is caused by the physical or sensory impairment. Is the person with the impairment able to complete routine daily personal care functions such as bathing and dressing (**Table 7–2**)? Is the person independently able to manage his or her home by making meals, cleaning, and completing other essential tasks? Or does the person with the impairment require assistance from other people for the completion of daily activities? Does the condition cause extreme limitation in personal activities and participation in society, or relatively little limitation in these domains (**Table 7–3**)? Can the person with the condition fully participate in social events or is the person marginalized because of his or her disability?

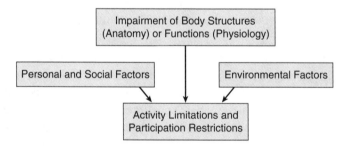

Figure 7–12 The relationship between impairments and disabilities (activity limitations and participation restrictions).

Table 7–2 Activities of daily living.

Activities of Daily Living (ADLs): Self-Care	Instrumental Activities of Daily Living (IADLs): Independence
Dressing	Shopping
Eating	Housekeeping
Ambulating (mobility)	Accounting (personal finances)
Toileting	Food preparation
Hygiene	Transportation

Table 7–3 Domains of activity and participation from the *International Classification of Functioning, Disability, and Health* (ICF).

Domain	Activities
Learning and applying knowledge	Watching, listening, learning to read, learning to write, learning to calculate, solving problems
General tasks and demands	Undertaking a single task, undertaking multiple tasks
Communication	Receiving spoken messages, receiving nonverbal messages, speaking, producing nonverbal messages, conversation
Mobility	Lifting and carrying objects, fine hand use (such as picking up objects or grasping them), walking, moving around using equipment (such as a wheelchair), using transportation
Self-care	Washing oneself (such as washing hands, bathing, and using a towel), caring for body parts (by brushing teeth, shaving, and grooming), toileting, dressing, eating, drinking, looking after one's own health
Domestic life	Acquisition of goods and services (such as by shopping), preparation of meals (such as by cooking), doing housework (such as cleaning house, washing dishes, doing laundry, and ironing), assisting others
Interpersonal interactions and relationships	Basic interpersonal interactions, complex interpersonal interactions, relating to strangers, formal relationships, informal social relationships, family relationships, intimate relationships
Major life areas	Informal education, school education, higher education, remunerative employment, basic economic transactions, economic self-sufficiency
Community, social, and civic life	Community life, recreation and leisure, religion and spirituality, human rights, political life and citizenship

Note: The ICF is a series of guidelines for assessing disability. For example, the ICF has codes for indicating changes in body structure such as total absence, partial absence, additional part, aberrant dimensions, discontinuity, or deviating position.

Source: Information from *International classification of functioning, disability, and health* (ICF). Geneva: WHO; 2001.

A second consideration is the environment and resources available for the person with a physical impairment. A person who uses a wheelchair may only have minor limitations in accessing buildings in South Korea, but may find it impossible to navigate the unpaved pathways of rural Kenya. An American with a visual impairment may have access to books through Braille editions, electronic magnifiers, and books on tape, but a similarly impaired person in Sierra Leone may not have access to any of these tools. Poverty also limits access to resources, and disabled people and their families are more likely to be poor than people without disabilities. Disabilities are expensive because there are direct costs related to treatment, the disabled person may be unable to work, and caregivers may have to limit their paid employment and home productivity or hire others to provide care. Disabled people may also have fewer opportunities to escape poverty because they are often denied access to education, employment, and public services. A safe physical environment (**Table 7–4**) and a strong social

Table 7–4 Environmental characteristics that relate to activities and participation.

Environment	Environmental Characteristics
Products and technology	Products for personal consumption (food, medicines), for personal use in daily living, for personal indoor and outdoor mobility and transportation, for communication; design, construction, and building materials of buildings for public use and buildings for private use
Natural environment and human-made changes to the environment	Climate, light, sound
Support and relationships	Immediate family, friends, acquaintances, peers, colleagues, neighbors, community members, people in positions of authority, personal care providers and personal assistants, healthcare professionals
Attitudes	Individual attitudes of immediate family members, friends, personal care providers and personal assistants, healthcare professionals; societal attitudes; social norms, practices, and ideologies
Services, systems, and policies	Housing, communication, transportation, legal, social, health, education and training, labor and employment

Source: Information from *International classification of functioning, disability, and health* (ICF). Geneva: WHO; 2001.

support system are key to preventing disability for older adults and for maximizing the activities and social participation of all who have impairments and disabilities.[20]

A third way to measure disability is based on the duration of the impairment. Is the condition permanent or short term? A person with a severe spinal cord injury will probably have life-long paralysis, but a broken bone will heal. Here, too, there are significant differences between high-income and low-income populations. Some conditions that are considered permanent disabilities in low-income regions are preventable or treatable in other parts of the world. Cataracts are the most common cause of blindness in older adults, but can be surgically corrected. Arthritis (swelling of the joints) may not be able to be cured, but the pain of arthritis can be managed with medications. Infections like onchocerciasis (river blindness) and trachoma that can cause blindness can be prevented or treated early so that they do not progress to an advanced stage.

Adults and children of all ages who have physical impairments can benefit from access to appropriate physical therapy, occupational therapy, speech therapy, and other types of rehabilitation. For example, people who have had a stroke can re-learn language and self-care skills, especially if they receive therapy within days after the stroke. Access to assistive medical devices, such as prosthetics for people with a missing arm or leg, orthotics and braces for people with various types of musculoskeletal disorders, hearing aids, and glasses, is also crucial. Most importantly, people with physical impairments and disabilities benefit from being included to the fullest extent possible in the activities of their families and communities.

7.8 DEMENTIA

Dementia is a term used to describe a gradual decline in cognitive function that usually presents as severe memory loss combined with other symptoms such as impaired judgment, personality changes, inappropriate behavior, difficulty with language, and/or confusion. The most common type of dementia is Alzheimer's disease, which is associated with anatomical changes in the brain, including the formation of beta-amyloid plaques and neurofibrillary tangles. Dementia may limit the ability of an older adult to live independently and may cause significant stress for those caring for a loved one with the disorder.

The risk of dementia increases significantly with age. About 5% to 10% of the disability in adults ages 60 and older is attributable to dementia, with much higher rates for the oldest adults.[7] More than 25 million adults worldwide currently have dementia, and that count will increase significantly in the coming decades.[21]

7.9 SCREENING AND EARLY DETECTION

Screening is a type of secondary prevention in which an entire well-defined group of people is encouraged to be tested for a disease based on evidence that members of the population are at risk for the disease and that early intervention improves health outcomes. The goal of screening programs is to diagnose cases of the disease at an early, more treatable stage and/or to identify people who have risk factors for the disease so that they can take preventive measures (**Figure 7–13**).

A good screening test will yield a high proportion of correct results (true positives and true negatives) and a very low proportion of erroneous results (false positives and false negatives). In other words, a good screening test should have a high sensitivity and a high specificity (**Figure 7–14**). The **sensitivity** of a test is the proportion of people who truly have the disease who test positive for the disease. The **specificity** of a test is the proportion of people who are truly free of the disease who test negative for it. A test is usually considered to be a relatively reliable tool, one that makes a correct diagnosis most of the time, if it has a sensitivity of at least 95%

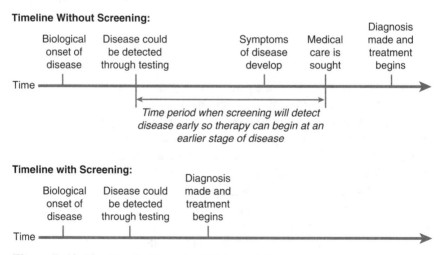

Figure 7–13 Timeline for the natural history of disease.

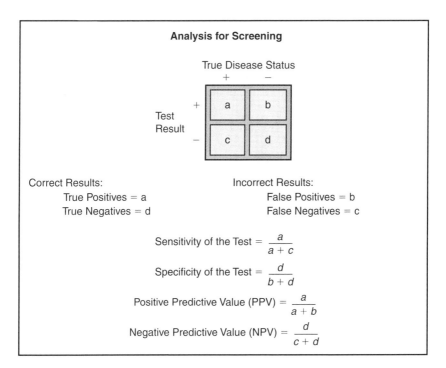

Figure 7–14 Validity of screening tests.

and a specificity of at least 80%. Ideally both of these values will exceed 99%. The **positive predictive value (PPV)** is the proportion of people who test positive for the disease who truly have disease, and the **negative predictive value (NPV)** is the proportion of people who test negative for the disease who truly do not have disease. These values are based in part on the prevalence of the disease in the population being tested. A test will have a higher PPV in a population with a high prevalence of disease than in one with a lower prevalence rate.

For many screening tests there is not one obvious cut-off point to distinguish between a person with disease and a person without disease. For example, hypertension could be defined as having a systolic blood pressure (SBP) greater than 160 mm Hg, or it could be defined more expansively as having an SBP greater than 140 mm Hg. Using a cut-off of 140 mm Hg would result in a much higher prevalence of hypertension than using a cut-off of 160 mm Hg. The people who design and implement screening tests do their best to determine the level at which the risk of disease is sufficient to declare that the person should be classified as having the condition. For some diseases, especially those with no treatment or treatment that is

Table 7–5 Questions to ask before starting a screening program.

Is the disease life threatening?

Is the disease common in the target population?

Is there an early asymptomatic stage of the disease that could be detected through screening?

Is the test for early disease valid? (Does it have high sensitivity and high specificity?)

Is the test acceptable to the target population?

Is there an acceptable treatment for individuals found to have the disease?

Are facilities for further testing and for treatment available to the target population?

---

expensive and potentially harmful, it is better to have a high threshold for declaring that a person has the condition. For others it is better to have a low threshold, especially when early intervention can prevent serious complications, as is the case for hypertension and diabetes.

Decisions about whether to implement a screening program and which population subgroups to target are made by health professionals, policymakers, and communities after considering the most important local health conditions. Diseases that are part of screening programs are usually severe, relatively common, and treatable. Screening for these types of conditions is considered to be a cost-effective way to diagnose people in the early, often asymptomatic stages of disease when treatment is easier and cheaper (**Table 7–5**). In developed countries, common types of screening tests include mole checks for skin cancer, Pap smears for cervical cancer, mammograms for early detection of breast cancer or precancerous lesions, digital rectal exams for prostate cancer, vision screening (including pressure tests for glaucoma), routine blood tests (for early detection of anemia, high cholesterol, high blood sugar, or other abnormalities), and routine blood pressure checks. Screening in low-income countries is more often geared at children and pregnant women, who are regularly weighed and examined, but adults in these areas would also benefit from improved access to routine screening for chronic diseases.

7.10 PLANNING FOR AGING POPULATIONS

A **population pyramid** displays the number of males and females by age group in a population. Low-income countries usually have a population pyramid with a wide base (many children) that gradually narrows in older age groups (**Figure 7–15**). These countries are often concerned about population growth and are taking measures to encourage decreased fertility rates. High-income countries often have low fertility rates that make the population "pyramid" look more like a cube (**Figure 7–16**). Some of these countries with narrow bases (few children), especially in Europe,

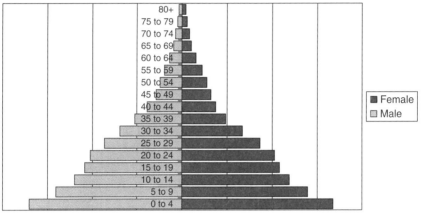

Figure 7–15 Population pyramid for Kenya in 2009.

Source: Data from *World development indicators database*. Washington DC: World Bank.

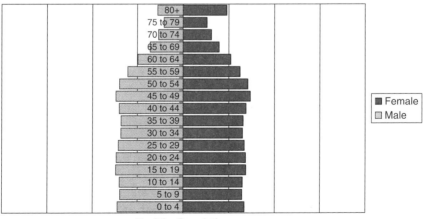

Figure 7–16 Population pyramid for the United States in 2009.

Source: Data from *World development indicators database*. Washington DC: World Bank.

Table 7–6 Aging indicators in 2010.

Country	USA	South Korea	Poland	Brazil	China	India	Kenya	Sierra Leone
Aging Index	66	71	92	27	43	17	6	4
Dependency Ratio	49	37	39	48	39	55	81	82
Elderly Support Ratio	5	7	5	10	9	13	21	29

Source: Data from Hughes BB, Kuhn R, Peterson CM, Rothman DS, Solórzano JR. Improving global health forecasting the next 50 years. Patterns of Potential Human Progress Series, Volume 3. Boulder CO: Paradigm Publishers; 2011.

face a shrinking population size and are concerned about who will care for the aging population as the ratio of older adults to working-age adults increases.

The data from these pyramids can be used to calculate a variety of indicators of population aging (Table 7–6). The aging index is usually calculated as the number of people age 65 or older for every 100 children under the age of 15. A higher aging index indicates a more aged population. Social support ratios like the dependency ratio indicate the number of dependent children and older people for every person of working age (often defined as people ages 15 through 64). The elderly support ratio is usually defined as the number of people ages 15 through 64 for every 100 people ages 65 and older in a population. Populations with relatively few working age adults for each older adult are more aged populations. (Because many older people remain active and economically independent, alternate measurements may include only dependent older people.) These population characteristics help social service providers and policymakers to understand the current needs of the populations they serve and to create plans that will help their populations prepare for the future.

Many older people contribute to families and communities by taking care of their grandchildren, providing training and guidance for younger employees, connecting younger generations to their cultural heritage, and sharing wisdom gained from decades of life experience. However, most older adults will eventually develop chronic health conditions that limit their independence. Staying with family when assistance with activities of daily living becomes necessary is often the preference of both older people and their families. In most of the world, care of the elderly is provided by spouses, children, and other family members, and institutionalization of older people is uncommon. But decreasing fertility rates mean that in many parts of the world there are fewer young people to care for older family members, and the increasing proportion of women who work outside the home also limits the number of people available to provide in-home care. Thus, an increasing proportion of older adults in a population puts stress on healthcare systems as well as on caregivers at home.

Few countries are prepared to care for a rapidly increasing number of older people with chronic illnesses and disabilities. In high-income countries, the growing proportion of older adults is already creating significant challenges for older adults, caregivers, health systems, and national pension systems. The national pension programs of many industrialized countries, especially in Europe, are on the verge of collapse because there are not enough young workers paying in to the programs to support retirees sufficiently. The retirement age is being increased and benefits are being cut. In developing countries where retirement accounts and pension plans are not the norm, aging is also expected to become a major social issue. The migration of young rural people to cities means that adult children often live far from their aging parents and cannot provide daily care, and few families have the ability to hire additional caregivers or nursing assistants. The ability to support older persons will become a significant concern in Latin America and much of Asia in the coming decades. All countries need to begin planning for the care of aging populations.[22]

7.11 DISCUSSION QUESTIONS

1. What have you gained from interactions with older adults? What have you contributed to enriching the lives of older adults?
2. How many years do you expect to live? What factors contribute to your estimation of your life expectancy?
3. What do you think will be the cause of your death? Why do you think that?
4. What are steps you can take now that will help you to live a long, healthy life? What are steps you can take now to minimize the likelihood of various types of chronic diseases and disabilities when you become an older adult?

5. What are some examples of health screening tests recommended for people of your age and sex? Do you adhere to these recommendations? Why or why not?

6. How have the older members of your family been cared for as they aged? Have they moved into an assisted living facility, moved in with their children or grandchildren, or made alternate arrangements? How did family and financial considerations play into these decisions?

7. What do you think your preferences for care will be when you are older? What factors might prevent you from receiving this type of care?

REFERENCES

1. *World development indicators database.* Washington DC: World Bank.
2. Hughes BB, Kuhn R, Peterson CM, Rothman DS, Solórzano JR. *Improving global health forecasting the next 50 years.* Patterns of Potential Human Progress Series, Volume 3. Boulder CO: Paradigm Publishers; 2011.
3. United Nations Department of Economic and Social Affairs. *World population ageing 2009.* New York: UN; 2010.
4. *The global burden of disease: 2004 update (April 2011 update).* Geneva: WHO; 2011.
5. *Active ageing: a policy framework.* Geneva: WHO; 2002.
6. Mackay J, Mensah GA. *Atlas of heart disease and stroke.* Geneva: WHO and U.S. CDC; 2004.
7. *The global burden of disease: 2004 update.* Geneva: WHO; 2008.
8. Ferlay J, Shin HR, Bray F, Forman D, Mathers C, Parkin DM. *GLOBOCAN 2008 v1.2: Cancer Incidence and Mortality Worldwide.* Lyon: IARC; 2010.
9. Ferlay J, Shin HR, Bray F, Forman D, Mathers C, Parkin DM. Estimates of worldwide burden of cancer in 2008: GLOBOCAN 2008. *Int J Cancer.* 2010;12:2893–2917.
10. Jemal A, Bray F, Center MM, Ferlay J, Ward E, Forman D. Global cancer statistics. *CA Cancer J Clin.* 2011;61:69–90.
11. Kamangar F, Dores GM, Anderson WF. Patterns of cancer incidence, mortality, and prevalence across five continents: defining priorities to reduce cancer disparities in different geographic regions of the world. *J Clin Oncol.* 2006;24:2137–2150.
12. Parkin DM, Bray F, Ferlay J, Pisani P. Global cancer statistics, 2002. *CA Cancer J Clin.* 2005; 55:74–108.
13. *Global status report on noncommunicable diseases 2010.* Geneva: WHO; 2011.
14. Mannino DM, Buist AS. Global burden of COPD: risk factors, prevalence, and future trends. *Lancet.* 2007:370:765–773.
15. Shaw JE, Sicree RA, Zimmet PZ. Global estimates of the prevalence of diabetes for 2010 and 2030. *Diabetes Res Clin Pract.* 2010;87:4–14.
16. van Dieren S, Beulens JW, van der Schouw YT, Grobbee DE, Neal B. The global burden of diabetes and its complications: an emerging pandemic. *Eur J Cardiovasc Prev Rehabil.* 2010;17(suppl):S3–S8.
17. Resnikofff S, Pascolini D, Mariotti SP, Pokharel GP. Global magnitude of visual impairment caused by uncorrected refractive errors in 2004. *Bull World Health Organ.* 2008;86:63–70.

18. *State of the world's sight: VISION 2020: the right to sight 1999–2005.* Geneva: WHO; 2005.
19. Mathers C, Smith A, Concha M. Global burden of hearing loss in the year 2000. Global Burden of Disease 2000 Study Working Paper. Geneva: WHO; 2003.
20. *International classification of functioning, disability, and health* (ICF). Geneva: WHO; 2001.
21. Ferri CP, Prince M, Brayne C, et al.; Alzheimer's Disease International. Global prevalence of dementia: a Delphi consensus study. *Lancet.* 2005;366:2112–2117.
22. *Why population aging matters: a global perspective.* Washington DC: U.S. Department of State and U.S. National Institute on Aging; 2007.

CHAPTER 8

The Environmental Context
of Health

Public health emphasizes the importance of safe home, work, and community environments. Reliable access to clean drinking water, a toilet, and fuel is critical for human health. Minimizing exposure to hazards and injuries at work is also essential for safety and well-being.

8.1 ENVIRONMENTAL AND OCCUPATIONAL HEALTH

Humans have long recognized the environment's role in disease etiology. Nearly 2500 years ago, Hippocrates, a Greek physician, catalogued environmental, dietary, behavioral, and constitutional conditions linked to health, and wrote that "from these things we must proceed to investigate everything else."[1] The **germ theory** of disease did not become widely accepted until the late 1800s, but for many centuries before microscopes allowed people to see pathogens, communities recognized that some illnesses were linked to environmental exposures, and they took care to dispose of human waste, to protect water sources, and to bury the carcasses of diseased animals.

Public health efforts in the 19th century focused primarily on environmental sanitation, with special attention aimed at reducing epidemics thought to be associated with urban crowding and its associated grime.[2] For most of the 1800s, the prevailing theory of disease causation in Western countries was that epidemics were spontaneously generated from "miasma atmospheres" that occurred in places with poor sanitation and the accompanying foul odors of poorly managed waste.[3] For example, during serious cholera outbreaks in England in the mid-1800s, investigators (led by William Farr, a respected health statistician) found a higher infection rate in places of low altitude, especially places near marshes that had an abundance of foul-smelling gases, and the **miasma** theory of disease blamed the spread of cholera on contact with those offensive gases.[4] This was a reasonable conclusion because the people who lived in the gassy, marshy areas were the same people who drank the bacterium-infected water that was the true cause of the outbreak (as determined by John Snow, one of the founders of modern epidemiology, who traced the source of one outbreak in London back to one very specific source, the Broad Street water pump).

By the middle of the 20th century, most medical scientists had shifted their efforts from the identification of social and environmental risk factors for disease to the identification of specific infectious agents and genes.[5] But even with the emphasis on immunology and genetics, one of the biggest public health breakthroughs in the 20th century was a series of studies published in the 1950s that confirmed that cigarette smoking was a major cause of lung cancer, emphysema, and cardiovascular disease.[6] Later studies indicated that exposure to secondhand smoke was an additional risk factor for lung disease.[7]

Today's scientists, health professionals, and health consumers agree that there are many social and behavioral, environmental, and biological contributors to disease. Good hygiene (like frequent handwashing) and the avoidance of known environmental hazards are important for preventing a host of diseases, and environmental health continues to play a very important role in public health and safety.

Modern environmental health scientists assess the impact of people on their environment and the impact of the environment on human health, specializing in areas like air quality, food protection, radiation protection, solid waste management, hazardous waste management, water quality, noise control, environmental management of recreational areas, housing quality, and animal and vector (insect) control. A major goal of environmental health is to understand the conditions that contribute to disease so that diseases can be prevented. For example, environmental health scientists may start with questions like "What are the health effects of smog (or contaminated water, acid rain, the thinning of the ozone layer, or the spraying of pesticides on crops)?" and then use the answers they find to promote changes in environmental health laws that regulate air quality, water quality, the disposal of waste, or chemical use.

Environmental health looks at all aspects of the physical environment— where people live and work and the materials used to construct these buildings, what people eat and where that food comes from, the source and quality of the drinking water, the quality of the air that is breathed, and the length and route of workers' commutes. A great deal of environmental research focuses on identifying environmental risk factors for cancer and for chronic diseases like asthma and arthritis. This research has shown, for example, that exposure to ultraviolet light from the sun and tanning beds contributes to the development of skin cancer and that air pollutants contribute to the development of lung cancer.

The physical environment also impacts health behavior. A recent study of global cancer mortality estimated that 35% of cancer deaths were due to just nine lifestyle and environmental factors: overweight and obesity, low fruit and vegetable intake, physical inactivity, smoking, alcohol use, unsafe sex, urban air pollution, indoor smoke from household use of solid fuels, and contaminated injections in healthcare settings.[8] Some of these factors, like air pollution and indoor smoke, are clearly environmental. Others are related both to the environment and to social, behavioral, and economic factors. Fruit and vegetable intake is easier for people who live where they can grow their own produce and harder for people who live in cities where produce is expensive and may not be fresh. A person who lives in an unsafe neighborhood may feel threatened when outdoors and may not have the space to be active indoors, so physical activity is curtailed.

Some environmental health researchers focus on issues related to geography, geology, and climate. Health risks are often tied to the local climate, whether the location is desert, tropical, artic, or something more moderate. Types of vegetation and animals that are native to particular climates, weather patterns and temperature, altitude, geologic formations (like volcanoes and earthquake fault lines), soil types, and other factors can influence risk for both communicable and noncommunicable diseases. For example, older people who live at high altitudes and have had long-term exposure to ultraviolet light, wind, and dust are at risk for developing a pterygium, a triangular growth that starts on the white part of the eye but may eventually cover the pupil and cause blindness. And malaria is a risk only for people who live in a climate that can support the lifecycle of the mosquitoes that spread the malaria parasites.

Most environmental health experts focus on aspects of health related to the home, workplace, or community. Occupational and industrial health specialists spend their time assessing and mitigating workplace hazards, which may mean measuring noise levels in a factory and issuing appropriate ear protection or making sure that people who spend their days in front of a computer have ergonomically designed chairs and are taking steps to minimize repetitive motion injuries. Other occupational and industrial health specialists focus on potential hazards in the home environment, such as lead paint, radon, and mold; they might also assess community risks, such as garbage dumps and runoff into waterways.

8.2 THE HOME ENVIRONMENT

Environmental health is also concerned with the health and safety of the home environment. Most buildings contain potential health hazards. Construction materials may be harmful, such as paint that contains lead (which can cause mental impairment in children who ingest paint chips) or insulation that contains asbestos (which can increase the risk of some types of lung cancer). Electrical wiring installed incorrectly may lead to the risk of electrocution. Windows without screens may let insects in, and poorly insulated and sealed walls and ceilings may not protect residents from cold and precipitation. Some residences may have high levels of radon, the second most common cause of lung cancer after tobacco, or may be infested with cockroaches, termites, or rats. There may also be hazardous chemicals stored in kitchens, bathrooms, garages, and sheds, and these substances, such as cleaning agents, fertilizers, and motor oil, may create new dangers when they are stored or disposed of improperly.

All of these conditions may be potentially hazardous, but in some ways it is a luxury to be able to worry about these household threats. For many people in the world, the most important household considerations are shelter, water, sanitation, and fuel for heat and cooking. A shelter is a dwelling that provides at least some protection from the sun, rain, wind, and other elements. At the outskirts of large cities in low-income parts of the world, large shantytowns built from cardboard may spring up overnight to accommodate rural-to-urban migrants. These may eventually be replaced with shacks built from blocks or bricks with a tin or asbestos roof, or replaced with sturdier houses constructed from cement, but once a minimal sort of protection is built the focus of the new resident is on finding a source of safe water for drinking and washing, a place away from the home that can be used to dispose of human waste, and a source of fuel for cooking.

Contaminated water, poor sanitation and hygiene, and inadequate management of human and animal waste are all associated with an increased risk of diarrheal diseases and other infections. Air pollution, including the indoor air pollution caused by cooking over open fires, is associated with acute respiratory infections, chronic respiratory diseases, and some types of cardiovascular disease and cancer. Increasing access to healthy housing, clean water supplies, sanitation facilities, and clean air and fuel improves the health of families and communities.

8.3 DRINKING WATER

Everyone needs access to an adequate supply of clean water. In addition to water for drinking and cooking, each person also needs water for hygiene (handwashing and bathing) and cleaning (washing clothes, cleaning cooking pots, and cleaning homes). Increased access to water is associated with improved health, as the incidence of diarrheal and other infectious diseases decreases when more water is available for hygiene. Another important household benefit of gaining access to an improved water source is that it saves a lot of time. When water sources are far from the home, women and children may spend several hours each day walking to a water source, waiting for their turn to fill a container, and walking home. The time saved could be used for other activities, which may be social, educational, or health oriented (such as cooking nutritious food, sleeping, or cleaning). There are at least five key aspects of water access: quality, quantity, proximity, reliability, and cost.

Quality: Water must be clean enough to drink safely. It needs to be free of bacteria, viruses, and parasites that can cause infection, and must also be free of harmful chemicals and sediments. The water should not appear cloudy, dirty, or strangely colored, so that it does not cause problems with cooking (such as giving food a strange flavor, color, or texture) or washing.[9] Ideally, the water should be drawn from a protected source, which means that people should not wash clothes or bathe near where drinking water is collected, and animals, sewage, and garbage should be kept away from the water source. Table 8–1 lists examples of improved and unimproved drinking water sources.[10]

Table 8–1 Examples of improved and unimproved drinking water sources.

Improved Drinking Water Sources	*Unimproved Drinking Water Sources*
• Piped water into home or yard	• Unprotected well
• Public tap or standpipe	• Unprotected spring
• Tube well or borehole	• Surface water (water from a river, dam, lake, pond, stream, canal, or irrigation channel)
• Protected dug well	• Water from vendors (like tanker trucks or carts with a small tank or drum)
• Protected spring	• Some bottled water
• Rainwater collection	

Source: Information from *Progress on sanitation and drinking water: 2010 update.* Geneva: UNICEF/WHO Joint Monitoring Programme for Water Supply and Sanitation; 2010.

Quantity: Enough water must be available so people can stay hydrated and clean. The average minimum amount of water needed by one person each day for survival purposes is about 15 to 20 liters (about 4 to 5 gallons): about 1 to 3 liters for drinking, 2 to 3 liters for food preparation and cleanup, 6 to 7 liters for personal cleanliness, and 4 to 6 liters for laundry.[11] Table 8–2 summarizes the levels of water access worldwide and shows that a minimum of 50 liters (13 gallons) of water per person per day is recommended for healthy living. About 1 in 7 people worldwide are in the "No access" category of the table.[12] The average American uses about 100 gallons daily for domestic purposes.[13]

Proximity: To be considered accessible, the water source must be close enough to the home so that distance does not prevent people from accessing the water they need. At best, water is piped directly to an individual house. However, many improved water systems instead simply bring clean water closer to homes via a public community standpost (standpipe), borehole, or protected (and lined) dug well. In some places it is possible for households to supplement their water access by collecting and storing rainwater for drinking and domestic use. Ideally, a safe drinking water source should be within 1 kilometer (about 0.6 miles) of a home.[14]

Reliability: The water source must be available and functioning all the time, or the household must have access to adequate water storage and water treatment methods such as filtering, boiling, and using chemicals like chlorine. One way to ensure that water systems can be maintained is to use **appropriate technology** that is simple enough that broken equipment, like water pumps, can be repaired by local residents cheaply and quickly.

Cost: Water must be affordable enough that people have access to at least the minimum amount of water necessary for healthy living. This does not mean that water must be free. Households that use a community water system may be asked to pay a reasonable fee for use so that the system can be maintained. These fees also promote water conservation if they are tied to the amount of water drawn from the pump by a household. In most cases, community water fees are minimal and are recognized as essential for keeping the water system running. However, when public water supplies are not available and exorbitant prices are charged for bottled water, the cost of water severely limits access to it.

Access to water is a requirement for life, so water access is a significant concern for the many people in Africa and the Middle East and parts of Asia and Latin America who have limited access to an improved water source (**Figure 8–1**),[10] especially those in rural areas

Table 8-2 Water service level (quantity, proximity, and quality) and health effects.

Service Level	Quantity (per person per day)	Proximity	Drinking Needs Met?	Hygiene Needs Met?	Level of Health Concern
No access	May be less than 5 liters	More than 1 km or 30 minutes round trip	Neither quantity nor quality ensured	No because only available at source	Very high
Basic access	About 20 liters	Between 100 and 1000 meters or 5 to 30 minutes round trip	Quantity ensured but quality not ensured	Yes for hand washing and food hygiene; no for laundry and bathing	High
Intermediate access	About 50 liters	Water delivered through one tap that is within 100 meters or 5 minutes round trip	Quantity and quality usually assured	Yes	Low
Optimal access	About 100 liters	Continuous supply through multiple taps	Quantity and quality ensured	Yes	Very low

Source: Data from Howard G, Bartram J. Domestic water quantity, service level and health. Geneva: WHO; 2003.

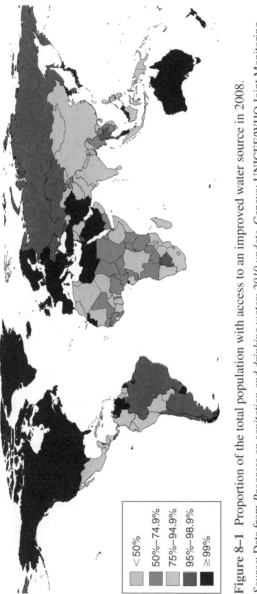

Figure 8–1 Proportion of the total population with access to an improved water source in 2008.

Source: Data from *Progress on sanitation and drinking water: 2010 update.* Geneva: UNICEF/WHO Joint Monitoring Programme for Water Supply and Sanitation; 2010.

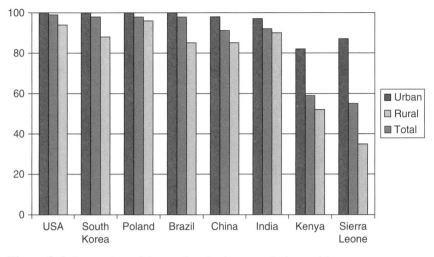

Figure 8–2 Proportion of the rural and urban populations with access to an improved drinking water source in 2010.

Source: Data from *Progress on sanitation and drinking water: 2012 update*. Geneva: UNICEF/WHO Joint Monitoring Programme for Water Supply and Sanitation; 2012.

(**Figure 8–2**).[12] In most of North America and Europe, both urban and rural households have access to tap water. In many other world regions, however, less than 90% of the urban population and less than 40% of the rural population has access to an improved water source, even though this proportion has increased significantly in recent decades (**Figure 8–3**).[12]

Only 2.5% of the world's water is freshwater rather than saltwater, and two-thirds of that freshwater is in glaciers. The main sources of freshwater for human use are rainwater, surface water (such as water from streams and rivers), and ground water (which is accessed by drilling wells). About 70% of freshwater used every year is put toward agricultural uses such as irrigation and livestock production,[15] and there are increasing demands for agricultural, industrial, and domestic water use as the world population grows. These are exacerbated when surface water becomes contaminated by agricultural runoff, human waste, and other pollutants, and when ground water becomes depleted and causes rivers, wetlands, and lakes that depend on the ground water to dry out. Water scarcity is becoming a major concern in many parts of the world, especially for small island nations and for the desert countries of the Middle East and North Africa

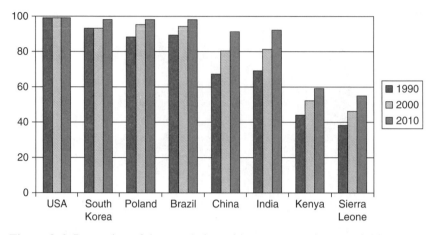

Figure 8–3 Proportion of the population with access to an improved drinking water source by decade between 1990 and 2010.

Source: Data from *Progress on sanitation and drinking water: 2012 update.* Geneva: UNICEF/WHO Joint Monitoring Programme for Water Supply and Sanitation; 2012.

where internal freshwater resources are extremely limited. Countries with less than 200 cubic meters of renewable freshwater resources (internal surface water plus groundwater fed by rainfall in that country) per person face ongoing challenges (**Table 8–3**).[15] As the demand for water increases, everyone needs to be concerned about the availability of freshwater resources.

8.4 SANITATION

Sanitation is the disposal of human excreta. There are several types of sanitation facilities that can be used for safe waste disposal (**Table 8–4**).[12] One of the most basic sanitation systems is a simple pit latrine, which is a hole in the ground covered by an outhouse or encircled by a privacy blind. In many communities, ownership of a latrine is a sign of prestige, besides providing safety, cleanliness, comfort, privacy, and protection from dangers at night and from snakes. A slightly more advanced ventilation-improved pit (or VIP) latrine vents fumes away from the outhouse and keeps flies out of it. Pour-flush systems require some water for washing away the waste. Septic tanks and sewer connections are

Table 8–3 Internal freshwater resources per person for countries with less than 200 m^3 of renewable freshwater resources per capita and for featured countries in 2007.

Country/Territory	Region/Type	Freshwater Resources per Capita (cubic meters)
Kuwait	Middle East	0
Bahrain	Middle East	5
Egypt	North Africa	22
United Arab Emirates	Middle East	34
Qatar	Middle East	49
The Bahamas	Small Island Nation	60
Yemen	Middle East	94
Libya	North Africa	97
Saudi Arabia	Middle East	99
Maldives	Small Island Nation	100
Israel	Middle East	104
Jordan	Middle East	120
Malta	Small Island Nation	123
Mauritania	North Africa	127
Singapore	Small Island Nation	131
Kenya	East Africa	548
India	South Asia	1134
South Korea	East Asia	1338
Poland	Europe	1406
China	East Asia	2134
USA	North America	9344
Sierra Leone	West Africa	29518
Brazil	South America	48498

Source: Data from *Little green data book 2011.* Washington DC: World Bank; 2011.

Table 8–4 Examples of improved and unimproved sanitation facilities.

Improved Sanitation Facilities	Unimproved Sanitation Facilities
• Connection to a public sewer system	• Open defecation in a field, street, body of water, or other place
• Connection to a septic system	• Bucket or bag
• Pour-flush latrine	• Open pit latrine
• Ventilated-improved pit (VIP) latrine	• Flush or pour-flush toilet that drains to the street, yard, an open sewer, a ditch, a drainage way, or another location
• Composting toilet	
• Simple pit latrine	• Public or shared latrine

Source: Information from Progress on sanitation and drinking water: 2012 update. Geneva: UNICEF/WHO Joint Monitoring Programme for Water Supply and Sanitation; 2012.

more advanced sanitation technologies. Advanced sanitation facilities are common in North America and Europe, but rare in many other regions (**Figure 8–4**).[12]

About half of the people who live in developing countries do not have access to even the simplest improved sanitation facility, such as a pit latrine, and must practice **open defecation** (**Figure 8–5**).[12] Rural residents may be able to go to a defecation site away from their living areas. Urban residents without access to a latrine often have no choice but to defecate on the street or into a bag that is thrown at the side of the street (a waste disposal method that is sometimes called a "flying toilet"). A desire for privacy means that many people, especially women, wait until dark to defecate, even though it is often dangerous for them to be out at night.

People who do not have an improved sanitation system are at increased risk for infectious diseases that are spread through contact with feces. The factors that contribute to diarrheal diseases have sometimes been described using the "six Fs": feces, fields, fluid, fingers, food, and flies.[16] When *feces* are not properly disposed of, they can contaminate *fields* (soil) and *fluids* (bodies of water). The fecal matter can then get onto hands, especially the hands of young children who frequently touch the ground, and *fingers* transport the fecal matter to *food* if hands are not washed before preparing food or before eating. *Flies* can also spread feces to food and water, and flies thrive where fecal matter is in the open. The risk of diarrheal disease increases when there is not enough *fluid* (water) to wash hands often.

The presence of feces near homes significantly increases the risk of bacterial, viral, and protozoal diarrheal diseases and helminthic (worm)

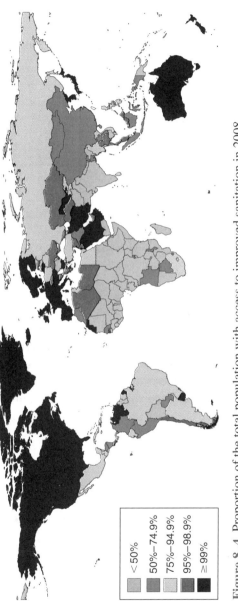

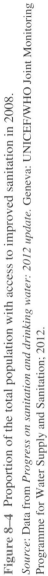

Figure 8–4 Proportion of the total population with access to improved sanitation in 2008.

Source: Data from *Progress on sanitation and drinking water: 2012 update.* Geneva: UNICEF/WHO Joint Monitoring Programme for Water Supply and Sanitation; 2012.

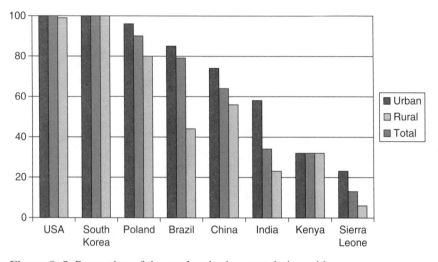

Figure 8–5 Proportion of the rural and urban population with access to an improved sanitation facility in 2010.

Source: Data from *Progress on sanitation and drinking water: 2012 update.* Geneva: UNICEF/WHO Joint Monitoring Programme for Water Supply and Sanitation; 2012.

infections. Intestinal worm infections can be treated through the periodic distribution of de-worming medicines to school-age children and other at-risk population groups, but improved sanitation is a necessity for preventing new infections and reinfections. The best programs for reducing diarrhea and parasitism combine improved water and sanitation systems with health education to promote frequent handwashing and consistent use of latrines instead of open defecation.[17] Improved sanitation facilities, which are becoming more common around the world (**Figure 8–6**),[12] must provide privacy, safety, and comfort, and must be kept clean.[16]

8.5 FUEL AND INDOOR AIR QUALITY

Energy is necessary for at least three important purposes: cooking food and boiling water for safe consumption, providing a source of heat when outdoor temperatures are low, and providing a source of light at night. More than 20% of the world's people do not have electricity in their homes (**Figure 8–7**).[18,19] Households without electricity usually rely on solid fuels (like wood, charcoal, coal, dung, and crop waste) for most of their energy needs. These may be supplemented by the use of candles and kerosene lamps for light.

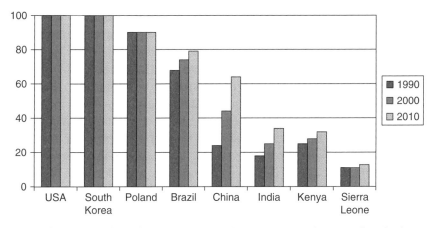

Figure 8–6 Proportion of the population with access to an improved sanitation facility by decade between 1990 and 2010.

Source: Data from *Progress on sanitation and drinking water: 2012 update*. Geneva: UNICEF/WHO Joint Monitoring Programme for Water Supply and Sanitation; 2012.

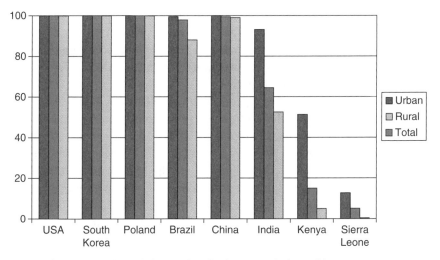

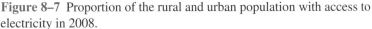

Figure 8–7 Proportion of the rural and urban population with access to electricity in 2008.

Source: Data from *World energy outlook 2010*. New York: International Energy Agency (IEA); 2010; and Legros G, Havet I, Bruce N, Bonjour S. *The energy access situation in developing countries: a review focusing on the least developed countries and sub-Saharan Africa*. New York: UNDP and WHO; 2009.

All fuels that are burned for energy release air pollutants, including the fuels that provide energy for electricity. (Worldwide, coal is the most commonly used source of fuel for electricity.[18]) But solid fuels used in homes are particularly unhealthy because they are usually burned in open fires or in simple stoves that release most of the smoke from burning into the home. The pollutants in smoke from burning solid fuels include carbon monoxide, sulfur oxides, nitrogen oxides, aldehydes, and polyaromatic compounds.[20] These chemicals can cause lung disease by triggering inflammation, damaging the cells that line the respiratory tract, and impairing immune response. The smoke also contains particulate matter that can get deep into the lungs. Indoor air pollution is responsible for about 1.5 million deaths worldwide every year[21,22] because it increases the risk of pneumonia and other respiratory diseases in children and increases the risk of chronic obstructive pulmonary disorder (COPD) and lung cancer in adults.[23] The risks associated with indoor air pollution levels are particularly high for women and young children who spend several hours a day near fires while cooking.

Use of solid fuels can have other negative health effects. Children are at risk for burns from falling into open fires or knocking over pots of boiling water. Women and children often spend hours each week collecting sticks and brush to use as fuel, and they are susceptible to injuries related to carrying heavy loads over uneven and uncleared terrain. As sources of biomass close to the home are used up, they must travel further distances to find fuel. There are also environmental consequences: burning of solid fuels contributes to outdoor air pollution, and the demand for wood and charcoal contributes to deforestation.

There are several ways that people without electricity can reduce their exposure to indoor air pollution.[24] One is to use improved cooking devices such as those that have flues to divert pollutants out of the home and those that use alternative energy sources (like solar panels) that create less smoke. A second is to increase ventilation or move the kitchen to the outside of the home. (Obviously, relocating the kitchen does not help minimize the cook's exposure if the outside cooking area does not have a good ventilation system.) A third is to change behaviors, like taking care to keep children away from smoke and using pot lids to conserve heat.

For those who are able to access electricity, there are additional health benefits besides cleaner indoor air. For example, refrigeration allows for safer food storage and the use of a radio or television allows for health and safety messages such as advertisements for immunization campaigns, information about handwashing and other disease prevention techniques, and alerts about potential natural disasters such as oncoming hurricanes to be quickly received. Ideally, electricity can be produced by renewable sources that minimize air pollution and other types of environmental damage.

8.6 THE WORK ENVIRONMENT

Occupational health was one of the first public health specialty fields.[25] In 1713, Bernardino Ramazzini published *Diseases of Workers*, a book that detailed the environmental hazards encountered in 52 occupations, listing poisoning, respiratory diseases, problems related to prolonged postures and repetitive tasks, and psychological stress as some of many on-the-job threats to health. In 1753, James Lind published the results of an experiment that supported the hypothesis that sailors could prevent scurvy if they carried citrus fruit with them on long journeys.[26] (After this discovery, sailors were sometimes called "limeys" for the citrus fruit carried on ships.) In 1775, Percivall Pott identified chimney soot as the cause of elevated rates of scrotal cancer in chimney sweeps.[27] The coal tar in chimneys is carcinogenic, and because sweeps rarely bathed or changed their trousers they had nearly constant exposure to the carcinogen. New occupational risks continue to be identified today.

Every worker may face a particular mix of biological, chemical, physical, mechanical, and psychosocial challenges at work. Some occupations carry specific risks. Those who work with heavy machinery are at risk for crush wounds from moving parts. Those exposed to loud noises are at risk for permanent hearing impairment. Medical workers are at risk for contracting infectious diseases from needlesticks and contact with body fluids. Some workers who have long-term exposure to industrial chemicals are at increased risk for developing certain types of cancers. Office workers are at risk for repetitive strain injuries, such as carpal tunnel syndrome, that can develop after performing the same tasks over and over. All workers may be subject to stress that can impair mental health.

The International Labor Organization (ILO) estimates that each year nearly 300 million workers miss at least 4 days of work due to an on-the-job injury and about 2 million people die as a result of job-related diseases, including more than 350,000 who die from injuries sustained at work.[28] Workplace hazards are estimated to be responsible for 37% of back pain, 16% of hearing loss, 13% of COPD, 11% of asthma, 9% of lung cancers, 8% of injuries, and 2% of leukemias worldwide.[29] Many of these injuries and deaths could be prevented if worksite managers and government officials enforced compliance with safety regulations.

8.7 TOXICOLOGY

Toxicology is the study of the harmful effects that chemicals and other environmental hazards like radiation can have on living things. Toxicologists study the way variations in exposure frequency (how often a person is exposed), duration (the length of exposure at a given time), and dose (the amount of hazardous substance contacted) influence health. They also assess the various exposure routes (like inhalation, ingestion, and absorption through the skin) and pathways (through air, water, food, soil, or other mechanisms) related to hazardous exposures. Substances identified as **carcinogens** (which can cause genetic mutations that lead to cancer), **teratogens** (which can cause birth defects), or other hazards can be regulated or banned. Hazardous exposures include radiation, chemical pollutants, and toxic substances like PCBs (polychlorinated biphenyls), dioxins, asbestos, lead, mercury, cadmium, organic solvents, and pesticides. Many of these are released into the environment through industrial activities. Some of the most common toxic substances are listed in **Table 8–5**.[30]

Hazardous substances are estimated to cause more than 400,000 deaths each year, including 100,000 occupational deaths from asbestos and 70,000 poisoning deaths due to agricultural pesticides.[31] Although these hazardous substances are used and produced in industrial settings in both developed and developing countries, workers in developing countries have greater risks from them. Many highly toxic agents that have been banned from use in the United States and other industrialized nations are still used in low-income nations. Occupational regulations in low-income countries are rarely enforced, so workers generally have very little access to protective gear and safety training. And in low-income countries where jobs are scarce, workers may have to choose between repeated exposure to very high doses of dangerous chemicals and being unemployed.

Ecotoxicology examines the impact of toxic exposures on populations, communities, and ecosystems. When industrial accidents occur, they do not just affect people who work at the site of an incident. The pollutants, toxins, and other substances released into air or water as a result of an accident can affect the local community and may spread to a much larger area. The radioactivity released during the meltdown of the nuclear reactor at Chernobyl in Ukraine (then part of the U.S.S.R.) in April 1986 spread a radioactive cloud across most of Europe. One health-related outcome of the meltdown was an increase in the incidence of thyroid cancer among children in the most contaminated regions.[32] An accident at a chemical

Table 8–5 Top hazardous substances in the United States in 2007.

	Substance	Uses
1	Arsenic	Used to make "pressure-treated" lumber, as a pesticide for cotton plants, and in copper and lead smelting
2	Lead	Used in production of batteries, ammunition, metal products (solder and pipes), and devices to shield x-rays; released from the burning of fossil fuels and during mining and manufacturing; used in some gasoline, paints, caulks, and ceramic products
3	Mercury	Used in thermometers, dental fillings, batteries, and some antiseptic creams and ointments
4	Vinyl chloride	Used to make polyvinyl chloride (PVC), plastic products like pipes, wire and cable coatings, and packaging materials
5	Polychlorinated biphenyls (PCBs)	Used as coolants and lubricants in transformers, capacitors, and other electrical equipment
6	Benzene	Used to make other chemicals that form plastics, resins, nylon and synthetic fibers, rubbers, lubricants, dyes, detergents, drugs, and pesticides
7	Cadmium	Extracted during production of metals like zinc, lead, and copper for use in batteries, pigments, metal coatings, and plastics
8	Polycyclic aromatic hydrocarbons (PAHs)	A group of over 100 different chemicals that are formed during incomplete burning of coal, oil, gas, garbage, tobacco, charbroiled meat, and other organic substances; also found in coal tar, crude oil, creosote, roofing tar, some medicines and dyes, plastics, and pesticides

Source: Information from *2007 CERCLA (Comprehensive Environmental Response, Compensation, and Liability Act) priority list of hazardous substances*. Atlanta, GA: U.S. Agency for Toxic Substances and Disease Registry; 2007.

plant in Bhopal, India, in December 1984 released liquid and vapor methyl isocyanate. Several thousand people died when they were exposed to the fumes, some in their beds and others in the street after they staggered out of their homes to try to escape from the chemical. Hundreds of thousands of people sustained lung injuries.[33]

Another example of widespread environmental damage that can be created by human activities is air pollution, which can be produced by transportation (exhaust from cars and trucks), power plants (which burn coal and oil to produce electricity), industrial processes, forest fires, and the disposal of solid waste. The substances released into the air from these processes include carbon monoxide, sulfur oxides, hydrocarbons, nitrogen dioxide, and particulates of solid or liquid substances that are small enough to remain suspended in the air for long periods of time and are easily moved by wind. Poor air quality can cause reduced visibility and unpleasant odors, interfere with plant growth and agricultural quality, and endanger health by irritating the eyes and respiratory tract, increasing the risk of asthma, and exacerbating symptoms of chronic diseases like cardiovascular diseases, COPD, and anemia.[34]

Many countries from all income levels have passed occupational and environmental health and safety laws as well as laws intended to reduce new pollution. And because pollutants and hazardous materials produced in one place can end up affecting people thousands of miles away, several international regulations and guidelines are intended to protect the environment as well as human health. For example, the Kyoto Protocol, an agreement made under the Framework Convention on Climate Change, asks countries to commit to voluntarily reduce their emissions of carbon dioxide, methane, nitrous oxide, and other greenhouse gases.

8.8 COMMUNITIES AND ENVIRONMENTAL HEALTH

Rural and urban households, businesses, and communities are inextricably linked to one another because everyone who lives or works in a community shares the same air, water, and other environmental exposures. Thus, it is advantageous to all parties when everyone works together to protect their communities and to promote health. Relatively simple examples of community environmental health action include community support for enforcement of transportation policies that protect pedestrians and bicyclists and voluntary organizations that maintain recreational space to promote physical activity. Sometimes community health problems call for more dramatic and far-reaching solutions. Two examples, arsenic poisoning from tube wells in Bangladesh and the debate over the use of DDT for malaria control, highlight different approaches to community health action.

In Bangladesh, surface water is often contaminated with feces from humans, cattle, and water buffaloes, so an initiative begun by UNICEF in the 1970s promoted the installation of tube wells that tap ground water. Only after millions of hand-pump tube wells had been dug did geologists determine that the wells extract water that flows through fluvial deposits that contain arsenopyrites. As a result, the concentration of arsenic in water from these wells is often tens of times higher than the recommended maximum exposure (10 μg/l, as advised by the World Health Organization).[35] Millions of Bangladeshis are at risk for arsenicosis, chronic arsenic poisoning from drinking contaminated water over a long period of time.[36] The most visible symptom is a change in skin color (hyperpigmentation) and the formation of hard skin patches (keratosis), but arsenicosis can also cause skin cancer and cancers of the lung, kidney, and bladder; liver damage; gangrene; and peripheral vascular disease.

An initial solution is to promote the use of a low-cost filter system that can remove arsenic from drinking water, but because even a very low-cost filter is more expensive than many Bangladeshi families can afford—and because the filters produce toxic waste, so they are at best only a temporary solution—other steps are needed. The amount of arsenic in each well varies widely, so workers are testing wells and then painting green handles on safe pumps and red handles on contaminated pumps.[37] Another solution is to collect rainwater during the rainy season or dig deeper wells that bypass the geologic formations that contain arsenic. There is no one approach that will work for all communities, so local communities must be involved in making decisions about what will work best for their geologic, social, and economic situations.

Many more communities around the world struggle against malaria, a mosquito-borne parasitic infection. In the middle part of the 20th century, DDT (dichloro-diphenyl-trichloroethane) was sprayed in large quantities over cities and crops to control malarial mosquitoes in the United States and other countries. DDT does not easily degrade—it is a persistent organic pollutant (POP)—so it builds up in the food chain, killing birds and fish. The United States banned DDT in 1972 (in large part because of the uproar caused by Rachel Carson's book *Silent Spring*, which had been published in 1962), and many other countries, both developed and developing, also enacted DDT bans. The DDT ban led to a drastic increase in the incidence of malaria in many countries.

In recent years, many communities in malaria-endemic areas have begun using DDT in homes. The environmental persistence that makes DDT an environmental hazard when it is sprayed outdoors makes it appealing for in-home use as an insecticide. DDT sticks to the walls so that pesticides only need to be used once or twice a year. Spraying a tiny amount of DDT on the walls of houses kills mosquitoes that land on the walls, but it seems to be harmless to humans and other animals. DDT is also cheaper and more effective than most other pesticides.

In 2001, a global treaty sponsored by the United Nations Environment Programme (UNEP) and many private environmental organizations banned 11 other POPs, but made a special exemption for indoor public health use of DDT.[38] Use of the chemical is now limited, but not banned. DDT is not a cure-all. It only protects people from bites while they are indoors, and some mosquitoes are resistant to the effects of DDT. Still, the World Health Organization now endorses the use of **indoor residual spraying (IRS)** for mosquito control in areas that have endemic or epidemic malaria transmission, and DDT could contribute, if used correctly, to preventing millions of malaria deaths.[39] Although still controversial, the re-implementation of minimal use of DDT for home protection may end up being an example of how people with different views on the risks and benefits of an environmental intervention can find a middle ground that is acceptable to most parties involved.

8.9 DISCUSSION QUESTIONS

1. What are some of the safety hazards in your home? What do you do to minimize the risk from these exposures?
2. What environmental hazards might be present in your water, food, and air? What can you do to minimize your exposures? What concerns must be addressed at the population level?
3. If the water fountain at your local grocery store was your nearest source of clean water, how would you have to change your schedule and habits to accommodate this? How much time would you lose each day to waiting in line, transporting water, and otherwise meeting your water needs?
4. How would your daily activities change if you did not have access to a modern sanitation system?
5. If you had to choose whether you would have running water in (or at least near) your home or electricity in your home, which would be your priority? Why?
6. What are the occupational risks associated with your chosen profession?
7. How might companies working in your community be harming the environment? What are local companies doing to help promote a healthier environment?

8. What are some examples of local and national organizations that focus on the environment or on environmental health? What steps do these organizations recommend individuals and families take to help foster a healthy environment? What volunteer opportunities do these organizations provide?

REFERENCES

1. Schettler T. *Toward an ecological view of health: an imperative for the twenty-first century.* Concord CA: The Center for Health Design; 2006.
2. Shryock RH. The early American public health movement. *Am J Public Health.* 1937;27:965–971.
3. Susser M, Susser E. Choosing a future for epidemiology: I. Eras and paradigms. *Am J Public Health.* 1996;86:668–673.
4. Bingham P, Verlander NQ, Cheal MJ. John Snow, William Farr and the 1849 outbreak of cholera that affected London: a reworking of the data highlights the importance of the water supply. *Public Health.* 2004;118:387–394.
5. Pearce N. Traditional epidemiology, modern epidemiology, and public health. *Am J Public Health.* 1996;86:678–683.
6. Doll R, Hill AB. Lung cancer and other causes of death in relation to smoking. *Br Med J.* 1956;2:1071–1081.
7. Hackshaw AK, Law MR, Wald NJ. The accumulated evidence on lung cancer and environmental tobacco smoke. *BMJ.* 1997;315:980–988.
8. Danaei G, Vander Hoorn S, Lopez AD, Murray CJ, Ezzati M; Comparative Risk Assessment collaborating group (cancers). Causes of cancer in the world: comparative risk assessment of nine behavioural and environmental risk factors. *Lancet.* 2005;366:1784–1793.
9. *Guidelines for drinking water quality,* 4th edition. Geneva: WHO; 2011.
10. *Progress on sanitation and drinking water: 2010 update.* Geneva: UNICEF/WHO Joint Monitoring Programme for Water Supply and Sanitation; 2010.
11. *Water for life: community water security.* New York: Hesperian Foundation and UNDP; 2005.
12. *Progress on sanitation and drinking water: 2012 update.* Geneva: UNICEF/WHO Joint Monitoring Programme for Water Supply and Sanitation; 2012.
13. *Estimated use of water in the United States in 2005* (circular 1344). Reston VA: U.S. Geolgcial Survey; 2009.
14. Howard G, Bartram J. Domestic water quantity, service level and health. Geneva: WHO; 2003.
15. *Little green data book 2011.* Washington DC: World Bank; 2011.
16. Conant J, Fadem P. *Community guide to environmental health.* Berkeley CA: Hesperian Foundation; 2008.
17. Mara D, Lane J, Scott B, Trouba D. Sanitation and health. *PLoS Med.* 2010;7:e1000363.
18. *World energy outlook 2010.* New York: International Energy Agency (IEA); 2010.
19. Legros G, Havet I, Bruce N, Bonjour S. *The energy access situation in developing countries: a review focusing on the least developed countries and sub-Saharan Africa.* New York: UNDP and WHO; 2009.

20. Zhang J, Smith KR. Indoor air pollution: a global health concern. *Br Med Bull.* 2003;68:209–225.

21. Smith KR, Mehta S. The burden of disease from indoor air pollution in developing countries: comparison of estimates. *Int J Environ Health.* 2003;206:279–289.

22. Bonjour S, Prüss-Üstün A, Rehfuess E. *Indoor air pollution: national burden of disease estimates.* Geneva: WHO; 2007.

23. Fullerton DG, Bruce N, Gordon SB. Indoor air pollution from biomass fuel smoke is a major health concern in the developing world. *Trans R Soc Trop Med Hyg.* 2008;102:843–851.

24. Bruce N, Rehfuess E, Mehta S, Hutton G, Smith K. Indoor air pollution. In: Jamison DT, Breman JG, Measham AR, et al., editors. *Disease control priorities in developing countries*, 2nd edition. Washington DC: Oxford University Press; 2006.

25. Abrams HK. A short history of occupational health. *J Public Health Policy.* 2001;22:34–80.

26. Hughes RE. James Lind and the cure of scurvy: an experimental approach. *Med Hist.* 1975;19:342–351.

27. Waldron HA. A brief history of scrotal cancer. *Br J Ind Med.* 1983;40:390–401.

28. Al-Tuwaijri D, Fedotov I, Feitshans I, et al. *Beyond deaths and injuries: the ILO's role in promoting safe and healthy jobs.* Geneva: ILO; 2008.

29. Fingerhut M, Nelson DI, Driscoll T, et al. The contribution of occupational risks to the global burden of disease: summary and next steps. *Med Lav.* 2006;97:313–321.

30. *2007 CERCLA (Comprehensive Environmental Response, Compensation, and Liability Act) priority list of hazardous substances.* Atlanta GA: U.S. Agency for Toxic Substances and Disease Registry; 2007.

31. *World Day for Safety and Health at Work 2005: a background paper.* Geneva: ILO; 2005.

32. Shibata Y, Yamashita S, Masyakin VB, Panasyuk GD, Nagataki S. 15 years after Chernobyl: new evidence of thyroid cancer. *Lancet.* 2001;358:1965–1966.

33. Mehta PS, Mehta AS, Mehta SJ, Makhijani AB. Bhopal tragedy's health effects: a review of methyl isocyanate toxicity. *JAMA.* 1990;265:2781–2787.

34. Brunekreef B, Holgate ST. Air pollution and health. *Lancet.* 2002;360:1233–1242.

35. Smith AH, Lingas EO, Rahman M. Contamination of drinking-water by arsenic in Bangladesh: a public health emergency. *Bull World Health Organ.* 2000;78:1093–1103.

36. Chakraborti D, Rahman MM, Das B, et al. Status of groundwater arsenic contamination in Bangladesh: a 14-year study report. *Water Res.* 2010;44:5789–5802.

37. Ahmed M, Jakariya M, Quaiyum M, Mahmud SN. An implementation guide for the Arsenic Mitigation Program. Dhaka: BRAC; 2002.

38. Sadasivaiah S, Tozan Y, Breman JG. Dichlorodiphenyltrichloroethane (DDT) for indoor residual spraying in Africa: how can it be used for malaria control? *Am J Trop Med Hyg.* 2007;77(6 suppl):249–263.

39. *World malaria report 2010.* Geneva: WHO; 2010.

CHAPTER 9

Control of Infectious Diseases

Bacteria, viruses, and parasites cause a variety of severe diseases. Approaches for the prevention and control of these infections must be tailored to the type of infection, the usual mode of transmission, and the technologies and other resources that are available.

9.1 GLOBAL INFECTIOUS DISEASES

Most North Americans and Europeans consider cancer, heart disease, or diabetes to be their number one health concern. Few mention infectious diseases as a top priority, except when a major infectious disease outbreak is getting a lot of media attention. This happens occasionally when there are new fears about the emergence of a particularly bad influenza strain or there is an outbreak linked to a food product or restaurant chain. These worries usually fade quickly. But in many parts of the world infectious diseases remain responsible for a large proportion of deaths of children, the poor, and other vulnerable population groups (**Figure 9–1**).[1] This fact alone is a very good reason to care deeply about developing new methods for prevention and treatment of infections and increasing access to these technologies. Everyone also needs to be concerned about infectious diseases because they can spread and adapt quickly, and they have the potential to affect nearly everyone. Infectious diseases are spread through social networks, and the web of human contacts is becoming more and more complex as modern transportation allows people and products to travel to almost anywhere in the world within a day. Global health professionals must know how infectious diseases are transmitted and how they can be contained.

187

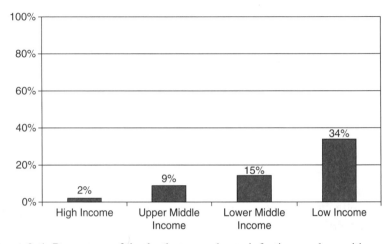

Figure 9–1 Percentage of deaths that were due to infectious and parasitic diseases in 2008, by country income level.

Source: Data from *The global burden of disease: 2004 update*. Geneva: WHO; 2008.

9.2 AGENTS OF INFECTION

There are many different types of pathogens that can cause infection, including bacteria, viruses, parasites, and fungi. Different infectious agents pose different risks and require different methods of prevention and treatment.

9.2.A Bacteria

Bacteria are microscopic, single-celled organisms that are found nearly everywhere on the planet, from the arctic tundra to hot springs deep in the ocean. Bacteria can be differentiated based on their shapes, such as rods (bacilli), spheres (cocci), and spirals (spirochetes, vibrios, and spirilla), by relative size (although all are very small), and by the amount of a substance called peptidoglycan in their cell walls. When stained with a special dye, the peptidoglycan on the surface of Gram-positive bacteria will bond to the stain. Gram-negative bacteria have an outer membrane over the peptido-glycan layer so the dye will not bond.

Bacteria play an important role in decomposition and chemical recycling, in the fixation of nitrogen into plants, and in the production of alcohol and foods like cheese and yogurt. Millions of helpful bacteria line the digestive tracts and other surfaces of humans, crowding out harmful bacteria. However, many types of bacteria can cause disease, like some strains of *E. coli*, which can cause diarrhea, and *Staphylococcus*, which can cause skin disease.

Bacteria cause illness in a variety of ways. For example, illness from a bacterial infection may be due to bacterial endotoxins that are released when the bacteria die and disintegrate. Many gastrointestinal diseases are the result of endotoxins being released from Gram-negative bacteria. Some bacteria produce exotoxins like the one that causes botulism, which can lead to severe illness and death in people who eat food from cans that are contaminated with the toxin. Tetanus toxin from *Clostridium tetani* spores can cause spasms and death. The toxin enters the body when a person sustains a puncture wound (often referred to as "stepping on a rusty nail") or gives birth in unsanitary conditions, but disease can be prevented with an immunization. Several other bacterial diseases are also vaccine-preventable, including whooping cough, pneumococcal pneumonia, and bacterial meningitis. Most bacterial infections can be cured with antibiotics, although a growing number of **pathogenic** (disease-causing) bacteria are becoming resistant to treatment with common antibiotics.

9.2.B Viruses

Viruses are extremely tiny, and because they are acellular (not cells) they are not considered to be alive. They can only replicate by invading the cells of a living host and taking control of the cells' nuclei. When a virus enters the body, spikes on the outer part of the virus, called a capsid, attach to the surface of a human cell. The outside of the virus is shed and the genetic material from inside the virus penetrates the cell and travels to the nucleus, where the virus takes command and directs the infected cell to make many new copies of the virus. The newly formed virus copies travel to the edge of the cell and enter new capsids. When released from the cell, the new virus particles travel to other parts of the body, infecting other cells, or are shed from the body to infect other people.

The body will recover from most viral infections on its own, but some viruses lead to chronic infections, such as HIV and the hepatitis C virus. Viral infections cannot be cured by antibiotics. Treating viral infections inappropriately by prescribing antibiotics poses a serious threat to global health by contributing to the development of antimicrobial resistance. For some types of viral infections, it is possible to take drugs that reduce the number of virus particles present in the body and that help mitigate symptoms.

For example, antiviral drugs can slow the progression of HIV infection, suppress the lesions caused by the herpes virus, and make influenza infections less severe. However, the better option is to take steps to prevent contracting a virus. Many viral infections can be prevented by vaccines, including polio, hepatitis B, rotavirus, human papillomavirus (HPV), measles, and chickenpox, and personal health practices such as handwashing and covering one's mouth when sneezing or coughing can limit transmission of many other viruses.

9.2.C Parasites

Parasites are eukaryotic organisms that survive by living off of a host. A eukaryote consists of a complex cell or cells that have a membrane-bound nucleus. Bacteria and viruses are not eukaryotes, but fungi, plants, and animals are. Some parasites only minimally affect their hosts, but others can cause serious illness or disability. There are two main types of eukaryotic parasites that affect human health: protozoa and helminths.

Protozoa are single-celled organisms that have animal-like characteristics and often live in water. *Paramecium* and *Amoeba*, which are often used as samples under microscopes in biology classes, are common protozoa. Protozoa are classified based on how they move and on the characteristics of their lifecycles. For example, flagellates have a "tail" that assists with motion, ciliates have rows of hair-like projections that help the organism to move, and apicomplexa (including the parasites that cause malaria, cryptosporidiosis, and toxoplasmosis, which can be acquired from contact with cat litter and can cross the placental barrier and cause congenital infection in the fetus) have complex life cycles involving both sexual and asexual reproduction.

Helminths are **endoparasitic** worms that live inside the body of the host. (Protozoa are also endoparasitic. In contrast, lice and the mites that cause scabies are **ectoparasitic** animals that live on the exterior surface of the body.) Helminths are classified by shape as well as by their lifecycles. Nematodes are roundworms, cestodes are tapeworms, and trematodes are flukes (flatworms). Helminths can be acquired by walking barefoot in contaminated soil, wading in contaminated water, ingesting contaminated food or water, and even by being bit by worm-infested insects. Some worms are microscopic, but others grow to be several inches—or even several feet—long as they mature in the human body.

Antiparasitic medications will kill many parasites, but may not be effective against all life stages of the parasites, and drug resistance is becoming a concern for many types of parasite infections.

9.2.D Fungi

Fungi come in many forms, including molds and yeasts. Fungi are important decomposers used to make bread, wine, and cheese, but some are pathogenic. Fungal conditions frequently occur after the bacteria that normally live in or on the body are disturbed by antibiotic use or immunosuppression. For example, the fungus *Candida albicans* is normally found on human skin, especially around moist areas like the mouth, groin, and underarms, and sometimes an overgrowth of *Candida*, called candidiasis, occurs and presents as thrush (a white coating on the tongue), a vaginal yeast infection, or diaper rash. Other examples of fungal infections include histoplasmosis, which is spread through animal droppings, *Pneumocystis carinii* (PCP) pneumonia, which is common among individuals with advanced HIV infection, and dermatomycoses (fungal diseases of the skin) like ringworm and athlete's foot. Fungi thrive in moist, dark places, and are especially common in the tropics.

9.2.E Prions

Prions, or "proteinaceous infectious particles," appear to cause some types of very rare degenerative nervous system diseases called transmissible spongiform encephalopathies (TSEs). Proteins are the building blocks of cells, tissues, and organs. Normal proteins are chains of amino acids that are folded into complex shapes. Mutant prion proteins lose their shapes by unraveling and straightening out. A single mutant prion appears to be able to cause the normal proteins near it to also unravel. In "mad cow disease" (bovine spongiform encephalopathy, or BSE), the brains of cows become spongy as their brain proteins unravel. The equivalent disease in humans is called Creutzfeldt-Jakob Disease (CJD). Infections are thought to be acquired through the ingestion of brain and nervous tissue from infected animals. Although cooking food at sufficient temperatures will kill most bacteria and parasites, heat will not kill prions because the proteins are already denatured (unraveled).

No treatment is available, so prevention is essential. Keeping livestock healthy protects humans from the risk of acquiring prions from animal-based food products. Livestock can be protected by making sure that animal feeds do not include animal proteins that could be contaminated with nervous tissue.

9.3 EXPOSURE, INFECTION, AND DISEASE

The **natural history** of an infectious disease describes the usual timeline from exposure to a particular agent to infection to either recovery or death (**Figure 9–2**).

Not all exposures to an infectious agent cause an infection. Some individuals may be more vulnerable to infections when the ability of their immune systems to fight off infection is weakened by age, malnutrition, cancer treatments, immunosuppressive drugs, or existing infections with other pathogens. Other individuals may be protected from new infections by previous infections (and resulting immunity), by immunization, or by genetics. And some potentially infectious agents do not have genetic characteristics that allow the agent to easily infect people or easily make them sick. **Infectivity** is the capacity of an infectious agent to cause infection in a susceptible human (a person who does not already have immunity to the infection). Measles has a high infectivity rate because a high proportion of the susceptible individuals exposed to measles become infected. In contrast, leprosy has a low infectivity rate and does not easily spread to susceptible people who do not have prolonged contact with an infectious person.[2] Infectivity is sometimes measured by calculating the **secondary attack rate**, which is the average number of other people that one contagious person infects.

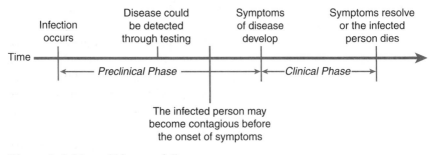

Figure 9–2 Natural history of disease.

An **infection** occurs when an infectious agent begins to reproduce inside a person. This usually causes an immunologic response specific to the agent, and that response can often be detected through laboratory testing. Many infections have a **latent phase** (also called an **incubation period**) that occurs immediately after infection. During this stage, the infectious agent multiplies in the host but the infected individual does not feel sick, even if he or she is contagious and able to spread the infection to others. Laboratory tests that detect early-stage infection can be critical for halting the spread of infection during outbreaks and for treating patients before they develop severe disease.

Disease occurs when an infected person develops symptoms or illness. Not all infections cause disease. For example, most children who are infected with the hepatitis A virus remain asymptomatic (do not show disease) even though they develop lifelong immunity to the disease following their infection,[3] and nearly one-third of the world's population has been infected with tuberculosis (TB), but only about 10% of those infected will develop symptoms of TB disease in their lifetimes.[4] **Pathogenicity** is the capacity of an infectious agent to cause disease in an infected human, and it is measured by the proportion of individuals with laboratory-confirmed infection who become ill.

In those who do develop symptomatic disease, there are three possible outcomes: death, recovery with immunity, or recovery without immunity (**Figure 9–3**). For nearly all infections, the recovery rate is extremely high. The body's immune system will fight off most infections even if they are left untreated, and once symptoms begin, most people with severe illnesses will seek medical care and be treated for the infection if an effective therapy is available. However, in some cases an infection will be fatal with or without medical intervention. **Virulence** is the ability of an infectious agent to

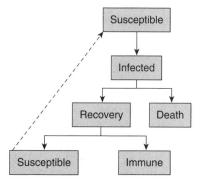

Figure 9–3 Outcomes for an infected individual.

cause severe disease or death in a host, and it is measured by the proportion of severe or fatal cases among all people who have the disease. A virulent infection will have a high **case fatality rate**. For example, rabies is an extremely virulent infection because no one who is bitten by a rabid animal survives without postbite vaccination treatment (called **post-exposure prophylaxis**, or PEP).

Some infections cause **acute** (short-term) disease, like influenza and the rhinoviruses that cause colds. Other infections cause **chronic** (long-term) disease, like HIV and *Helicobacter pylori*, a bacterial infection that can cause stomach ulcers. Chronic infections can increase susceptibility to other infections, and some chronic infections may also increase the risk of cancer. For example, hepatitis C virus increases the risk of liver cancer, chronic schistosomiasis (a helminth infection) increases the risk of bladder cancer, and HPV can cause cervical cancer.

Many infections spark an immune process that forms "memory" antibodies in the blood that allow the body to quickly destroy any new pathogens of the same type that invade the body in the future. These types of infections are good candidates for vaccine development. Recovery from other infections may provide no protective immunity against future infections. These types of infections are not likely to be controlled through immunization, so prevention must focus on avoidance of exposure.

9.4 INFECTIOUS DISEASE TRANSMISSION

An infectious agent can be transmitted to a susceptible human through several different **modes of transmission**.

Direct transmission, also called person-to-person transmission, occurs when a susceptible person touches an infectious person's blood or other body fluids and then touches his or her mouth, eyes, nose, or another **portal of entry**. (Sometimes direct transmission also occurs when a susceptible person is close enough to a sick person to breathe in the droplets expelled when a sick person coughs, sneezes, or breathes, or to have those droplets land on their skin or eyes.) Direct transmission can also occur through sexual contact. Frequent handwashing and use of personal protective equipment such as gloves and condoms can help prevent direct transmission.

Airborne transmission occurs when pathogens are aerosolized or suspended in the air and people breathe in that contaminated air. Influenza, colds, and TB are examples of airborne infectious diseases. To prevent a contagious person from spreading an airborne infection to susceptible people, it may be necessary to treat the patient in **isolation** by limiting his or her contact with others and by protecting other people from the air exhaled by the sick person. Facemasks can also help protect people from contracting airborne infections.

Vectorborne infections are spread by insect **vectors** like mosquitoes or ticks. Malaria, Lyme disease, and dengue fever are all transmitted through insect bites. Control of vectorborne diseases can be at least partially attained through the use of insecticides or other methods of reducing the insect population. Preventing insect bites reduces the risk of susceptible humans becoming infected, and reducing insect bites also lowers the likelihood of an infected human passing the infectious agent to susceptible insects.

Animals can play a role in the infection transmission process. Rodents are frequent carriers of infections such as plague and typhus fever, which are both spread by ticks that live on those rodents. Livestock may be carriers of infectious agents such as the ones that cause African sleeping sickness (which is spread by tsetse fly bites). In some cases, animals may directly transmit infectious agents to humans. For example, rabies is spread through the saliva of infected mammals, some infectious agents that cause diarrhea can be passed from livestock and pets to people, and most strains of influenza that affect humans originate in bird or mammal populations.

Many diarrheal infections are acquired through the ingestion of contaminated food or water. **Fecal–oral transmission** occurs when a person ingests products contaminated with fecal material from animals or humans. Cholera is a waterborne infection, and many infectious agents that cause diarrhea (such as *Salmonella* and *Shigella*) are spread through ingestion of fecally contaminated food. Indirect transmission can also occur as a result of contact with inanimate objects (called **fomites**), such as doorknobs, that serve as vehicles of transmission.

Some infections, such as HIV, have **vertical transmission**, also called **mother-to-child transmission (MTCT)**, because the agent can be passed from a mother to her fetus during pregnancy or delivery or to her baby through breastmilk.

To control infectious diseases in a population, several other aspects of transmission must be considered. The **reservoir** is the environmental home for an infectious agent. Some infections, like smallpox and measles, only occur in humans. Infectious diseases that usually occur only in humans are called **anthroponoses**. Some infectious agents, like the ones that cause West Nile virus, rabies, and influenza, can affect many types of animals. Infectious diseases that usually occur in animals and only occasionally infect humans are called **zoonoses**. Other infectious agents have an environmental reservoir and live in the soil (like hookworm) or water (like cholera). Controlling an infectious disease may require controlling animal populations (if that is possible), altering the environment to reduce the exposure of humans to pathogens, and educating individuals and communities about how to reduce their risk of infection.

The **cycle of infection** describes how an infectious agent cycles between different species. Measles and gonorrhea cycle only between humans, so the cycle of infection is human–human–human. Vectorborne infections like malaria have a human–insect–human cycle. Some infectious agents cycle between humans and the environment, such as cholera and hookworm. Zoonoses may have a vertebrate–vertebrate–vertebrate cycle, which on occasion can become a vertebrate–vertebrate–human cycle, as happens with rabies. Or a zoonotic disease may have an animal–insect–animal cycle that occasionally affects a human. Some infectious agents have much more complex cycles and undergo life stages in several different animal hosts and perhaps also in the environment. For example, schistosomiasis cycles from snails (which serve as an **intermediate host** for the *Schistosoma* parasite) into water into humans (which serve as the **definitive host** in which the parasites reach sexual maturity), then eggs are released from humans back into water and back into snails and the cycle begins again. Each host in the cycle of infection must be considered for inclusion in an infection control plan.

9.5 DIARRHEAL AND FOODBORNE DISEASES

Infectious diseases—illnesses caused by communicable pathogens—are often classified based on the primary symptoms they cause (such as diarrhea or respiratory disease), the mode of transmission (such as vectorborne or sexually transmitted), or by other key features of the infection or the resulting disease.

Most diarrheal infections and other forms of infectious gastroenteritis are spread by fecal–oral transmission (**Table 9–1**). For example, *Escherichia coli* bacteria are spread via fecal contamination of food and water, including swimming pools that are not properly maintained, and by person-to-person contact. Although many strains are not harmful, some are deadly, like *E. coli O157:H7*, which can cause bloody diarrhea and kidney failure (hemolytic uremic syndrome). Cholera, another bacterial infection, is also spread through contaminated water, and because the

Table 9–1 Examples of diarrheal and foodborne diseases.

Disease	Agent Name	Type of Agent
Amebiasis (amoebiasis)	*Entamoeba histolytica*	Protozoan (ameboid)
Balantidiasis (balatidiosis)	*Balantidium*	Protozoan (ciliated)
Bacillus cereus food intoxication	*Bacillus cereus*	Bacterial enterotoxin
Botulism	*Clostridium botulinum*	Bacterial toxin
Brucellosis	*Brucella abortus, Brucella melitensis*	Bacterium
Campylobacter enteritis	*Campylobacter jejuni*	Bacterium
Cholera	*Vibrio cholerae*	Bacterium
Clostridium perfringens food intoxication	*Clostridium perfringens*	Bacterial enterotoxin
Cryptosporidiosis	*Cryptosporidium*	Protozoan (sporozoan)
Cyclosporiasis	*Cylclospora cayetanensis*	Protozoan (sporozoan)
Escherichia coli	*Escherichia coli*	Bacterium
Giardiasis	*Giardia*	Protozoan (flagellate)
Helicobacter pylori	*Helicobacter pylori*	Bacterium
Hepatitis A	Hepatitis A virus	Virus (picornavirus)
Listeriosis	*Listeria monocytogenes*	Bacterium
Norovirus	Noroviruses	Virus (calicivirus)
Paratyphoid fever	*Salmonella* paratyphi	Bacterium
Rotavirus	Rotavirus	Virus (reovirus)
Salmonellosis	*Salmonella*	Bacterium
Shigellosis	*Shigella*	Bacterium
Staphylococcal food intoxication	*Staphylococcus aureus*	Bacterial enterotoxin
Typhoid fever	*Salmonella* typhi	Bacterium

Source: Information from Heymann DL, editor. *Control of communicable diseases manual*, 19th edition. Washington DC: American Public Health Association; 2008.

bacteria can live in harsh environments, like ocean water and sewage, and can survive for long periods of time, cholera outbreaks have occurred in many parts of the world in recent years. Cholera infection causes severe watery diarrhea, and death can occur if rehydration and electrolyte balance cannot be maintained through fluid replacement. Typhoid, paratyphoid, shigellosis, salmonellosis, and campylobacteriosis are also bacterial infectious diarrheal diseases spread through ingestion of fecally contaminated food and water or the transfer of fecal matter from the hand to the mouth.

Protozoan infections can also be spread through food and water that has been contaminated with animal feces. A 1993 outbreak of cryptosporidiosis in Wisconsin, in the United States, was caused by a failure of the water treatment system. The outbreak caused more than 100 deaths in the city of Milwaukee and made more than 400,000 people sick.[5] Amoebic dysentery and giardiasis cause hundreds of thousands of people around the world to become sick each year.

Viruses are even more common as a cause of diarrhea. For children, rotavirus is the most common cause of severe diarrhea.[6] Rotavirus is now vaccine-preventable, but the vaccine is not available in every part of the world. For adults, a variety of viruses, including noroviruses (often associated with cruise ship outbreaks), can cause outbreaks of gastroenteritis.

While most diarrheal infections are short-term ones, some can become chronic diseases. For example, brucellosis (also called undulant fever) can be transmitted to humans through unpasteurized dairy products, and if untreated the infection may cause chronic, cyclic fevers. Untreated *Helicobacter pylori* infection is associated with stomach ulcers.

Effective methods for the prevention of diarrheal diseases include safe food handling, frequent handwashing, consistent access to clean drinking water, and community-wide sanitation. These practices can also help prevent foodborne infections that do not cause diarrhea, such as listeriosis, which can be acquired from processed meats and other foods and can cause miscarriages, stillbirths, and preterm delivery if pregnant women contract the infection.

9.6 RESPIRATORY DISEASES

Upper respiratory infections like colds and lower respiratory infections like pneumonia are often caused by viruses (**Table 9–2**). Pneumonias caused by influenza viruses and other influenza-like illnesses (ILIs) are a

Table 9–2 Examples of infectious respiratory diseases.

Disease	Agent Name	Type of Agent
Aspergillosis	*Aspergillus*	Fungus
Blastomycosis	*Blastomyces dermatitidis*	Fungus
Coccidioidomycosis (Valley fever)	*Coccidioides immitis*	Fungus
Cryptococcosis	*Cryptococcus neoformans*	Fungus
Diphtheria	*Corynebacterium diphtheriae*	Bacterium
Group A strep	*Streptococcus pyogenes*	Bacterium
Hantavirus	Hantavirus	Virus (bunyavirus)
Hendra virus	Hendravirus	Virus (paramyxovirus)
Hib	*Haemophilus influenzae* type b	Bacterium
Histoplasmosis	*Histoplasma capsulatum*	Fungus
Influenza	Influenza virus	Virus (orthomyxovirus)
Klebsiella pneumonia	*Klebsiella pneumoniae*	Bacterium
Legionellosis (Legionnaires' disease, Pontiac fever)	*Legionellae*	Bacterium
Mycoplasma pneumonia	*Mycoplasma pneumoniae*	Bacterium
Nipah virus	Nipah virus	Virus (paramyxovirus)
Pertussis (whooping cough)	*Bordatella pertussis*	Bacterium
Pneumococcus	*Streptococcus pneumoniae*	Bacterium
Psittacosis	*Chlamydia psiattaci*	Bacterium
Rhinitis (common cold)	Rhinoviruses	Virus
Q fever	*Coxiella burnetii*	Bacterium
Tuberculosis	*Mycobacterium tuberculosis*	Bacterium

Source: Information from Heymann DL, editor. *Control of communicable diseases manual*, 19th edition. Washington DC: American Public Health Association; 2008.

particular global concern. Other viral pneumonias, such as those caused by hantavirus, can also spark outbreaks.

Bacterial respiratory diseases are also common. Pneumococcus and *Haemophilus influenzae* type B (usually shortened to "Hib") are both vaccine-preventable infections but continue to cause many child deaths around the world each year. Some respiratory infections can cause long-term damage. Strep throat, an illness caused by a type of Group A *Streptococcus*, is a common childhood infection that if left untreated can lead to complications such as scarlet fever or rheumatic fever, a condition that may cause permanent damage to the valves of the heart. Tuberculosis infections can cause chronic illness and require months or years of antibiotic treatment.

Fungal and parasitic causes of pneumonia are relatively uncommon compared to bacterial and viral respiratory infections, but they also occur.

Most respiratory infections are acquired through the air. Pertussis, spread via the inhalation of droplets suspended in the air, is a vaccine-preventable bacterial infection characterized by whooping sounds made when people with the disease inhale during severe coughing fits. Legionellosis, also called Legionnaires' disease (for severe disease) or Pontiac fever (for milder disease), is acquired through the inhalation of moistened water from air conditioners and hot tubs (spas). Psittacosis, also called parrot fever, is acquired when bird owners inhale the dried bird droppings of infected pets.

Prevention methods for respiratory infections include isolating infected persons, reducing exposure to smoke (which damages the respiratory tract and increases susceptibility to respiratory diseases), vaccinating members of vulnerable population groups, and encouraging frequent handwashing and the covering of the nose and mouth when coughing or sneezing.

9.7 VECTORBORNE DISEASES

A wide variety of insect vectors can transmit infectious agents to humans, including various types of mosquitos, flies, fleas, lice, and ticks (**Table 9–3**).

Several types of bacterial and rickettsial infections are spread by the bites of infected ticks and fleas, including Lyme disease, Rocky Mountain spotted fever, bartonellosis, and typhus. (Rickettsia are a special type of bacterium.) The "Black Death" of medieval Europe was a type of plague (a bacterial infection that still exists today), and it killed one-quarter to one-half of the population of affected cities. The usual symptoms of bubonic plague are severely swollen lymph nodes and pain, but some

Table 9–3 Examples of vectorborne (insect-spread) diseases.

Disease	Agent Name	Type of Agent	Vector
African sleeping sickness (African trypanosomiasis)	*Trypanosoma brucei*	Protozoan (flagellate)	Tsetse flies (*Glossina*)
Babesiosis	*Babesia*	Protozoan (sporozoan)	Ticks
Bartonellosis	*Bartonella bacilliformis*	Bacterium	Sand flies (*Lutzomyia*)
Chagas disease (American trypanosomiasis)	*Trypanosoma cruzi*	Protozoan (flagellate)	Kissing bugs (*Reduviidae*)
Chikungunya fever	Chikungunya virus	Virus (togavirus)	Mosquitoes
Crimean-Congo hemorrhagic fever	Crimean-Congo hemorrhagic fever virus	Virus (bunyavirus)	Ticks
Dengue fever	Dengue virus	Virus (flavivirus)	Mosquitoes
Ehrlichiosis	*Ehrlichia*	Bacterium	Ticks
Japanese encephalitis	Japanese encephalitis virus	Virus (flavivirus)	Mosquitoes (*Culex*)
Leishmaniasis (Kala azar)	*Leishmania*	Protozoan (flagellate)	Sandflies
Loiasis (African eyeworm)	*Loa loa*	Helminth (filarial nematode)	Deer flies (*Chrysops*)
Lyme disease	*Borrelia burgdorferi*	Bacterium	Ticks (*Ixodes*)
Lymphatic filariasis	*Wuchereria bancrofti, Brugia malayi, Brugia timori*	Helminth (filarial nematode)	Mosquitoes
Malaria	*Plasmodium*	Protozoan (sporozoan)	Mosquitoes (*Anopheles*)
Plague	*Yersinia pestis*	Bacterium	Fleas
Rift Valley fever	Rift Valley fever virus	Virus (bunyavirus)	Mosquitoes

(Continues)

Table 9–3 *(Continued)*

Disease	Agent Name	Type of Agent	Vector
River blindness (onchocerciasis)	*Onchocerca volvulus*	Helminth (filarial nematode)	Blackflies (*Simulium*)
Rocky Mountain spotted fever	*Rickettsia rickettsii*	Bacterium (rickettsia)	Ticks
Tularemia	*Francisella tularensis*	Bacterium	Ticks and others
Typhus fever	*Rickettsia prowazekii*	Bacterium (rickettsia)	Fleas, lice, and mites
Viral encephalitis	Eastern equine encephalitis, Western equine encephalitis, Venezuelan equine encephalitis, and others	Virus (togavirus)	Mosquitoes
West Nile virus	West Nile virus	Virus (flavivirus)	Mosquitoes (*Culex*)
Yellow fever	Yellow fever virus	Virus (flavivirus)	Mosquitoes (*Aedes*)

Source: Information from Heymann DL, editor. *Control of communicable diseases manual*, 19th edition. Washington DC: American Public Health Association; 2008.

cases develop a more severe pneumonic plague. Plague is transmitted to humans by a rodent flea.

Viruses spread by **arthropods** such as insects and arachnids (spiders, ticks, mites) are called **arboviruses** (short for arthropod-borne viruses). Dengue fever is spread by the bites of infected *Aedes* mosquitoes that thrive in urban areas. West Nile virus is spread by *Culex* mosquitoes, and typically affects animals but may also cause disease in humans. Yellow fever, Japanese encephalitis, Rift Valley fever, and Venezuelan equine encephalitis are other examples of arboviral diseases.

Vectorborne protozoan infections (including the *Plasmodium* parasite that causes malaria, which is transmitted by the bite of infected *Anopheles* mosquitoes) are of particular global health interest. Three examples of these protozoan infections highlight the diversity of these infectious diseases and the vectors that spread them.

African sleeping sickness (trypanosomiasis) is spread by the bite of infected tsetse flies and can cause chronic fevers and headaches that lead to paralysis and death. The infection primarily affects livestock, but outbreaks among humans can occur. Without early treatment, infection with African trypanosomiasis is fatal.[7]

Chagas disease, also called American sleeping sickness (and also caused by a trypanosome), is spread by "kissing bugs" that live in the cracks of low-quality houses in South America and Central America. The insects emerge at night to take bloodmeals from sleeping people. The feces of the insects contain parasites that can enter the bloodstream through the wound left after the bloodmeal. Within a few days, a sore may develop at the site of the bite, which is often near the eye. About one-third of people who are infected develop a chronic infection that can cause severe damage to the heart and digestive tract.[8]

Leishmaniasis is spread by female phlebotomine sandflies, which need blood from a human or other mammal in order to develop their eggs. There are several forms of leishmaniasis. The cutaneous form produces skin lesions and can lead to permanent disfigurement. The mucosal form causes lesions on the mucous membranes of the nose, mouth, and throat. The visceral form, also known as kala azar, causes chronic fevers, weight loss, anemia, and swelling of the spleen and liver, leading to death within a few years if left untreated.[9]

Helminths can also be transmitted by insect bites. Two examples of vectorborne worm infections are onchocerciasis and lymphatic filariasis.[10] Onchocerciasis, also known as river blindness, is caused by a filarial (threadlike) parasite spread by the bite of infected black flies in parts of Africa and the Americas. Adult worms form nodules under the skin and release new immature worms (microfilariae) into surrounding tissues. If the nodules form near the eyes and the infection is not treated, the result can be blindness. Lymphatic filariasis (LF), also caused by a filarial infection, is transmitted by several different mosquito species. Extreme swelling of body parts (often an arm, leg, or scrotum) can occur when worms block the flow of lymph (tissue fluid) out of body tissues. LF can cause a condition called elephantiasis when a limb swells and develops a coarse texture similar to that of an elephant's leg. More than 100 million people worldwide are infected with the worms that cause LF.[11]

Prevention of vectorborne infections includes minimizing insect bites through the use of barriers (such as bednets and protective clothing) and chemical repellents, using insecticides to reduce insect populations, and modifying the environment to limit insect breeding grounds (such as by draining swamps or by removing old tires and other items that can house pools of standing water). Control of animal populations and waste management that keeps rodents and other mammals away from humans can also help to control the spread of infections that are transmitted by insects that live on mammals.

9.8 SEXUALLY TRANSMITTED INFECTIONS (STIS)

Sexually transmitted infections (STIs) are spread by intimate contact (Table 9–4).

Bacterial STIs can be treated with antibiotics if an infected person knows that he or she has been infected, but many infections remain undiagnosed and untreated, and they can cause chronic health problems. Gonorrhea and chlamydia are both often asymptomatic (causing no symptoms) but if untreated they can cause pelvic inflammatory disease (PID), which can lead to pain and to infertility in women. Syphilis can be treated in the early stages when there is a chancre or rash, but if left untreated it may cause weakened arterial walls and nervous system impairment.

Table 9–4 Examples of sexually transmitted infections.

Disease	Agent Name	Type of Agent
Chlamydia	Chlamydia trachomatis	Bacterium
Gonorrhea	Neisseria gonorrhoeae	Bacterium
Hepatitis B	Hepatitis B virus	Virus (hepadnavirus)
Herpes	Herpes simplex virus	Virus (herpesvirus)
HIV	Human immunodeficiency virus	Virus (retrovirus)
Phthiriasis	Phthirus pubis	Crab lice
Syphilis	Treponema pallidum	Bacterium
Trichomoniasis	Trichomonas vaginalis	Protozoan (flagellate)
Warts	Human papillomavirus (HPV)	Virus (papillomavirus)

Source: Information from Heymann DL, editor. Control of communicable diseases manual, 19th edition. Washington DC: American Public Health Association; 2008.

Several STIs are caused by viruses, including HIV, herpes, hepatitis B virus (HBV), and HPV, which causes genital warts and increases the risk of cervical cancer. Vaccines for HBV (which is also spread through vertical transmission and contact with blood) and HPV are now available in some countries, but no successful vaccine has been developed for HIV or herpes. No cure for these infections has been discovered, so once a person is infected he or she will always have the infection. Some drugs, like interferon, can help suppress some viral infections, but drugs will not cure viral infections.

A few parasites, such as the *Trichomonas* protozoan and pubic lice, are also transmitted through sexual contact.

STIs can be prevented by abstinence from sexual activity, the use of barriers such as condoms that limit direct contact with body fluids (although some infections may occur even with condom use), and treatment of infected individuals so that they do not transmit the infection to sexual partners.

9.9 NEGLECTED TROPICAL DISEASES (NTDS)

Neglected tropical diseases (NTDs) are infectious diseases that primarily affect the poorest regions of the world (many of which are located in the tropics) and have not been a priority for funding agencies, pharmaceutical companies, or global policymakers.[12] Several of the diseases mentioned in previous sections are considered to be NTDs, including African trypanosomiasis, Chagas disease, leishmaniasis, lymphatic filariasis, and onchocerciasis (river blindness). Other NTDs that are now receiving special attention from researchers and public health partnerships include dracunculiasis (Guinea worm) and schistosomiasis, along with several very common intestinal worm infections (including ascariasis, hookworm, and trichuriasis).

Guinea worm disease is an extremely painful condition. People become infected by drinking water that contains water fleas infected with Guinea worm larva. A mature Guinea worm may grow inside the body to up to 3 feet in length, and once the worm is mature it may crawl down the inside of an infected person's leg and emerge from a painful blister near the foot. The worm can also emerge from a wrist or another body part. It can take weeks for the worm to be extracted from the body, and a person with an emerging Guinea worm is usually unable to work during this time because of pain. The worm cannot simply be pulled out of the body, because if it breaks and part of the worm is left inside the body a serious infection can result. Instead, the worm is often tied to a stick, which is used to coil the Guinea worm as it slowly makes its way out of the human's body, at a rate of an inch or so per day. Many people with an emerging worm only feel relief from pain by putting their feet in cool water, but this causes the worm to release eggs and can contaminate drinking water supplies. There is no drug for dracunculiasis, but the prevalence of the disease is decreasing as use of water filters becomes more common. Found primarily in western and central Africa, the ultimate goal is to eradicate Guinea worm disease.[13]

Schistosomiasis, sometimes called bilharziasis, is a type of flatworm that can enter the body through the skin and can then migrate to the bladder or intestines, where the worms can cause scarring. There are several different kinds of schistosomiasis that can be found in Africa, the Middle East, Latin America, Asia, and the Pacific. In each species, the worms infect both snails and humans, and the parasite cycles between these two species. Eggs released into water from the urine or feces of infected people can infect snails living in the water. After the worms undergo several developmental stages in snail hosts, the mature larvae are released into water and seek entry into the skin of humans who are wading in the water while fishing, washing clothes, bathing, or swimming. An effective drug called praziquantel cures the infection, but people who are treated for schistosomiasis are immediately susceptible to new infection when they come into contact with contaminated water. Molluscicides are sometimes used to kill the snails that live in infested waters, but snails will eventually move back into the waters, and new snail habitats are created when dams and irrigation systems are built. The prevalence of schistosomiasis increased drastically when the Aswan Dam was built on the Nile River in Egypt, when dams were built on the Senegal and Volta Rivers and other locations in West Africa, and when small dams and irrigation projects have been introduced into villages in many parts of the world.[14] The complex lifecycle of the worm makes control of schistosomiasis a challenge.[15]

Ascariasis (roundworm), hookworm, and trichuriasis (whipworm) are the three most common **soil-transmitted helminth (STH)** infections, and nearly 1 billion people worldwide have at least one of these parasites living in their bodies (**Figure 9–4**).[16,17] All STHs are contracted via contact with soil mixed with feces that contain worm eggs. Ascariasis is the most common helminth infection in the world and occurs when a person ingests eggs from *Ascaris lumbricoides*. The larvae hatch in the small intestine, penetrate the intestinal wall, and travel through the blood to the lungs, where they may be coughed up and swallowed and then develop in the intestines into mature, egg-producing worms. Adult worms in the intestine may grow to more than

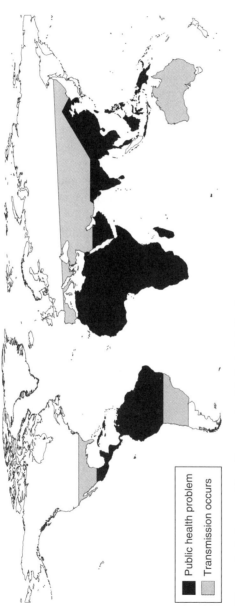

Figure 9–4 Areas with soil-transmitted helminth infections.

Source: Data from *Geographical distribution and useful facts and stats.* Geneva: WHO Partners for Parasite Control.

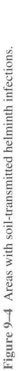

a foot in length, and eggs passed in the stool may lead to infection in others if open defecation is practiced. Hookworm is most often acquired by walking barefoot through contaminated soil because the larvae can penetrate human skin. After passing through the bloodstream, heart, and lungs, the adult worms migrate to the gut and latch on to the intestinal wall, causing bleeding and increasing the risk of anemia, especially in children. When the eggs that cause trichuriasis are swallowed, they mature in the colon. Trichuriasis can cause digestive system symptoms. Deworming medications (such as albendazole and mebendazole) are available for all three of these infections, but re-infection can occur quickly when eggs from the worms remain in the local environment. Mass drug administration, in which whole communities routinely receive antihelmthic drugs once or twice a year, is the primary current approach to STH prevention and control.[18]

People can become hosts to other types of roundworms and also pinworms, flatworms (which include blood, liver, lung, and intestinal flukes), tapeworms (which can be found in beef, pork, and fish), and other kinds of worms (Table 9–5). Worms contracted from contaminated soil, water, food, or feces may take up residence in the intestine, liver, lungs, blood, or other body parts, including, sometimes, the brain. Intestinal worms increase the risk of malnutrition because nutrients from food go to the worms instead of the human host.

Three bacterial NTDs are also receiving new attention: leprosy, trachoma, and Buruli ulcer (*Mycobacterium ulcerans* infection). Leprosy, more formally called Hansen's disease, used to be a relatively common, disfiguring disease, and people who contracted it were often ostracized

Table 9–5 Examples of helminth diseases.

Disease	Agent Name	Type of Helminth	Transmission
Angiostrongyliasis	*Parastrongylus*	Nematode	Ingestion of undercooked mollusks
Ascariasis	*Ascaris lumbricoides*	Nematode: roundworm	Ingestion of soil or food contaminated with feces
Clonorchiasis	*Clonorchis sinensis*	Trematode: liver fluke	Ingestion of undercooked freshwater fish
Diphyllobothriasis	*Diphyllobothrium*	Trematode: tapeworm	Ingestion of undercooked freshwater fish

(Continues)

Table 9–5 *(Continued)*

Echinococcosis	*Echinococcus granulosus*	Trematode: tapeworm	Contact with dogs
Enterobiasis	*Enterobius vermicularis*	Nematode: pinworm	Ingestion of food contaminated with feces
Fascioliasis	*Fasciola*	Trematode: liver fluke	Ingestion of undercooked aquatic plants
Fasciolopsiasis	*Fasciolopsis buski*	Trematode: liver fluke	Ingestion of undercooked aquatic plants
Guinea worm disease (dracunculiasis)	*Dracunculus medinensis*	Nematode: Guinea worm	Ingestion of infected water fleas
Hookworm	*Ancylostoma, Necator americanus*	Nematode: hookworm	Skin contact with contaminated soil
Hymenolepiasis	*Hymenolepsis nana*	Trematode: tapeworm	Ingestion of food contaminated with feces
Paragonimiasis	*Paragonimus*	Trematode: lung fluke	Ingestion of undercooked freshwater crabs
Schistosomiasis (bilharziasis)	*Schistosoma*	Trematode: blood fluke	Contact with bodies of water that are home to infected snails
Strongyloidiasis	*Strongyloides*	Nematode: threadworm	Skin contact with contaminated soil
Taeniasis (cysticercosis)	*Taenia solium, Taenia saginata*	Trematode: tapeworm	Ingestion of undercooked pork, beef, or other meat
Toxocariasis	*Toxocara*	Nematode: round worm	Ingestion of soil or food contaminated with feces
Trichinosis (trichinellosis)	*Trichinella spiralis*	Nematode: threadworm	Ingestion of undercooked pork or other meat
Trichuriasis	*Trichuris trichiura*	Nematode: whipworm	Ingestion of soil contaminated with feces

Source: Information from Heymann DL, editor. *Control of communicable diseases manual*, 19th edition. Washington DC: American Public Health Association; 2008.

by their communities, but it is now able to be controlled with antibiotic treatment.[19] Trachoma blindness, caused by poor facial hygiene, remains the leading infectious cause of blindness in the world, but the number of new cases each year has been decreasing with improved access to water for washing.[20] *Mycobacterium ulcerans* causes deep ulcers, and the means of transmission remains poorly understood.[21]

9.10 OTHER INFECTIOUS DISEASES

A wide range of infections not listed in the previous tables also cause diseases of global concern (**Table 9–6**). These include various causes of encephalitis and meningitis, hemorrhagic fevers, skin lesions, and other diseases.

9.11 INFECTION CONTROL AND PREVENTION

Individuals, communities, public health organizations, and governmental agencies all have a role to play in the control and prevention of infectious diseases. Individuals contribute to reducing the burden of infectious disease by engaging in healthy behaviors such as washing hands frequently and staying home from work or school when sick. Communities play key roles in environmental health, making sure that water supplies are kept clean and that mosquito populations are controlled. At the national and international levels, scientists, policymakers, and others work together to create and disseminate technologies such as new vaccines and to track and address emerging infectious disease problems.

9.11.A Behavior Change

The **Health Belief Model** proposes that the decision of an individual to engage in a healthier behavior is dependent on the person's perceptions about his or her susceptibility to a disease, the severity of the disease, the ability of the behavior to effectively prevent the disease, the barriers to implementing a change, and the cost–benefit ratio for taking action.[22] Health education is essential for helping individuals to make better assessments about their risk of infection and disease and about the benefits of behavior change. Health behaviorists and educators often

Table 9–6 Examples of other infectious and parasitic diseases.

Disease	Agent Name	Type of Agent	Key Feature
Acanthamebiasis	*Acanthamoeba*	Protozoan	Can cause encephalitis
Anthrax	*Bacillus anthracis*	Bacterium	Spread by spores
Buruli ulcer	*Mycobacterium ulcerans*	Bacterium	Causes severe skin lesions
Candidiasis	*Candida albicans*	Fungus	Causes thrush, vaginal yeast infections, and skin infections
Chickenpox / Shingles	Varicella-zoster virus (VZV)	Virus (herpesvirus)	Causes skin lesions
Cytomegalovirus	Cytomegalovirus (CMV)	Virus (herpesvirus)	Maternal infections can harm fetuses
Dermatophytosis (tinea, (dermatomycosis)	Several	Fungus	Causes ringworm and athlete's foot
Ebola-Marburg hemorrhagic fevers	Ebola virus, Marburg virus	Virus (filovirus)	Cause hemorrhagic fevers
Hansen's disease (Leprosy)	*Mycobacterium leprae*	Bacterium	Causes skin lesions and nerve damage
Hepatitis C	Hepatitis C virus	Virus (flavivirus)	Causes liver damage
Lassa fever	Lassa virus	Virus (arenavirus)	Can cause hemorrhagic fever
Leptospirosis	*Leptospira*	Bacterium	Can cause organ failure and hemorrhage
Measles	Measles virus	Virus (paramyxovirus)	Rash and risk of severe complications
Meningococcal infection	*Neisseria meningitides*	Bacterium	Causes meningitis

(Continues)

Table 9–6 *(Continued)*

Disease	Agent Name	Type of Agent	Key Feature
Mononucleosis	Epstein-Barr virus	Virus (herpesvirus)	Causes chronic fatigue
Mumps	Mumps virus	Virus (paramyxovirus)	Causes swelling of the salivary glands
Naegleriasis	*Naegleria fowleri*	Protozoan	Can cause encephalitis
Pediculosis	*Pediculus*	Lice	Head and body lice
Polio (poliomyelitis)	Poliovirus	Virus (picornavirus)	Can cause paralysis
Rabies	Rabies virus	Virus (rhabdovirus)	Causes fatal encephalitis
Rubella (German measles)	Rubella virus	Virus (togavirus)	Maternal infections can harm fetuses
Scabies	*Sarcoptes scabiei*	Mite	Causes skin lesions
Staph infections	*Staphylococcus aureus*	Bacterium	Usually cause skin lesions, but can cause severe disease
Tetanus	*Clostridium tetani*	Bacterium	Spread by spores; causes painful muscle contractions
Toxoplasmosis	*Toxoplasma gondii*	Protozoan (sporozoan)	Maternal infections can harm fetuses
Trachoma	*Chlamydia trachomatis*	Bacterium	Can cause blindness
Transmissible spongiform encephalopathies (Creutzfeldt-Jakob disease, kuru)	—	Prion protein	Cause degenerative brain damage
Viral meningitis	Several types of viruses	Virus	Causes brain inflammation

Source: Information from Heymann DL, editor. *Control of communicable diseases manual*, 19th edition. Washington DC: American Public Health Association; 2008.

refer to a triad of *k*nowledge, *a*ttitudes (or beliefs), and *p*ractices (or behaviors), which is sometimes shortened to **KAP**. Once individuals understand why a behavior is healthy and believe that it is worth the effort to make a change, it is easier for them to choose to engage in healthier behaviors.

There are hundreds of relatively simple healthy behaviors that reduce the risk of an individual contracting an infectious disease, including washing hands often, following safe food handling and storage guidelines, receiving an annual influenza vaccine, wearing protective clothing when walking in wooded areas (to prevent insect bites), using a condom when engaging in sexual activity, avoiding unclean needles for injections, and wearing shoes when walking outside. There is an equally long list of the actions individuals can take to avoid passing an infection on to others, including avoiding open defecation, covering coughs and sneezes, sleeping under a bednet when sick with a vectorborne infection, and completing full courses of prescribed antibiotics.

However, the ability to practice these healthy behaviors is not merely a function of knowledge and attitudes. Access to the necessary tools and resources is also essential. Teenagers who want to practice safer sex will not be able to do so if they cannot acquire condoms. Employees with influenza who want to stay home so they do not risk making co-workers sick may not have that option if there is no sick leave policy that protects them from losing their jobs when they miss a day of work. Thus, community organizations and governments that help to increase access to health resources and that create policies to facilitate healthier behaviors are also essential to the success of behavior change campaigns.

9.11.B Environmental Control

Local environmental control activities can help reduce the incidence rate for a variety of infectious diseases. For example, community prevention efforts for dengue fever focus on eliminating the standing water where the *Aedes* mosquitoes that transmit the four serotypes of the virus breed.[23] (No successful vaccine exists yet, as it is very difficult to develop a vaccine that is effective against all four serotypes.) Any small body of standing water, such as water that collects in old cans and discarded tires, can become a breeding ground. A single family that does not clean up its yard can put a whole neighborhood at risk, so all households in a community must be involved in dengue prevention projects.

Communities can also reduce infection transmission by increasing drinking water quality and the amount of water available to each person, ensuring access to sanitation facilities, promoting proper waste management, implementing policies that reduce air pollution, reducing mosquito populations through water drainage and insecticides, and controlling rodent and snail populations. Additionally, local and national governments can implement food safety regulations, enforce zoning laws that restrict the number of individuals who can share a dwelling unit, require pet vaccination, and take other steps to minimize the infectious disease risks in the natural and built environments.

9.11.C Vaccination

Immunization programs can be a key tool for preventing and containing epidemics of vaccine-preventable diseases. Immunizations are usually developed by partnerships of scientists, clinicians, public health professionals, and others who represent for-profit pharmaceutical companies, nonprofit health organizations, and governments. These teams work together to select target diseases, to create and test new vaccines, to identify and educate the populations that would most benefit from the vaccine, and to manufacture and deliver the vaccines to those populations.

A vaccine is usually made from either a weakened (attenuated) version of the infectious agent or from an inactive virus or killed bacterium. The vaccine prompts the body's immune system to create special "memory cells" specific to the surface proteins contained in the vaccine. When a vaccinated person is later exposed to that same infectious agent in a live or active form, the body's immune system is able to quickly identify the agent and disable it before it has a chance to multiply. Vaccination, like a "real" infection, creates **active immunity** because the body has a lasting memory of the infection. (**Passive immunity** is acquired through breastmilk or immunoglobulin shots and lasts only a few months.)

When individuals receive a vaccination, they are not just protecting themselves from disease, they are also protecting the people around them. Reducing the proportion of a population that is susceptible to an infection protects the whole population (including those who are unable to receive vaccines, perhaps because of an allergy to a vaccine component or because of another medical condition). Suppose that during an outbreak each infected person exposes about 10 other people to the infection. In a completely susceptible population, all 10 of the exposed people might become infected, and each of those 10 people could spread the infection to many others. But if 80% of the members of the population have been vaccinated, only two of the initial 10 contacts are likely to result in infection, and those two newly infected people will not be able to spread the infection to many others. **Herd immunity** helps contain epidemics.

9.11.D Drug Therapy

Antibacterial and antiparasitic medications that cure infections are a central part of many infectious disease control programs. (Antiviral drugs that suppress viral infections, but do not cure them, can also be helpful for disease control.) Besides being healthier themselves, individuals who receive drug therapy have a reduced risk of spreading infection to others. At the population level, **mass drug administration (MDA)**, the routine distribution of antibiotics or antiparasitics to populations with high a prevalence of treatable infections, is often used to deworm schoolchildren as part of treatment and control programs for intestinal worms and schistosomiasis. MDA is also part of onchocerciasis (river blindness) control programs. The main limitation of MDA for these helminth control programs is that the children and other medication recipients are almost immediately susceptible to reinfection. To be effective, MDA must be accompanied by health education and environmental hygiene programs.

A second concern of drug therapy more generally is drug resistance, which is now seen for a variety of infectious agents, including methicillin-resistant *Staphylococcus aureus* (MRSA), which often causes skin infections, multidrug-resistant tuberculosis (MDR-TB), and drug-resistant gonorrhea. Bacteria (and some other types of infectious agents) are usually susceptible to certain types of antimicrobials, and will be killed when they are exposed to correct doses of the right classes of these medications. But a growing number of these agents have developed resistance to at least some of the types of antibiotics that were once effective against them.[24] Resistance develops because of changes in the pathogen's genes. One of the main causes of the development of **antimicrobial resistance** seems to be the misuse of antibiotics. If someone has a mild bacterial infection, such as bronchitis or a mild ear infection, and takes antibiotics for only a few days rather than finishing the entire prescription, or if that person skips a few doses, that person will have killed off the susceptible, weaker bacteria, but the hardier bacteria will survive. This is a process that biologists call **selection**. The remaining bacteria may have developed resistance to the misused drug, which means that it will be harder for that person to fight off the infection with common antibiotics. Worse yet, that person could also spread this hardier strain to other people, for whom the common first-line antibiotics will not work at all. Another misuse of antibiotics is taking the drugs for viral infections like the common cold. The individual taking the drugs is not being helped by the antibiotic, and instead is killing off the body's helpful bacteria and allowing potentially harmful bacteria that are already in the body to proliferate. These stronger bacteria may develop drug resistance, necessitating that the infected person take yet another antibiotic.

9.11.E Surveillance

Surveillance systems track infectious disease reports from hospitals and other information sources to look for patterns and possible outbreaks or **clusters** of disease, which occur when there is an unusually high incidence of disease in a particular place (spatial clustering) or time (temporal clustering). Surveillance systems, which are usually run by governments, use continuous monitoring in a population so that changes can be detected quickly and appropriate control measures can be implemented.

It is not necessary to track an entire population. Usually several representative clinics or communities will be selected to participate in **sentinel surveillance**, which is when information from continuous monitoring at several selected "sentinel" sites is used to alert public health officials to possible changes in community health status. If an outbreak is suspected, a more rigorous investigation involving additional sites can be conducted. **Passive surveillance** that collects reports of notifiable disease diagnoses from medical laboratories and **active surveillance** in which public health officials contact healthcare providers to ask about whether they are seeing particular types of disease are other means of collecting surveillance data.

The health statistics collected as part of surveillance allow communities, states and provinces, and nations to know what diseases are common in their populations and to recognize when an unusual health situation has developed. Without baseline data about incidence and prevalence, it is impossible to know if unusual numbers of cases are being diagnosed. An **endemic** disease is always present in a population. An **epidemic** (or **outbreak**) occurs when a disease is occurring more often than usual and there are more than a few sporadic occurrences of disease. A **pandemic** is a worldwide epidemic, like some influenza epidemics.

9.11.F Elimination and Eradication

Infection **control** measures like behavior change, environmental and vector control, vaccination, and mass drug administration can be used to limit the incidence of infection in a local area. When control measures remove all risk of new infection in a region, **elimination** of the infection from that area has been achieved.

When aiming for elimination, it may be necessary during outbreaks to track down and **quarantine** (limit the movement of) ill individuals and all of their primary contacts and secondary contacts (people contacted by primary contacts) in order to contain an outbreak. This was done in China during the 2003 SARS outbreak, and it helped to stop the spread of the virus.[25]

For some infections, it is possible, at least in theory, to completely eradicate the infectious agent. **Eradication** is achieved when there is no risk of infection or disease anywhere in the world even in the absence of immunization or any other control measures. To be a candidate for eradication, the infectious agent must usually meet several criteria. There must be an intervention, such as a vaccine, that effectively interrupts the chain of transmission. If a vaccine is used as part of the eradication strategy, the vaccine should confer lifelong or long-term immunity to the infection. The disease must be highly pathogenic so that people who contract the disease have obvious symptoms and can be easily tracked. Additionally, eradication is more likely when the infection only occurs in humans. If both humans and animals serve as hosts for the infection, it may be impossible to monitor and contain all human and animal cases.

Not all infections are appropriate candidates for eradication. Eradication campaigns require lots of staff and structural support for intense weeks or months of mass immunization and for many years of follow-up surveillance. Because it takes a great deal of time, money, and organizational sophistication to achieve eradication, only diseases that are severe and for which there is a high likelihood of a successful campaign are targeted for eradication. A global eradication campaign cannot begin unless there is widespread political commitment to achieving success and a support system to ensure completion.[26]

The only infectious disease eradicated thus far is smallpox. A massive worldwide immunization campaign that included re-vaccination in areas where any new case of smallpox occurred led to the successful eradication of the disease in 1979. (Because several laboratories kept samples of smallpox virus, the disease is not considered to be extinct. Eradication is complete when an infectious agent is no longer found in nature. **Extinction** is complete when an agent no longer exists in nature or in the laboratory.)

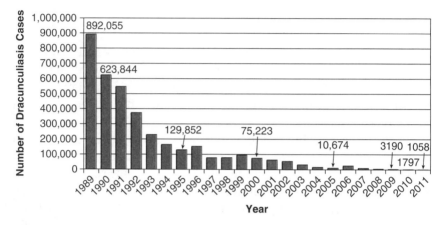

Figure 9–5 Worldwide dracunculiasis (Guinea worm) incidence.

Data from Monthly report on dracunculiasis cases, January–December 2010. *Wkly Epidemiol Rec.* 2011;86:91–92; and Dracunculiasis eradication: global surveillance summary, 2006. *Wkly Epidemiol Rec.* 2007;82:133–140; and Dracunculiasis eradication: global surveillance summary, 2005. *Wkly Epidemiol Rec.* 2006;81:173–182; and *Guinea-worm disease: countdown to eradication.* Geneva: WHO; 2012.

Polio is scheduled for eradication soon, if the global immunization plan is continued until no cases of polio exist.[27] Dracunculiasis (Guinea worm disease) is also nearing eradication. Although there is no vaccine for dracunculiasis, education programs that emphasize filtering drinking water to remove the water fleas that carry the worm larvae and that teach infected people to stay out of water so they do not pass worm eggs to susceptible water fleas have contributed to a rapid decline in the number of cases reported each year. Prior to the start of the global eradication program there were estimated to be more than one million new cases each year, but by 2005 there were only about 10,000 cases annually, and by 2010 there were fewer than 2000 cases worldwide (**Figure 9–5**).[28–31] Other infectious diseases are being considered for future eradication efforts.

9.12 DISCUSSION QUESTIONS

1. The most common infections in high-income countries tend to be caused by bacteria and viruses. Are you surprised by how many diseases world-wide are caused by parasites?

2. Epidemiologists use an "agent-host-environment" triad (sometimes adding "vector" as a fourth category) to explore the factors that contribute

to infectious disease in communities. Describe the "AHE" factors that are associated with a selected diarrheal infection, a respiratory infection, a vectorborne infection, and an STI. How do the AHE factors differ for the four diseases you selected? What do the AHEs indicate about disease control and prevention strategies?

3. The tables in the chapter classify bacteria, viruses, and other agents by categories like "causes diarrhea" and "vaccine-preventable." What are some other ways that the infectious agents listed in these tables could have been arranged?

4. Of all the infectious diseases mentioned in this chapter, which one would you most like to eradicate? Why?

5. What are some specific behavioral changes you can make and actions you can take that will reduce your risk of acquiring infections?

6. What are some infectious diseases that are *endemic* in your community? What are some *epidemics* that have occurred recently?

7. What infectious diseases meet the criteria for eradication and would be good candidates for a global eradication campaign?

REFERENCES

1. *The global burden of disease: 2004 update*. Geneva: WHO; 2008.
2. Heymann DL, editor. *Control of communicable diseases manual*, 19th edition. Washington DC: American Public Health Association; 2008.
3. Jacobsen KH, Koopman JS. Declining hepatitis A seroprevalence: a global review and analysis. *Epidemiol Infect.* 2004;133:1005–1022.
4. Young DB, Perkins MD, Duncan K, Barry CE III. Confronting the scientific obstacles to global control of tuberculosis. *J Clin Invest.* 2008;118:1255–1265.
5. Mac Kenzie WR, Hoxie NJ, Proctor ME, et al. A massive outbreak in Milwaukee of *Cryptosporidium* infection transmitted through the public water supply. *N Engl J Med.* 1994;331:161–167.
6. Parashar UD, Burton A, Lanata C, et al. Global mortality associated with rotavirus disease among children in 2004. *J Infect Dis.* 2009;200(suppl 1):S9–S15.
7. Brun B, Blum J, Chappuis F, Burri C. Human African trypanosomiasis. *Lancet.* 2010;375:148–159.
8. Rassi A Jr, Rassi A, Marin-Neto JA. Chagas disease. *Lancet.* 2010;375:1388–1402.
9. Bern C, Maguire JH, Alvar J. Complexities of assessing the disease burden attributable to leishmaniasis. *PLoS Negl Trop Dis.* 2008;2:e313.
10. Taylor MJ, Hoerauf A, Bockarie M. Lymphatic filariasis and onchocerciasis. *Lancet.* 2010;376:1175–1185.
11. Bockarie MJ, Pederson EM, White GB, Michael E. Role of vector control in the global program to eliminate lymphatic filariasis. *Annu Rev Entomol.* 2009;54:469–487.
12. Feasey N, Wansbrough-Jones M, Mabey DCW, Solomon AW. Neglected tropical diseases. *Br Med Bull.* 2010;93:179–200.

13. Cairncross S, Muller R, Zagaria N. Dracunculiasis (Guinea worm disease) and the eradication initiative. *Clin Microbiol Rev.* 2001;15:223–246.

14. Steinmann P, Keiser J, Bos R, Tanner M, Utzinger J. Schistosomiasis and water resources development: systematic review, meta-analysis, and estimates of people at risk. *Lancet.* 2006;6:411–425.

15. King CH. Toward the elimination of schistosomiasis. *N Engl J Med.* 2009;360:106–109.

16. Bethony J, Brooker S, Albonico M, et al. Soil-transmitted helminth infections: ascariasis, trichuriasis, and hookworm. *Lancet.* 2006;367:1521–1532.

17. *Geographical distribution and useful facts and stats.* Geneva: WHO Partners for Parasite Control.

18. Hotez PJ, Fenwick A, Savioli L, Molyneux DH. Rescuing the bottom billion through control of neglected tropical diseases. *Lancet.* 2009;373:1570–1575.

19. Suzuki K, Akama T, Kawashima A, Yoshihara A, Yotsu RR, Ishii N. Current status of leprosy: epidemiology, basic science and clinical perspectives. *J Dermatol.* 2012;39:121–129.

20. Mariotti SP, Pascolini D, Rose-Nussbaumer J. Trachoma: global magnitude of a preventable cause of blindness. *Br J Ophthalmol.* 2009;93:563–568.

21. Merritt RW, Walker ED, Small PL, et al. Ecology and transmission of Buruli ulcer disease: a systematic review. *PLoS Negl Trop Dis.* 2010;14:e911.

22. Redding CA, Rossi JS, Rossi SR, Velicer WF, Prochaska JO. Health behavior models. *Int Electron J Health Educ.* 2000;3(SI):180–193.

23. Gubler DJ. The changing epidemiology of yellow fever and dengue, 1900 to 2003: full circle? *Comp Immunol Microbiol Infect Dis.* 2004;27:319–330.

24. Goldbert DE, Siliciano RF, Jacobs WR. Outwitting evolution: fighting drug-resistant TB, malaria, and HIV. *Cell.* 2012;148:1271–1283.

25. Ou J, Li Q, Zeng G, Dun Z, Qin A. Efficiency of quarantine during an epidemic of severe acute respiratory syndrome—Beijing, China, 2003. *Morb Mortal Wkly Rep.* 2003;52:1037–1040.

26. Knobler S, Lederberg J, Pray LA, editors. *Considerations for viral disease eradication: lessons learned and future strategies.* Workshop Summary: Forum on Emerging Infections, Board on Global Health, Institute of Medicine, National Academy of Sciences. Washington DC: National Academy Press; 2002.

27. Larson HJ, Ghinai I. Lessons from polio eradication. *Nature.* 2011;473:446–447.

28. Monthly report on dracunculiasis cases, January–December 2010. *Wkly Epidemiol Rec.* 2011;86:91–92.

29. Dracunculiasis eradication: global surveillance summary, 2006. *Wkly Epidemiol Rec.* 2007;82:133–140.

30. Dracunculiasis eradication: global surveillance summary, 2005. *Wkly Epidemiol Rec.* 2006;81:173–182.

31. *Guinea-worm disease: countdown to eradication.* Geneva: WHO; 2012.

CHAPTER 10

Global Infectious Disease Initiatives

HIV/AIDS, tuberculosis, and malaria are among the infectious diseases that cause the most deaths worldwide each year. These infections and others are the target of special global health initiatives that aim to prevent, diagnose, and treat as many cases as possible.

10.1 COMPARISON OF HIV, TB, AND MALARIA

The "big three" infectious diseases of greatest concern to people living in most low- and middle-income countries are HIV/AIDS, tuberculosis (TB), and malaria. A comparison of these three (**Table 10–1**) highlights some of the challenges of global infectious disease control initiatives: each of the infections is caused by a different type of agent, each has a distinct primary mode of transmission, and each causes hundreds of thousands of deaths each year.[1] Several major global health initiatives seek to address these "big three" diseases, and others are targeting influenza and other infections. This chapter highlights these key infectious diseases and the efforts being made to reduce the global burden from them.

10.2 HIV/AIDS

Human immunodeficiency virus (HIV) is a viral infection spread when body fluids like blood, semen, vaginal fluid, or breastmilk are exchanged during sexual contact, the sharing of needles used to inject drugs, or by mother-to-child transmission (MTCT) during childbirth or breastfeeding. HIV is not transmitted through casual contact like shaking hands, sharing eating utensils, or using the same toilet, and transmission of HIV through blood transfusions is rare now that donated blood and blood products can be tested for HIV. The virus destroys specialized white blood cells, such

221

Table 10–1 Comparison of HIV/AIDS, tuberculosis, and malaria.

Disease	HIV/AIDS	Tuberculosis (TB)	Malaria
Type of infectious agent	Virus	Bacterium	Protozoan
Infectious agent	Human immunodeficiency virus (HIV)	Mycobacterium tuberculosis	Several types of Plasmodium
Primary mode(s) of transmission	Sexual contact and injecting drug use	Airborne by droplet spread	Mosquito bites
Can it be cured with medication?	No	Yes	Yes
Number of adult and child deaths worldwide in 2008	1,800,000	1,300,000	800,000
Proportion of all deaths worldwide in 2008	3.1%	2.4%	1.5%
Number of deaths of children under 5 years of age in 2008	190,000	60,000	710,000
Proportion of all under-5 child deaths in 2008	2.3%	0.7%	8.5%

Source: Data from The global burden of disease: 2004 update (May 2011 update). Geneva: WHO; 2011.

as CD4$^+$ T cells, that are needed by the immune system to fight infection. (Nearly all HIV work focuses on HIV virus type 1, or HIV-1. There is also an HIV-2 virus. HIV-2 accounts for only a small fraction of the HIV cases in the world, and occurs primarily in West Africa. HIV-2 progresses more slowly and causes milder symptoms than HIV-1.[2])

Acquired immunodeficiency syndrome, abbreviated as AIDS, is a **syndrome** (a collection of symptoms) that occurs as a result of the destruction of immune system cells by the HIV virus. Because AIDS is a syndrome and not an infectious agent, a person cannot "catch" AIDS from someone else. A person can become infected with HIV, and that infection can cause AIDS to develop. The constellation of diseases that occur in people with AIDS, such as *Pneumocystis carinii* pneumonia (PCP) and

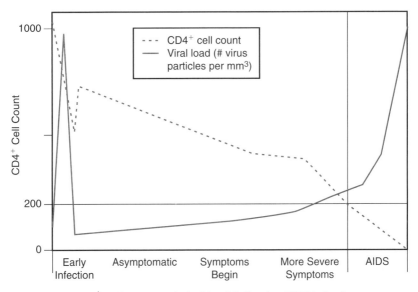

Figure 10–1 CD4$^+$ cell count and viral load following HIV infection.

Kaposi's sarcoma, are called **opportunistic infections (OIs)** because they only occur when the body's immune system is weakened enough to give the infectious agents an opportunity to invade. The most common OIs in low-income countries include tuberculosis, bacterial pneumonia, chronic diarrhea, and fungal infections such as *Cryptococcus*.[3]

A person newly infected with HIV may experience flu-like symptoms for a few days or weeks, but is often asymptomatic (**Figure 10–1**). During this stage, the newly infected individual still has a normal number of CD4 cells, but there is a high viral load in the blood (many virus particles per cubic millimeter) and it is possible to transmit the virus.[4]

The World Health Organization (WHO) identifies four clinical stages of HIV infection and AIDS disease that follow primary infection (**Table 10–2**).[3] In stages 1 and 2, which can last from a few weeks to more than 20 years, the infected person is asymptomatic or has only minor symptoms like skin infections and recurrent respiratory infections. Stage 3 is marked by more severe symptoms like recurrent respiratory infections, persistent fevers, tuberculosis, mouth ulcers, and the loss of more than 10% of body weight due to chronic diarrhea. The CD4 count begins to fall and the viral load in the blood begins to rise. In stage 4, serious opportunistic

Table 10–2 WHO staging system for HIV infection and disease based on clinical classification.

	Primary HIV Infection	Clinical Stage 1	Clinical Stage 2	Clinical Stage 3	Clinical Stage 4 (AIDS)
HIV-associated symptoms	Asymptomatic	Asymptomatic	Mild	Advanced	Severe
Weight	Normal	Normal	Loss of less than 10% of body weight	Loss of more than 10% of body weight	HIV wasting syndrome
Activity level	Asymptomatic	Asymptomatic, normal activity	Symptomatic, normal activity	Bed-ridden less than 50% of the day in the past month	Bed-ridden more than 50% of the day during the past month
Examples of common clinical conditions	Acute retroviral syndrome: flu-like symptoms about 2–4 weeks after initial infection that resolve within a few weeks	Persistent enlargement of lymph nodes in several parts of body	Minor skin problems (like fungal infections and mouth ulcers); upper respiratory infections	Chronic diarrhea, chronic fevers, thrush, pulmonary TB, severe bacterial infections like pneumonia and meningitis	Chronic diarrhea, chronic fevers, complex infections, and HIV-associated cancers

Source: Information from *Interim WHO clinical staging of HIV/AIDS and HIV/AIDS case definitions for surveillance: African Region* (WHO/HIV/2005.02). Geneva: WHO; 2005.

infections mark the onset of AIDS, and the CD4 count becomes very low (below 200 particles per mm^3) and may fall to undetectable levels.

There is currently no HIV vaccine and no drug that can cure an HIV infection. However, people who have HIV infection can take **antiretroviral drugs (ARVs)** to keep the viral count low and to slow the progression of symptoms. (Also, antiretroviral drugs given as post-exposure prophylaxis immediately after a known exposure, such as a nurse or doctor being stuck by a needle used on an HIV-infected patient, may lower the risk of the exposed person becoming HIV infected.[5]) The best current treatment for HIV infection is called **highly active antiretroviral therapy (HAART)**. HAART consists of combinations (sometimes called "cocktails") of several types of drugs, including reverse transcriptase inhibitors and protease inhibitors. The median survival time after infection with HIV if a person does not take HAART is about 10 years; after onset of clinical AIDS the expected survival without HAART is less than 2 years.[2] HAART prolongs both the duration of time between infection and the onset of clinical AIDS and the time between onset of AIDS and death, extending the lives of people with HIV infection by years or even decades.[6]

HAART does not work for all people with HIV because some cannot tolerate the side effects, some do not adhere to the treatment regimen and skip too many doses for the drugs to be effective, and some have a drug-resistant strain of HIV.[7,8] Even if the drugs do reduce the viral load, they do not cure the HIV infection or alleviate all symptoms. Once treatment is stopped, the levels of HIV in the blood may quickly rise.[9] Still, millions of people with HIV infection who would benefit from access to HAART do not have access to it because they cannot afford the treatment. Only about 47% of people with HIV infection worldwide are taking antiretroviral drugs.[10] Coverage rates range from only 10% in North Africa and the Middle East to 32% in East Asia, 37% in South Asia, 49% in sub-Saharan Africa, and 64% in Latin America.[10]

One of the alarming characteristics of HIV/AIDS is how quickly the epidemic emerged. The first cases of AIDS in the world were identified in the United States in homosexual men in 1981 (though cases in the United States and other parts of the world had probably occurred before the 1980s),[11] and by the early 1990s there were 10 million people worldwide living with HIV. By the mid-1990s there were 20 million people living with HIV. By the early 2000s more than 30 million people were living with HIV.[12]

HIV/AIDS now occurs in every part of the world, with some regions bearing a particularly heavy burden (**Table 10–3** and **Figure 10–2**), especially sub-Saharan Africa.[10,13] However, even within world regions, infection

Table 10–3 HIV/AIDS statistics in 2010.

Region	Prevalence of HIV Infection Among Adults (ages 15–49)	Number of Adults and Children Living with HIV	Proportion of Global HIV Cases in This Region	Proportion of Adults Living with HIV Who Are Women	Number of Adults and Children Newly Infected with HIV in 2010	Number of Adult and Child Deaths Due to HIV/AIDS in 2010	Proportion of Global HIV Deaths in This Region
Africa	4.7%	22,900,000	67%	59%	1,900,000	1,200,000	67%
The Americas	0.5%	3,000,000	2%	31%	170,000	96,000	2%
Europe	0.4%	2,300,000	4%	32%	190,000	99,000	4%
South and Southeast Asia	0.3%	3,500,000	10%	37%	210,000	230,000	13%
North Africa and the Middle East	0.2%	560,000	9%	40%	82,000	38,000	5%
East Asia and Oceania	0.1%	1,300,000	7%	28%	130,000	80,000	6%
TOTAL	0.8%	34,000,000	100%	50%	2,700,000	1,800,000	100%

Source: Data from Global HIV/AIDS response: progress report 2011. Geneva: WHO/UNAIDS/UNICEF; 2011.

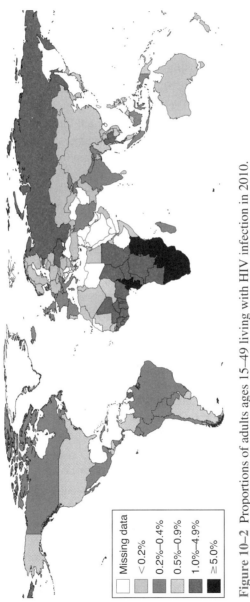

Figure 10–2 Proportions of adults ages 15–49 living with HIV infection in 2010.

Source: Data from *Report on the global AIDS epidemic 2010.* Geneva: UNAIDS; 2011.

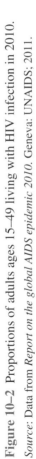

Missing data

<0.2%

0.2%–0.4%

0.5%–0.9%

1.0%–4.9%

≥5.0%

rates are not uniform. For example, the prevalence of HIV infection among reproductive-age adults in East and Southern Africa is about 7.1% while the rate in West and Central Africa is about 2.8%.[10]

Sub-Saharan Africa is home to just over 10% of the world's population, but about two-thirds of all people with HIV infection live in the region. Nearly 5% of African adults between 15 and 49 years old have contracted HIV, and in some southern African countries more than 25% adults of reproductive age (ages 15 to 49) are infected with HIV.[13] In the 1990s and early 2000s, AIDS caused life expectancy to plummet in many countries and changed the entire social structure in some parts of Africa.[14] Because nearly all infections and deaths occur in young- and middle-aged adults, older adults have been forced to take on the care of their sick adult children and their young grandchildren. If the grandparents are deceased or unable to care for children, **AIDS orphans** (children who have lost both parents, at least one to AIDS) often end up homeless and living on the street. The HIV incidence rate has decreased in most sub-Saharan African countries when compared to peak rates, and significantly increased access to ARVs has helped to reduce the number of deaths from HIV/AIDS each year. Still, nearly 23 million sub-Saharan Africans are living with HIV, and millions who would benefits from antiretroviral drugs do not have access to them.[10]

Anyone who is exposed to blood or body fluids can contract HIV. (This is why workers are often trained to use **universal precautions**, such as wearing gloves, when caring for a sick person or cleaning up a spill or soiled laundry.) People in some population groups—such as paid sex workers, men who have sex with men (MSM), injecting drug users (IDU), and prisoners—are at elevated risk because they may engage in high-risk behaviors that increase the likelihood of contact with blood and other body fluids. They also may have limited access to healthcare services because of discrimination. And many people are at risk because they have not been educated about HIV and HIV prevention, or do not take preventive measures because they do not think they are at risk. Health workers in all regions of the world must continue HIV/AIDS education initiatives because the incidence of new cases tends to increase when people stop worrying about their risk.

Women have greater biological and social risk of contracting HIV than men.[15] Anatomically, the walls of the vagina are thin and may tear during intercourse, facilitating the entrance of HIV into the bloodstream. Women are at least twice as likely as men to acquire HIV from an act of heterosexual intercourse. Socially, women marry at younger ages than men, may not have the power to demand condom use, and are more likely to be the victims of sexual violence. Among sub-Saharan Africans who are 15 to 24 years old, nearly three times more women than men have HIV infection.[10] In some places, the majority of women with HIV infection are married, and many of those women contracted HIV from their husbands. Women are often hesitant to ask their husbands and partners to use condoms, so programs that educate and encourage women and men to take measures to protect their health are important contributors to HIV prevention.

In 2010, about 3.4 million children (ages 0 to 14) worldwide were living with HIV, about 390,000 children became infected, and 250,000 children died of HIV.[10] The vast majority of these children were infected through MTCT. Babies can be infected by their mothers during pregnancy, the birth process, or breastfeeding. In the absence of any drug interventions, a baby born to an HIV-infected mother has about a 15% to 30% risk of contracting HIV during delivery.[16] The likelihood of transmission is much lower if the mother takes ARVs during pregnancy, because a woman with a low viral load has a lower risk of passing the virus to her baby during delivery.[17] When HAART is used, the risk of MTCT is about 2% or less.[18] Even when a mother has not taken ARVs during pregnancy, the risk of MTCT during delivery can be reduced to less than 5% if the woman is given a single dose of nevirapine at the start of labor and her baby is given a single dose of nevirapine after delivery.[19] (Zidovudine is also commonly used to prevent MTCT.)

HIV is excreted in breastmilk, and the risk of HIV infection in babies who are breastfed for several months can be as high as 25% to 45%.[16] The risk is highest in babies whose mothers are not on ARVs. Mothers with HIV infection are encouraged to use formula instead of breastmilk. However, many women living with HIV have no choice but to breastfeed their babies. Some cannot afford formula and others do not have reliable access to clean water. The risk of infant death due to diarrhea from unsafe water used to mix formula is often greater than the risk of contracting HIV through breastmilk, and women are often forced to make painful decisions about which risks they will expose their babies to.

The most important way to help control the HIV/AIDS pandemic is to emphasize prevention (**Table 10–4**).[10,20] One campaign uses ABC as a reminder to be *A*bstinent, to *B*e faithful if sexually active, and to consistently and correctly use a *C*ondom during every sex act. The ABC approach used in Uganda is often credited with reducing the prevalence of HIV by more than half in the 1990s.[21] The ABC approach works to prevent uninfected people from contracting HIV, and also helps keep people with HIV

Table 10–4 Preventive and treatment interventions for HIV/AIDS.

Preventive Interventions (Primary Prevention)	Treatment Interventions (Secondary Prevention)
• Safe sex, including condom use • Unused needles for drug users • Male circumcision • Treatment of other sexually transmitted infections (STIs) • Safe, screened blood supplies • Antiretrovirals (ARVs) in pregnancy to prevent mother-to-child transmission (MTCT) and after occupational exposure • Health education on abstinence, condom use, STI treatment, ARV use to prevent MTCT, feeding substitutions for mothers with HIV • HIV voluntary counseling and testing (VCT) so that people with HIV can take steps to prevent transmitting the virus to others • Use of universal precautions for safety when handling blood and other body fluids	• Treatment of opportunistic infections (OIs) • Co-trimoxazole prophylaxis • Highly active antiretroviral therapy (HAART) • Palliative care (pain management)

Source: Data from *Global HIV/AIDS response: progress report 2011.* Geneva: WHO/UNAIDS/UNICEF; 2011; and Wagstaff A, Claeson M, Hecht RM, Gottret P, Fang Q. Millennium Development Goals for health: what will it take to accelerate progress? In: Jamison DT, Breman JG, Measham AR, et al., editors. *Disease control priorities in developing countries*, 2nd edition. Washington DC: Oxford University Press and IBRD / World Bank; 2006.

infection healthy. Because HIV has a lot of genetic variability, people who are infected with HIV need to protect themselves against other subtypes of the virus. (Male circumcision has also recently been shown to significantly reduce the risk of HIV infection,[22] but it does not negate the need to use condoms as protection against HIV and other sexually transmitted infections.)

Several major global health initiatives are seeking to reduce the incidence of HIV infection and to prolong the healthy lives of those who do contract the virus. These include the work of PEPFAR, IAVI, The Global Fund, and others. PEPFAR (the U.S. President's Emergency Plan for AIDS Relief), initiated in 2004, provided ARVs to more than 3 million people worldwide in 2010 and is expanding its coverage.[23] The International AIDS

Vaccine Initiative (IAVI) is developing and testing several candidate HIV vaccines.[24] The Global Fund to Fight AIDS, Tuberculosis, and Malaria, funded by a variety of donor countries, foundations, private sector organizations, and other entities, provides financing to grant-receiving countries for programs those countries implement to address the "big three" diseases, including HIV.[25]

10.3 TUBERCULOSIS (TB)

Tuberculosis (TB) is caused by the bacterium *Mycobacterium tuberculosis*. TB can affect any part of the body, but it usually occurs in the lungs, a condition called pulmonary TB. TB used to be called consumption because people with the disease were "consumed" by it and developed a bloody cough, persistent fever, wasting, and pale skin.

A distinction is made between having TB infection (latent TB) and having TB disease (active TB). More than one-third of the world's population has been infected with the TB bacillus, but only about 5% to 10% of infected people will develop TB disease during their lifetimes.[26] *M. tuberculosis* is spread through the air, but only people with active TB disease are contagious. A person with untreated active TB may infect several other people each year, especially if they have frequent and prolonged interactions.[27]

Anyone can become infected with TB, although the rate of infection is higher among low-income individuals and those who are undernourished, have underlying medical conditions, smoke tobacco, and/or live or work in substandard facilities that are crowded and have poor ventilation that contributes to high levels of indoor air pollution.[28]

Infection rates are highest in Africa and Asia, but TB occurs in every part of the world (**Figure 10–3** and **Table 10–5**).[29] Each year about 10 million new cases of TB disease occur, about 12 million people are living with the disease, and more than 1 million people die of TB (not including those with HIV infection who die because of co-infection with TB).[29] The incidence rate has decreased in recent decades in most world regions, especially in higher-income areas, but the rate is increasing in sub-Saharan Africa (**Figure 10–4**).[30]

People with HIV infection are much more likely to develop active TB disease than people without HIV infection, and TB is a leading cause of death in people with AIDS. About 13% of people with TB disease worldwide also have HIV infection, but nearly 40% of sub-Saharan Africans with

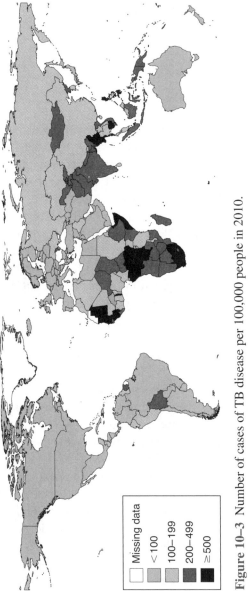

Figure 10–3 Number of cases of TB disease per 100,000 people in 2010.

Source: Data from *Global TB control report 2011.* Geneva: WHO; 2011.

Missing data
<100
100–199
200–499
≥500

Table 10-5 Global TB statistics in 2010.

	Incidence of New TB Disease per 100,000 People in 2010	Number of New Cases of TB Disease in 2010	Total Number of TB Cases in 2010	Mortality from TB per 100,000 People	Number of Deaths (excluding deaths from HIV/AIDS) in 2010	Proportion of Adults with TB Disease Who Have HIV Infection	Proportion of New TB Cases Who Have MDR-TB
Africa	276	2,300,000	2,800,000	30	250,000	39%	2%
South and Southeast Asia	193	3,500,000	5,000,000	27	500,000	5%	2%
North Africa and the Middle East	109	650,000	1,000,000	16	95,000	2%	3%
East Asia and Oceania	93	1,700,000	2,500,000	8	130,000	2%	5%
Europe	47	420,000	560,000	7	61,000	5%	12%
The Americas	29	270,000	330,000	2	20,000	13%	2%
TOTAL	128	8,800,000	12,000,000	15	1,100,000	13%	3%

Source: Data from Global TB control report 2011. Geneva: WHO; 2011.

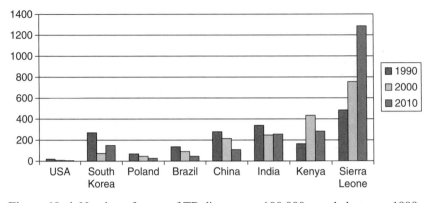

Figure 10–4 Number of cases of TB disease per 100,000 people between 1990 and 2010.

Source: Data from *Global TB control report 2011*. Geneva: WHO; 2011.

TB have HIV co-infection.[29] About one in four people with HIV/AIDS who die each year die due to TB infection.[31] Early diagnosis of TB can be critical for survival. One of the challenges of the relationship between TB and HIV, especially in sub-Saharan Africa, is that people with a lung infection may delay seeking treatment because they fear that a diagnosis of TB may be accompanied by a diagnosis of AIDS.[32] Delayed diagnosis creates an unnecessarily high risk of death from TB. People with an HIV infection can be successfully treated for TB, but they must be strong enough to survive several months of antibiotic treatment.[33]

The standard treatment regimen for TB involves taking a combination of up to five different drugs every day for six months or longer. The first two months are the most crucial, but following through with the full course of treatment is essential so that all of the bacteria, including the hardiest organisms, are killed. The protocol for treatment that the WHO recommends is called **directly observed therapy, short-course (DOTS)**. The key part of DOTS is the "directly observed" component. TB patients being treated under DOTS are required to have a trained observer watch them take their pills every day. This observer might be a doctor or nurse if the person is an inpatient or reports to a clinic for his or her daily treatment, a shopkeeper or other community leader, or a family member who is supervised by another community member. If the patient misses a dose, a public health worker will track the patient down and try to ensure compliance. (Some countries have public health laws stipulating that people who are not compliant with TB treatment can be hospitalized under guard or imprisoned for the duration of their treatment, but most do not enforce these regulations.) Still, the **case detection rate**, the proportion of those with TB disease who are diagnosed as having the disease, is low in many places. And among those who test positive for TB (either by sputum smear microscopy or by a laboratory culture test or molecular test) and begin treatment, the **default rate**, the proportion of people who are diagnosed but do not complete the full course of treatment, is high in some places.[29]

One of the problems that can result when people being treated for TB stop taking their drugs a few months into treatment is the emergence of multidrug-resistant TB (MDR-TB). MDR-TB that does not respond to standard antibiotic therapies is a growing problem. An estimated 3% of TB cases worldwide are resistant to at least one TB drug, but in some countries the proportion is much higher.[29] MDR-TB can be treated using a directly observed therapy approach (through a special protocol called DOTS-Plus), but the drugs are more expensive and the course of treatment is much longer, usually two years rather than six months. New concerns are arising about extensively drug-resistant TB (XDR-TB) and totally drug-resistant TB (TDR-TB).[34]

A vaccine called BCG (Bacillus Calmette-Guerin) is available and used in many countries, but it provides protection for only about half of the people who receive it.[35] The standard test for TB is the PPD test (also called the Mantoux test) in which a small amount of TB bacterial protein is injected under the skin and the reaction is monitored. A person with TB will have an immune response and develop a rash at the injection site. If a person has a positive PPD test, then a chest x-ray will be taken to look for pockets of infection. The person may also take a sputum test, in which the phlegm produced by deep coughs is analyzed for the presence or absence of TB bacteria. Some workplaces and schools require employees and students to prove that they do not have TB. One of the disadvantages of BCG is that people who have received BCG usually test positive on PPD tests, so more tests are required to prove that they do not actually have TB. Several new TB vaccines are being developed and tested, but are not yet ready for widespread use.

Several interventions help reduce the individual and public health burden of tuberculosis (**Table 10–6**).[20] Control of the spread of TB also requires structures to be in place to support diagnosis and treatment, including a supply chain that provides consistent access to all essential TB medications in every country and a reporting system that allows governments to track their progress toward improved prevention, diagnosis, and treatment.

Table 10–6 Preventive and treatment interventions for tuberculosis.

Preventive Interventions (Primary Prevention)	Treatment Interventions (Secondary Prevention)
• Directly observed treatment (DOTS) of contagious cases of TB to prevent transmission and emergence of drug-resistant strains • Testing and treatment of contacts • BCG immunization	• Directly observed treatment (DOTS) from diagnosis until cure • Early identification of cases with active TB disease

Source: Information from Wagstaff A, Claeson M, Hecht RM, Gottret P, Fang Q. Millennium Development Goals for health: what will it take to accelerate progress? In: Jamison DT, Breman JG, Measham AR, et al., editors. *Disease control priorities in developing countries*, 2nd edition. Washington DC: Oxford University Press and IBRD / World Bank; 2006.

Clinicians, public health workers, and members of communities with a high prevalence of TB play a critical role in local and national TB control by diagnosing, treating, and supporting individuals with TB disease. At the global level, TB control efforts are being led by the Stop TB Partnership, which brings together representatives from the WHO and other international agencies, national and subnational governmental organizations, foundations, nongovernmental organizations (including patient support networks), private sector entities (including pharmaceutical and diagnostic companies), and universities and research institutions. The aims of the Stop TB Partnership include expanding access to DOTS, improving treatment of TB-HIV co-infection, addressing MDR-TB, increasing the use of advanced laboratory tests for TB, and developing new TB vaccines, diagnostic tools, and medications.[36]

10.4 MALARIA

Malaria is a parasitic infection caused by protozoa of the *Plasmodium* species. There are five types of *Plasmodium* known to cause human infection: *Plasmodium falciparum*, *P. vivax*, *P. malariae*, *P. ovale*, and *P. knowlesi*. Infection with any of the five species can cause cyclic fevers, headaches, and joint pain, and can in some cases can cause organ failure and brain inflammation, especially in children. *P. falciparum* is generally the most serious infection, and it causes about 90% of malaria cases worldwide.[37]

The parasites are passed from one human to another by female *Anopheles* mosquitoes that need a bloodmeal in order to produce and lay eggs. The mosquitoes usually seek out bloodmeals between sunset and sunrise. Once a bloodmeal is taken, the mosquitoes deposit their eggs in water. Any places where water collects (ponds, lakes, puddles, and even buckets and old tires that might trap rainwater) can serve as mosquito habitats. Environmental changes related to road building, mining, logging, agriculture, and irrigation may also create breeding sites, further increasing the mosquito population.[38] The incidence of malaria varies seasonally, and generally increases during rainy seasons when mosquito populations increase.

The malaria parasite has a very complex lifecycle (**Figure 10–5**). A mosquito acquires *Plasmodium* infection by biting an infected human. After the malaria parasites undergo several stages of development in the gut of the mosquito, they travel to the salivary gland of the mosquito and are injected into a human during a bloodmeal. Once in the human body, the parasites move to the liver and reproduce rapidly. After several days the maturing parasites enter the bloodstream and invade red blood cells, the cells that carry oxygen throughout the body. The parasites grow and divide inside the red blood cells. Every 2 to 3 days (depending on the species of *Plasmodium*) the red blood cells rupture, releasing parasites and toxins into the bloodstream and causing fever, chills, and anemia. The cycle can continue for 10 to 14 days or longer if untreated.

Although anyone can contract malaria, children and pregnant women are most at risk for severe complications and death. Children with malaria are at risk for developing severe anemia and cerebral malaria, which

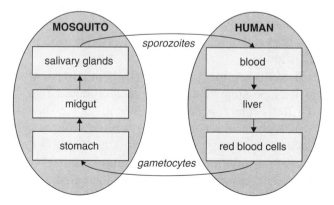

Figure 10–5 The life cycle of *Plamsodium.*

is characterized by coma and convulsions. If children survive cerebral malaria, they may have permanent brain damage and learning disabilities.[39] Adults who have grown up in endemic areas usually have some degree of resistance to severe malaria.[40] However, susceptibility to malaria increases during pregnancy, and complications are common because pregnant women are often anemic, having too few red blood cells to carry oxygen even before additional red blood cells are destroyed by *Plasmodium*.[41] As a result, babies born to mothers with malaria are at increased risk of low birthweight and other birth complications.[41]

Each bout of malaria causes several days or weeks of lost productivity in terms of absence from work or school and the inability to work growing food and around the home.[42] Infection is most common during the seasons when subsistence farmers grow and harvest their crops, and when malaria (or caring for people with malaria) keeps family members from being in the fields at this crucial time it can result in long-term undernutrition for all members of the household. A child may have several episodes of clinical malaria every year, and children carry the risk of long-term reductions in school performance due to missed class days and continued weakness from anemia. The cost of lost productivity due to malaria extends to whole countries as well. A world map of the distribution of the burden of malaria (**Figure 10–6**) looks very similar to a world map of the distribution of poverty.[42] Malaria-endemic countries also have lower rates of economic growth than countries without malaria.[43]

Several hundred million acute clinical cases of malaria occur each year, resulting in more than half a million deaths, mostly of children.[37] The countries with the highest burden from malaria are in sub-Saharan Africa, where more than 90% of malaria deaths occur; parts of Asia are also significantly affected (**Table 10–7**).[37] Most cases of malaria occur in the tropics, where mosquitoes survive year-round and environmental control of insect populations through spraying of insecticides and land and water management is limited.

Nearly half of the world's population lives in an area where malaria occurs, and it is possible that this percentage could rise.[44] Until the middle of the 20th century, malaria was endemic in the United States and Mediterranean, with cases reported as far north as Canada and Siberia. A massive insecticide spraying program led by the WHO in the 1950s and 1960s eliminated malaria from dozens of countries, but it is possible for a re-emergence to occur, especially because of increased concern over the environmental impact of spraying insecticides and the risk of mosquitoes developing insecticide resistance.[45]

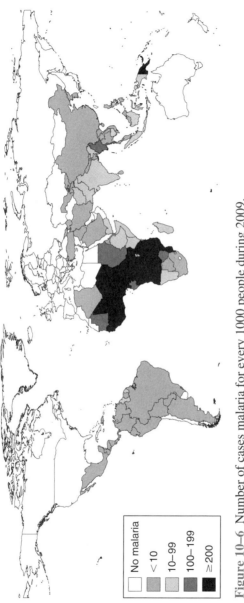

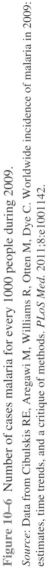

Figure 10–6 Number of cases malaria for every 1000 people during 2009.

Source: Data from Cibulskis RE, Aregawi M, Williams R, Otten M, Dye C. Worldwide incidence of malaria in 2009: estimates, time trends, and a critique of methods. *PLoS Med.* 2011;8:e1001142.

Table 10–7 Regional malaria burden in 2010.

	Estimated Number of Cases	Proportion of Global Clinical Malaria Cases in This Region	% of Malaria Caused by P. Falciparum	Estimated Number of Deaths from Malaria	Proportion of Global Malaria Mortality Burden in This Region
Africa	174,000,000	81%	98%	600,000	91%
South and Southeast Asia	28,000,000	13%	54%	40,000	6%
North Africa and the Middle East	10,000,000	5%	82%	15,000	2%
East Asia and Oceania	2,000,000	1%	77%	5,000	1%
The Americas	1,000,000	<1%	34%	1,000	<1%
Europe	200	0%	0%	0	0%
TOTAL	216,000,000	100%	91%	655,000	100%

Source: Data from World malaria report 2011. Geneva: WHO; 2011.

There are few antimalarial drugs that work today. For decades, the drug of choice for treating malaria was chloroquine, but in most parts of the world the common strains of malaria have become chloroquine-resistant and the drug is now ineffective. Strains of malaria are also becoming resistant to other drug options, such as sulfadoxone/pyrimethamine (also called SP or Fansidar) and artemisinin-based drugs.[46] The WHO strongly urges the use of **artemisinin-based combination therapy (ACT)**, which combines at least two different antimalarial drugs (such as artemether plus lumefantrine or artesunate plus mefloquine), because combination drugs slow the emergence of drug resistance.[47] Because the parasites that cause malaria are very complex organisms, developing new drugs (or developing a vaccine) is a considerable scientific challenge.

Prevention of malaria is of increasing importance as treatment is becoming more difficult (**Table 10–8**).[20] Although travelers from nonendemic areas to

Table 10–8 Preventive and treatment interventions for malaria.

Preventive Interventions (Primary Prevention)	Treatment Interventions (Secondary Prevention)
• Use of insecticide-treated bednets (ITNs)	• Rapid detection and early treatment of uncomplicated cases
• Indoor residual spraying (IRS) of insecticide in epidemic-prone areas	• Treatment of complicated cases such as cerebral malaria and severe anemia
• Intermittent presumptive treatment (IPT) of pregnant women (IPTp)	

Source: Information from Wagstaff A, Claeson M, Hecht RM, Gottret P, Fang Q. Millennium Development Goals for health: what will it take to accelerate progress? In: Jamison DT, Breman JG, Measham AR, et al., editors. *Disease control priorities in developing countries,* 2nd edition. Washington DC: Oxford University Press and IBRD / World Bank; 2006.

places where malaria is endemic generally take prophylactic (preventive) antimalarial drugs, these are not fully effective in preventing disease. More importantly, it is not realistic or healthy to encourage prophylactic use among people living in highly endemic areas. The cost would be high, the long-term effects of drug use could be potentially harmful, and widespread use of antiparasitic drugs would contribute to the development of drug-resistant *Plasmodium* at a time when many species are no longer susceptible to existing antimalarial drugs.

The only guaranteed way to prevent malaria is to avoid all mosquito bites. Because the mosquitoes that spread malaria bite primarily at dawn and dusk, the use of **insecticide-treated bednets (ITNs)** that put a mesh barrier between people and mosquitoes and also kill mosquitoes that are near the net is highly encouraged. Field studies of ITNs show a significant reduction in child mortality when bednets are used consistently.[48] It is also important for malaria patients to stay under a bednet so mosquitoes cannot bite them and become carriers of malaria. Many adults who have grown up in endemic areas continue to have parasitemia (malaria parasites in the blood) even when asymptomatic, so all people who live in at-risk areas, including both children and adults, should consistently use ITNs. ITNs must generally be re-dipped in a pyrethroid insecticide once or twice a year to maintain their effectiveness as insecticides, unless they are **long-lasting insecticide-treated nets (LLINs)** that remain effective for several years.[49]

Other barrier methods include wearing clothes that cover the arms and legs during the times of the day when mosquitoes are most likely to bite and having screens or curtains cover the windows and doors of houses when it is possible to do this. Insect repellents like "bug sprays" and mosquito mats and coils are also helpful, as is reducing pooled water near the home to minimize breeding areas. Additionally, indoor residual spraying (IRS) of insecticides can help to kill mosquitoes in the home. Unfortunately, most of the households at greatest risk for malaria have little or no money available to spend on malaria prevention.[50]

At the global level, the Roll Back Malaria (RBM) Partnership brings together the WHO, UNICEF, other multilateral organizations, national governments from malaria-endemic countries and donor countries, researchers, and representatives from foundations, nongovernmental organizations, academia, and the private sector in order to increase and sustain access to effective prevention and treatment technologies.[51] Other partnerships, such as the Medicines for Malaria Venture (MMV) and the Malaria Vaccine Initiative (MVI), are working to create new preventive, diagnostic, and treatment tools for reducing the burden of disease caused by malaria.[52]

10.5 INFLUENZA

Global health professionals are always concerned about the potential for a worldwide influenza outbreak. Influenza viruses cause fevers and respiratory disease, and they can exacerbate existing medical conditions (especially lung and heart diseases) and lead to pneumonia. ("Stomach flu" is not caused by influenza viruses.) Although the highest fatality rates from influenza are usually among the elderly and immunocompromised, anyone who contracts influenza can die from it. The most serious influenza pandemic in the 20th century occurred in 1918 and 1919 during World War I, and that strain killed a disproportionate number of young adults.[53]

Influenza viruses affect humans and also many types of animals, including chickens, ducks, pigs, horses, and even dogs, whales, and bats. Two main types of influenza viruses cause epidemics among humans, influenza A and influenza B. Influenza A viruses are further classified based on the types of surface antigens they present. The two key surface antigens for Influenza A are hemagglutinin (H) and neuraminidase (N). Influenza A strains are classified using abbreviations like H3N2 and H1N1 that are derived from the hemagglutinin and neuraminidase types. Surface antigens are proteins that are "read" by the body's immune cells. When an immune cell "reads" another cell that is part of the body, it recognizes that it is seeing itself. Immune cells can also recognize some of the infectious agents that the immune system has fought off before and can quickly respond to stop these infections from reoccurring. This kind of active immunity can result from either previous infection or from immunization.

All infectious agents, whether newly emerging or long established in a population, are constantly adapting and changing in ways that can make them more or less transmissible, infective, pathogenic, and virulent. Influenza viruses fool the bodies of their hosts by changing their surface antigens so that the hosts' immune systems cannot recognize them. There are two processes for changing surface antigens. **Antigenic drift** occurs when small genetic mutations bring about small changes in the antigens. Antigenic drift is why infection with one version of H3N2 influenza may not confer immunity to another form of H3N2. Antigenic drift makes it necessary to develop a new influenza vaccine every year. **Antigenic shift** occurs when two very different influenza viruses attack the same cell and the genetic material from both recombines to form a new type of influenza. Antigenic shift led to the emergence in 1997 in Southeast Asia of the H5N1 strain of avian influenza that spread rapidly through the bird population, affecting both domestic birds (like ducks and chickens) and wild migrating fowl. On occasion, a human becomes infected with one of these new strains of "bird flu" and becomes seriously ill. A pandemic may result if that strain develops the ability to be easily transmitted from human to human. A pandemic occurred in 2009 when a type of H1N1 "swine flu" began circulating widely in the human population.[54]

Influenza is a prime example of how global travel can contribute to the spread of newly mutated infectious agents. An infected person can fly to any part of the world in a day or two and spark a new epicenter of infection. On the other hand, global travel and communication may also help contain a pandemic by enabling medical equipment and knowledge to be quickly shared and public health officials to be immediately alerted to possible influenza outbreaks. During the 2009 H1N1 pandemic, revised International Health Regulations guided the coordinated global response to the outbreak. Countries reported cases of H1N1 to the WHO, and the WHO used its Pandemic Alert System to keep member nations and the public informed about the spread of the epidemic.[55] Coordinated vaccine capacity-building efforts initiated before the pandemic allowed pharmaceutical companies around the globe to expedite the development, testing, and manufacturing of H1N1 vaccines.[56] Local, national, and global preparedness plans implemented years before the emergence of H1N1 guided the response to the pandemic, and refined plans are available for implementation when the next major influenza pandemic emerges.

10.6 OTHER GLOBAL INFECTIOUS DISEASE INITIATIVES

A variety of additional global initiatives are seeking to control or eradicate other infectious diseases. Some of these programs are disease specific. For example, the Global Polio Eradication Initiative, a public–private partnership led by the WHO, UNICEF, the U.S. Centers for Disease Control and Prevention (CDC), and Rotary International, among others, has decreased the incidence of polio infection worldwide by 99% and hopes to achieve eradication within a few years.[57] Some initiatives are focused on technology. For example, the GAVI Alliance assists lower-income countries with gaining access to new vaccines as quickly as possible after they are developed, tested, and shown to be safe.[58] The specific vaccines GAVI helps countries to acquire are tailored to each partner country's needs.

A growing number of projects are targeting neglected tropical diseases (NTDs). The Carter Center, founded in 1982, is seeking to eradicate Guinea worm and to widely control river blindness, lymphatic filariasis, schistosomiasis, and trachoma in areas where these infections have been endemic.[59] In 2012, the Bill & Melinda Gates Foundation, several major pharmaceutical companies, and other partners announced a plan to seek to control 10 key NTDs (including leprosy, African sleeping sickness, Chagas disease, visceral leishmaniasis, and soil-transmitted helminths) by 2020.[60]

All of these disease control programs, and the ones for HIV/AIDS, tuberculosis, malaria, and influenza, require the financial, technical, and operational support of dozens of different players, including international and national governmental agencies, a variety of nongovernmental organizations, businesses, charitable foundations, scientists and other researchers, health professionals, and local volunteers. The success of these partnerships depends on the commitment all of the involved parties make to achieving public health goals.

10.7 DISCUSSION QUESTIONS

1. Most people with HIV infection would benefit from ARV therapy, but many do not have access to these drugs. What are some of the barriers to accessing these medications? What are some ways that these barriers can be overcome?
2. What are some of the factors contributing to the increase in HIV incidence and prevalence in some world regions and the decrease in other regions? How could additional infections be prevented?

3. What are some of the special populations at risk for HIV infection? What are some public health interventions that would reduce the infection rate in these populations?

4. What are some of the reasons why every country in the world needs to be concerned about TB?

5. Why does malaria continue to kill millions of children each year even though there are many tools available to prevent malaria infection? What additional steps can be taken to prevent malaria deaths?

6. Compare and contrast the global impact of HIV/AIDS, malaria, and TB.

7. How did you react to the emergence of the H1N1 strain of influenza? Did you alter your routines in any way? How will you react to the next strain of influenza that emerges?

8. How should individuals, households, communities, schools, and nations prepare for a possible influenza outbreak?

9. Visit the website for an organization or partnership seeking to control, eliminate, or eradicate a particular infectious disease. What progress is being made toward the organization's goal?

REFERENCES

1. *The global burden of disease: 2004 update (May 2011 update).* Geneva: WHO; 2011.
2. Jaffar S, Grant AD, Whitworth J, Smith PG, Whittle H. The natural history of HIV-1 and HIV-2 infections in adults in Africa: a literature review. *Bull World Health Organ.* 2004;82:462–469.
3. *Interim WHO clinical staging of HIV/AIDS and HIV/AIDS case definitions for surveillance: African Region* (WHO/HIV/2005.02). Geneva: WHO; 2005.
4. Daar ES, Little S, Pitt J, et al. Diagnosis of primary HIV-1 infection: Los Angeles County Primary HIV Infection Recruitment Network. *Ann Intern Med.* 2001;134:25–29.
5. Panlilio AL, Cardo DM, Grohskopf LA, Heneine W, Ross CS; U.S. Public Health Service. Updated U.S. Public Health Service guidelines for the management of occupational exposures to HIV and recommendations for postexposure prophylaxis. *MMWR Recomm Rep.* 2005;54(RR-9):1–17.
6. Hammer SM, Eron JJ Jr, Reiss P, et al. Antiretroviral treatment of adult HIV infection: 2008 recommendations of the International AIDS Society—USA panel. *JAMA.* 2008;300:555–570.
7. Ammassari A, Murri R, Pezzotti MP, et al. Self-reported symptoms and medication side effects influence adherence to highly active antiretroviral therapy in persons with HIV infection. *J Acquir Immune Defic Syndr.* 2001;28:445–449.
8. Unge C, Södergård B, Marrone G, et al. Long-term adherence to antiretroviral treatment and program drop-out in a high-risk urban setting in sub-Saharan Africa: a prospective cohort study. *PLoS One.* 2010;5:e13613.
9. García F, Plana M, Vidal C, et al. Dynamics of viral load rebound and immunological changes after stopping effective antiretroviral therapy. *AIDS.* 1999;13:F79–F86.

10. *Global HIV/AIDS response: progress report 2011.* Geneva: WHO/UNAIDS/UNICEF; 2011.
11. *Pneumocystis* pneumonia—Los Angeles, 1981. *MMWR Morb Mortal Wkly Rep.* 1981;30:250–252.
12. *AIDS epidemic update 2007.* Geneva: UNAIDS; 2007.
13. *Report on the global AIDS epidemic 2010.* Geneva: UNAIDS; 2011.
14. *Report on the global AIDS epidemic 2008.* Geneva: UNAIDS; 2008.
15. Higgins JA, Hoffman S, Dworkin SL. Rethinking gender, heterosexual men, and women's vulnerability to HIV/AIDS. *Am J Public Health.* 2010;100:435–445.
16. De Cock KM, Fowler MG, Mercier E, et al. Prevention of mother-to-child HIV transmission in resource-poor countries: translating research into policy and practice. *JAMA.* 2000;283:1175–1182.
17. Volmink J, Siegfried NL, van der Merwe L, Brocklehurst P. Antiretrovirals for reducing the risk of mother-to-child transmission of HIV infection. *Cochrane Database Syst Rev.* 2007;(1):CD003510.
18. Marseille E, Kahn JG, Mmiro F, et al. Cost effectiveness of a single-dose nevirapine regimen for mothers and babies to decrease vertical HIV-1 transmission in sub-Saharan Africa. *Lancet.* 1999;354:803–809.
19. McIntyre J. Strategies to prevent mother-to-child transmission of HIV. *Curr Opin Infect Dis.* 2006;19:33–38.
20. Jamison DT, Breman JG, Measham AR, et al., editors. *Disease control priorities in developing countries,* 2nd edition. Washington DC: Oxford University Press and IBRD/World Bank; 2006.
21. Murphy EM, Greene ME, Mihailovic A, Olupot-Olupot P. Was the "ABC" approach (abstinence, being faithful, using condoms) responsible for Uganda's decline in HIV? *PLoS Med.* 2006;3:e379.
22. Sawires SR, Dworkin SL, Fiamma A, Peacock D, Szekeres G, Coates TJ. Male circumcision and HIV/AIDS: challenges and opportunities. *Lancet.* 2007;369:708–713.
23. *The U.S. President's Emergency Plan for AIDS Relief: 7th annual report to Congress.* Washington DC: PEPFAR; 2011.
24. *2010 annual progress report.* New York: IAVI; 2011.
25. *Making a difference: global fund results report 2011.* New York: The Global Fund; 2011.
26. Dye C, Williams BG. The population dynamics and control of tuberculosis. *Science.* 2010;328:856–861.
27. Sepkowitz KA. How contagious is tuberculosis. *Clin Infect Dis.* 1996;23:954–962.
28. Lönnroth K, Jaramillo E, Williams BG, Dye C, Raviglione M. Drivers of tuberculosis epidemics: the role of risk factors and social determinants. *Soc Sci Med.* 2009;68:2240–2246.
29. *Global TB control report 2011.* Geneva: WHO; 2011.
30. Dye C, Lönnroth K, Jaramillo E, Williams BG, Raviglione M. Trends in tuberculosis incidence and their determinants in 134 countries. *Bull World Health Organ.* 2009;87:683–391.
31. Getahun H, Gunneberg C, Granich R, Nunn P. HIV infection-associated tuberculosis: the epidemiology and the response. *Clin Infect Dis.* 2010;50(suppl 3):S201–S207.
32. Storla DG, Yimer S, Bjune GA. A systematic review of delay in the diagnosis and treatment of tuberculosis. *BMC Public Health.* 2008:8:15.

33. Harries AD, Zachariah R, Corbett EL, et al. The HIV-associated tuberculosis epidemic: when will we act? *Lancet.* 2010;375:1906–1919.
34. Velayati AA, Masjedi MR, Farnia P, et al. Emergence of new forms of totally drug-resistant tuberculosis bacilli: super extensively drug-resistant tuberculosis or totally drug-resistant strains in Iran. *Chest.* 2009;136:420–425.
35. Colditz GA, Brewer TF, Berkey CS, et al. Efficacy of BCG vaccine in the prevention of tuberculosis: meta-analysis of the published literature. *JAMA.* 1994;27:698–702.
36. *Stop TB Partnership annual report 2010.* Geneva: WHO; 2010.
37. *World malaria report 2011.* Geneva: WHO; 2011.
38. Yasuoka J, Levins R. Impact of deforestation and agricultural development on anopheline ecology and malaria epidemiology. *Am J Trop Med Hyg.* 2007;76:450–460.
39. Idro R, Jenkins NE, Newton CR. Pathogenesis, clinical features, and neurological outcomes of cerebral malaria. *Lancet Neuro.* 2005;4:827–840.
40. Doolan DL, Dobaño C, Baird JK. Acquired immunity to malaria. *Clin Microbiol Rev.* 2009;22:13–36.
41. Desai M, ter Kuile FO, Nosten F, et al. Epidemiology and burden of malaria in pregnancy. *Lancet Infect Dis.* 2007;7:93–104.
42. Cibulskis RE, Aregawi M, Williams R, Otten M, Dye C. Worldwide incidence of malaria in 2009: estimates, time trends, and a critique of methods. *PLoS Med.* 2011;8:e1001142.
43. Sachs J, Malaney P. The economic and social burden of malaria. *Nature.* 2002;415:680–685.
44. Hay SI, Guerra CA, Tatam AJ, Noor AM, Snow RW. The global distribution and population at risk of malaria: past, present and future. *Lancet Infect Dis.* 2004;4:327–336.
45. Mendis K, Rietveld A, Warsame M, Bosman A, Greenwood B, Wernsdorfer WH. From malaria control to eradication: the WHO perspective. *Trop Med Int Health.* 2009;14:802–809.
46. Plowe CV. The evolution of drug-resistant malaria. *Trans R Soc Trop Med Hyg.* 2009;103(Suppl 10):S11–S14.
47. *Guidelines for the treatment of malaria, 2nd edition.* Geneva: WHO; 2010.
48. Lengeler C. Insecticide-treated bed nets and curtains for preventing malaria. *Cochrane Database Syst Rev.* 2004;(2):CD000363.
49. WHO Global Malaria Program. *Insecticide-treated mosquito nets: a WHO position statement.* Geneva: WHO; 2007.
50. Barat LM, Palmer N, Basu S, Worrall E, Hanson K, Mills A. Do malaria control interventions reach the poor? A view through the equity lens. *Am J Trop Med Hyg.* 2004;71(2 suppl):174–178.
51. *Roll Back Malaria global strategic plan 2005–2015.* Geneva: WHO; 2005.
52. Sachs JD. A new global effort to control malaria. *Science.* 2002;298:122–124.
53. Brundage JF, Shanks G. Deaths from bacterial pneumonia during the 1918–19 influenza pandemic. *Emerg Infect Dis.* 2008;14:1193–1199.
54. Novel Swine-Origin Influenza A (H1N1) Virus Investigation Team; Dawood FS, Jain S, et al. Emergence of a novel swine-origin influenza A (H1N1) virus in humans. *N Engl J Med.* 2009;360:2605–2615.
55. Gostin LO. Influenza A(H1N1) and pandemic preparedness under the rule of international law. *JAMA.* 2009;301:2376–2378.

56. Girard MP, Tam JS, Assossou OM, Kieny MP. The 2009 A (H1N1) influenza virus pandemic: a review. *Vaccine*. 2010;28:4895–4902.

57. Polio Global Eradication Initiative. *Annual report 2010*. Geneva: WHO; 2011.

58. *GAVI Alliance progress report 2010*. Washington DC: GAVI Alliance; 2010.

59. The Carter Center. *Annual report 2009–10*. Atlanta GA: The Carter Center; 2010.

60. Molyneux DH. The 'Neglected Tropical Diseases': now a brand identity; responsibilities, context and promise. *Parasit Vectors*. 2012;5:23.

CHAPTER 11

Global Nutrition

A nutritious diet is essential for health. In low-income regions, undernutrition due to too few calories, vitamins, and minerals is a major contributor to morbidity and mortality. In high- and middle-income countries, obesity is a significant and growing public health concern.

11.1 ESSENTIAL NUTRIENTS

Every person needs to eat on a regular basis to provide his or her body with energy and the materials needed to build and repair cells and tissues, fight infections, and stay warm. The body requires **macronutrients** such as carbohydrates, protein, and fats and oils in relatively large quantities because they provide energy. Small amounts of **micronutrients** like vitamins and minerals are also needed. This chapter begins with an overview of the nutrients that all people need, and then discusses the problems associated with taking in too few or too many calories and nutrients. Diseases associated with undernutrition and diseases associated with obesity are both major global health problems.

11.2 MACRONUTRIENTS

Carbohydrates are found in cereal grains like rice, maize, and wheat (the three most common staple foods in the world), in starchy roots like potatoes and yams, and in fruits and vegetables. Carbohydrates (also called **saccharides**) are chains of sugars. When the body requires a quick source of energy, the body's cells break down carbohydrates through a process called cellular respiration. Simple carbohydrates are made up of very short chains of sugars and are easily absorbed into the bloodstream. The lactose found in milk and the glucose and fructose found in fruits and honey are all simple sugars. Table sugar, or sucrose, is a disaccharide ("two sugar") composed of glucose and fructose. Complex carbohydrates (often classified as starches), such as those found in whole grain products like whole wheat bread and oatmeal, are made up of longer chains of sugars (polysaccharides) and take longer to digest, which is why eating complex carbohydrates keeps a person from feeling hungry longer than eating simple sugars. Fiber, found in unprocessed plant-based foods, is another type of carbohydrate and is essential for healthy digestion because it provides bulk that moves food material through the intestines. Nutritionists recommend that for most people 45% to 65% of calories taken in over a day should come from carbohydrates.[1]

Proteins are chains of **amino acids**. Amino acids from food are broken down and reassembled in the cells to form new proteins. The keratin that makes up hair and nails, the hemoglobin in blood that transports oxygen, the antibodies that help the body's immune system recognize and fight infection, the actin and myosin that contract and relax muscles, and the collagen in ligaments, tendons, and skin are all types of proteins. There are more than 20 different kinds of amino acids. Humans are unable to produce eight of these amino acids, and must acquire those **essential amino acids** from food. Proteins from animal-based foods are usually **complete proteins** that contain all of the essential amino acids. Plant proteins are usually incomplete proteins, but eating a diverse diet with a variety of **complementary proteins** like maize (corn) with beans or nuts and whole wheat bread can provide all of the amino acids in one meal. Nutritionists generally recommend that for most people 10% to 35% of daily calories should come from high-quality proteins.[1] In some regions of the world the typical diet includes too little protein, and this can cause health problems (**Figure 11–1**).[2]

Fats and oils are both types of **lipids**, or fatty acids, which are carbon-hydrogen chains with other chemical groups at the ends of the chains. **Fats** are lipids of animal origin like butter and lard that are solid at room temperature. **Oils** are lipids of plant origin like corn oil and olive oil that are liquids at room temperature. Lipids contain more energy per gram than any other biological molecule and provide long-term energy storage, insulation, protective padding around internal organs, and assistance with nutrient absorption. They are needed for the processing of some vitamins (A, D, E, and K), and are used by the body to make other compounds, such as steroid hormones (chemical messengers). Nutritionists recommend that about 20% to 35% of calories consumed in a day should come from healthy fats and oils.[1] In some parts of

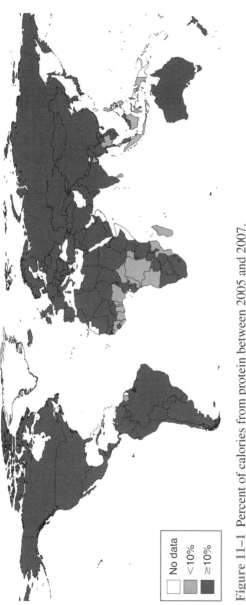
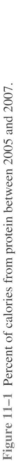

Figure 11–1 Percent of calories from protein between 2005 and 2007.

Source: Data from Food and Agriculture Organization (FAO) of the United Nations. *FAO statistical yearbook 2012.* Rome: FAO; 2012. Table 16: Dietary energy supplies and changes in dietary composition.

the world the average person takes in too few calories from fats and oils, while in other places the average daily intake far exceeds the recommended amount (**Figure 11–2**).[2]

Not all fatty acids are equally healthy. The relative healthiness of lipids is often related to the amount of hydrogen they contain. Unsaturated fatty acids contain at least one double bond in the carbon chain. Both monounsaturated fats like those found in olive oil, avocados, and nuts and the polyunsaturated fats in cold water fish like salmon (which contain omega-3 fatty acids) seem to be protective against heart disease.[3] Saturated fatty acids are found in meat, butter, and other animal products and can contribute to blocked arteries. The term **saturated fatty acid** refers to the fact that the molecule is "saturated" with hydrogen, meaning that no more hydrogen can be added to it because only single bonds exist between its carbon atoms. **Trans fats**, liquid oils that have been transformed into solid fats by adding hydrogen to them through the use of pressure, are found in margarine and processed foods and have been shown to raise "bad" (or "*l*ousy") LDL (low-density lipoprotein) cholesterol while depleting "good" (or "*h*ealthy") HDL (high-density lipoprotein) cholesterol. When the LDL/HDL ratio is high, the excess fat in the blood is deposited on the walls of blood vessels as plaque.[4] When there is a lot of plaque lining the blood vessels, the resulting atherosclerosis increases the risk of having a heart attack or stroke.

Water, though not a nutrient, is also an essential part of the diet. Every cell in the body needs a way to take in oxygen and nutrients along with a way to get rid of carbon dioxide and waste. Blood, which is about 92% water, is the medium for transporting gases, nutrients, and wastes throughout the body. Without adequate blood volume—without adequate water in the body—blood pressure drops and it is difficult for the body's cells to function. A person who loses a lot of blood due to an injury or a lot of water due to excessive vomiting or diarrhea can go into hypovolemic shock, shock caused by too little blood volume. Water also helps the body regulate its temperature by sweating and helps the body get rid of waste through urination and defecation. An adult loses about 2 to 3 quarts of water a day by urinating, sweating, and exhaling humidified air. More may be lost in hot climates, during intense physical activity, or when a person has diarrhea. This lost water must be replaced to avoid dehydration. Severe dehydration can cause an imbalance of the acids and bases in the blood, loss of muscle tone, organ failure (especially of the kidneys), and death.

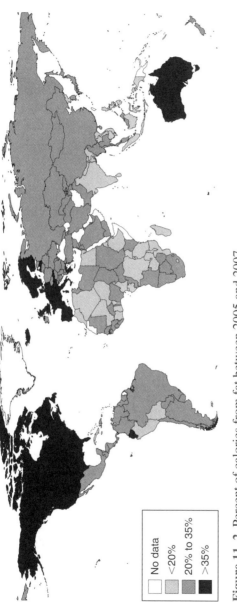

Figure 11–2 Percent of calories from fat between 2005 and 2007.

Source: Data from Food and Agriculture Organization (FAO) of the United Nations. *FAO statistical yearbook 2012.* Rome: FAO; 2012. Table 16: Dietary energy supplies and changes in dietary composition.

11.3 MICRONUTRIENTS

Vitamins act as regulators and help the body use energy. There are more than a dozen vitamins necessary for health, and most of them must be included in the diet. For example, folate (or folic acid) must be ingested daily because the chemical is not able to be stored by the body. Folic acid is necessary for growth and red blood cell production. Women of child-bearing age need to make sure that they have an adequate intake of folic acid, because deficiency during the first weeks of pregnancy is associated with neural tube defects in developing fetuses. (The most common neural tube defects are anencephaly, a fatal condition in which the brain fails to develop, and spina bifida, in which the spinal cord does not develop properly.) These defects occur very early in the pregnancy, usually before a woman knows she is pregnant, so it is recommended that all women who might become pregnant take a multivitamin. Vitamin C is another vitamin that must be part of the diet. It is an antioxidant that reduces free radicals (ions in the cells that may damage cell membranes), and it helps the body absorb iron and create collagen, which is essential for maintaining healthy gums, skin, and other tissues. A few vitamins can be produced by the body. For example, vitamin D, which is essential for bone strength, can be made by the body when the skin is exposed to sunlight (though some individuals require supplemental vitamin D in order to reach the recommended blood levels for the vitamin). **Table 11–1** summarizes the main functions of key vitamins and the problems that may occur when a person is vitamin deficient, such as pellagra, beriberi, scurvy, rickets, and osteomalacia.

Minerals help the body to build strong bones, transmit nerve signals, and maintain a normal heart rate, among other critical functions. Minerals like calcium, phosphorus, magnesium, sulfur, chloride, copper, selenium, and manganese must be taken in through the diet. Some minerals, like zinc, promote growth and wound healing. Others, like sodium and potassium, are electrolytes that contribute to maintaining blood chemistry, blood pressure, and, in the case of potassium, a regular heartbeat. Fluoride is essential for the development of strong teeth and bones, so some communities add fluoride to drinking water to ensure that children have an adequate intake of the mineral. As with any nutrient, either a deficiency or an excess of minerals can be harmful. Some people develop problems by overdosing on vitamin and mineral supplements. Others add too much salt to their foods, and excess sodium can increase the risk of high blood pressure in some adults. Even fluoride, which has dramatically improved

Table 11–1 Vitamin nutrients.

Vitamin	Key Function(s)	Problems of Deficiency
Biotin (vitamin B_7)	Metabolism	Skin rash; mental changes
Folate (vitamin B_9)	Cell production	Anemia; neural tube defects in babies born to mothers who are deficient
Niacin (vitamin B_3)	Metabolism; skin health; digestive and nervous system function	*Pellagra*: dark, peeling rash on skin exposed to sun; diarrhea; mental changes
Pantothenic acid (vitamin B_5)	Metabolism; red blood cell production	Paresthesia (numbness and tingling of limbs)
Pyridoxine (vitamin B_6)	Cell production	Anemia; seizures
Riboflavin (vitamin B_2)	Metabolism; skin and eye health	Cracked lips; mouth and throat sores; scaly skin
Thiamine (vitamin B_1)	Metabolism; nerve function	*Beriberi*: weakness; heart arrhythmias; heart failure
Vitamin A (retinol + carotene)	Eye, skin, and bone health; immune system function	Increased susceptibility to infection and death; night blindness; blindness
Vitamin B_{12}	Cell production	Anemia; mental changes
Vitamin C (ascorbic acid)	Collagen formation; metabolism; immune system function; antioxidant	*Scurvy*: bone pain; bleeding gums and loose tooth
Vitamin D	Bone growth and health	*Rickets* (in children): bowed legs or knock knees, spinal deformities, swollen bones in wrists, muscle weakness; *osteomalacia* (in adults): bone pain, fractures, muscle weakness
Vitamin E	Antioxidant	Anemia
Vitamin K	Blood clotting	Bleeding disorders

dental health, can cause weak bones and teeth if excess fluoride (fluorosis) replaces some of the calcium in teeth, stains teeth brown, and causes teeth to become pitted or break. Table 11–2 summarizes the main functions of key minerals and the problems associated with mineral deficiencies.

Table 11–2 Mineral nutrients.

Mineral	Key Function(s)	Problems of Deficiency
Calcium	Bone growth and health; blood production; muscle and heart function	Muscle cramps; heart arrhythmias; osteoporosis
Chloride	Cell function; digestive function	Electrolyte imbalance
Chromium	Glucose tolerance	Impaired glucose tolerance
Copper	Red blood cell production	Anemia
Fluorine	Formation and health of bones and teeth	Weak tooth enamel; dental caries (cavities); weak bones
Iodine	Making thyroid hormones that support growth and metabolism	Goiter (enlarged thyroid gland in neck); cretinism (a physical and mental developmental disorder); hypothyroidism (low energy, feeling cold, dry skin, constipation); impaired fetal development
Iron	Red blood cell production	Anemia and related fatigue
Magnesium	Bone health; heart, muscle, and nerve function; immune system function	Muscle weakness; heart arrhythmias; mental changes
Manganese	Cell function	Not known
Molybdenum	Cell function	Heart arrhythmias
Phosphorus	Bone growth and health	Muscle weakness; mental changes
Potassium	Cell function; muscle and nerve function	Fatigue; weakness; heart arrhythmias
Selenium	Cell function	Fatigue; weakness
Sodium	Cell function; muscle and nerve function	Muscle weakness; nausea; mental changes
Zinc	Child growth and development; healthy skin	Slow growth; slow wound healing; diarrhea

11.4 MEASURING NUTRITIONAL STATUS

Anthropometry is the measurement of the human body. Height, weight, waist circumference, body fat percentage, and other measurements can be useful indicators of whether a person is underweight or overweight. They can also be used to predict some health risks. For example, having a waist circumference greater than 35 inches for a woman or 40 inches for a man is associated with an increased risk of diabetes and heart disease.[5]

The **body mass index (BMI)** is often used to estimate the body composition of adults. The BMI is calculated by taking weight in kilograms and dividing it by the square of the height in meters.

$$BMI = \frac{weight\ (kg)}{height\ (m) \times height\ (m)} = 703 \times \frac{weight\ (lb)}{height\ (in) \times height\ (in)}$$

International classification schemes generally suggest that a BMI of less than 18.5 indicates underweight, a BMI of 18.5 to 25 is in the "normal" range, a BMI of greater than 25 indicates overweight, and a BMI greater than 30 indicates obesity.[6] The BMI has several limitations as a measure of health status. One is that the BMI does not consider the effect of body fat, so people who are trim but have a lot of muscle mass may be incorrectly classified as overweight. BMI also does not measure physical fitness levels, and people with "normal" weights may have poor cardiovascular endurance.

For children, the more accurate measures of healthy growth are weight-for-height, weight-for-age, and height-for-age. Additional measures, such as a child's arm circumference-for-age (the mid-upper arm circumference, or MUAC) and the child's head circumference-for-age, can also be useful for assessing growth.[7] Global growth standards for children from birth through 60 months are provided by the World Health Organization.[8] These growth charts can be used worldwide because scientific evidence shows that infants and children from geographically diverse regions experience very similar growth patterns when their health and nutritional needs are met.[9] However, one limitation of many growth standards for children is that they require caregivers to know the birth date of the child, and many children born at home or orphaned do not have a record of this date. When this information is not available, it can be difficult to determine if a child is growing well.

Figure 11–3 shows a sample weight-for-age chart for girls. The graph has age (in months) on the *x*-axis and weight (in pounds) on the *y*-axis. The graph allows a parent or healthcare worker to easily determine if a child of a particular age is underweight (below the 15th percentile) or severely

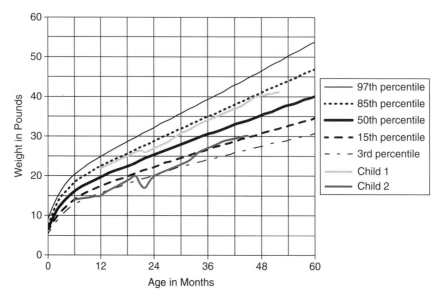

Figure 11–3 A sample child growth chart showing weight-for-age for girls from birth to age 5.

Source: Data for growth standards and percentile curves from WHO Child Growth Standards. *Length/height-for-age, weight-for-age, weight-for-length, weight-for-height and body mass index-for-age: methods and development.* Geneva: WHO; 2006.

underweight (under the 3rd percentile) for his or her age. The sample curve for "Child 1" shows a child of healthy weight. The sample curve for "Child 2" shows an underweight child. Both children lost weight just before their second birthdays, probably due to diarrheal disease. For "Child 1," this was a minor event that barely influenced her growth. For "Child 2," this bout of diarrhea pushed her into severe malnutrition and could easily have caused her death. Children should be weighed often, especially when they are very young, so that growth trends can emerge. A child like "Child 2" who loses weight or fails to gain weight needs extra medical attention.

11.5 UNDERNUTRITION

Undernutrition is malnutrition resulting from deficiencies in the amount of food or types of nutrients eaten or from poor absorption of the nutrients that have been consumed. For example, lack of protein in the diet means that the body does not have the amino acids it needs to repair itself, and too little fat in the diet means that fat-soluble vitamins (like vitamins A, D, and E) cannot be processed. To stay healthy, every human needs a diet that includes at least some carbohydrates, proteins, fats or oils, and a variety of vitamins and minerals. The total amount of energy, protein, and other nutrients needed by a person varies based on age, sex, body size, activity level, climate, and pregnancy and lactation status.

Many babies begin life undernourished, often as a result of their mothers being undernourished when they became pregnant and not taking in adequate nutritients during pregnancy.[10] **Low birthweight (LBW)** babies have an increased risk of breathing problems and other potentially life-threatening difficulties during their first weeks of life, and some of these children develop long-term impairments like learning disabilities, cerebral palsy, mental retardation, and visual or hearing impairment, especially if they have a very low birth weight.[11]

Undernourished children may have **stunting** (low height for age) and **wasting** (low weight for height). Some children develop **kwashiorkor** and have **edema** (swelling) of the arms, legs, and face; weak muscles; and pale hair and skin. Children with kwashiorkor may maintain a moderate weight and have a swollen belly. This is not because they are "fat." Instead, their nutrient-deficient bodies are retaining fluids (causing excess body weight) and the abdominal walls are so weak that the internal organs sag out. Kwashiorkor often develops in children who have been weaned early (frequently because of the birth of a younger sibling) and have a diet high in starch but low in protein. A child who has severe **protein-energy malnutrition (PEM)** may develop a condition called **marasmus** that is associated with very low weight, weakness, and the eventual shutdown of body systems. Children with marasmus look skeletal, have loose and wrinkled skin, and have too little energy to move or cry. Both marasmus and kwashiorkor increase susceptibility to infection and put children at risk for permanent disability and death.[12]

Even mild and moderate undernutrition can significantly increase the risk of illness and death due to diarrhea, acute respiratory infections, malaria, and measles.[13] At least one in five deaths of under-5 children can be attributed to undernutrition.[14] To reduce the risk of mortality, children with **severe acute malnutrition (SAM)** often require inpatient hospital care or intensive outpatient care as they receive therapeutic nutrition in the form of energy-dense, nutrient-enriched food (sometimes called "ready-to-use therapeutic food," or RUTF) and treatment for co-morbid infections.[15]

The statistics on childhood hunger are very concerning. About 42% of children in South Asia, 20% in sub-Saharan Africa, 11% in the Middle East and North Africa, and 10% in East Asia and the Pacific are moderately or severely underweight.[16] In total, more than 100 million children under 5 years of age worldwide are underweight (**Figure 11–4**),[17] including nearly 80 million children in Asia and 30 million in Africa.[14]

Undernutrition is closely associated with poverty. Poor children are much more likely than rich children to be underweight, and poverty creates a cycle of malnutrition and infectious disease that is hard to break. This can have long-term consequences. Adults who were undernourished as children tend to be shorter, less educated, less economically productive, and more likely to have LBW babies than adults who were not underfed in childhood.[18] And adults with reduced nutritional status, especially older adults, are at risk of decreased productivity and functioning, which can have a further negative effect on their children and families.[19]

11.6 HUNGER AND FOOD SECURITY

Food security exists when a household, or a larger population, has access to enough food that its residents can be healthy and productive at all times. Access to food means that individuals and households are able to produce, purchase, or otherwise acquire an adequate quantity, quality, and variety of food during the entire year.[20] In other words, food security is about the distribution and affordability of food as much as it is about food production. Residents of lower-income countries tend to spend a higher proportion of their incomes on food than those who live in higher-income countries (**Figure 11–5**).[21] Similarly, low-income households within a country usually spend a higher proportion of their resources on food than richer families do,[22] but they may still not be able to access enough safe, nutrient-rich food.[23]

Although some food insecurity issues are caused by natural and humanitarian disasters, most food insecurity is the result of chronic poverty. Households may experience long-term food insecurity, or they may have seasonal insecurity between growing seasons or during periods of underemployment or illness. Food insecurity exists in both low-income and high-income countries. For example, in the United States about 14.5% of households were food insecure at some point during 2010.[24] Many rural areas and low-income urban areas in the United States are said to be **food deserts** with very limited access to healthy food.[25] Members of food

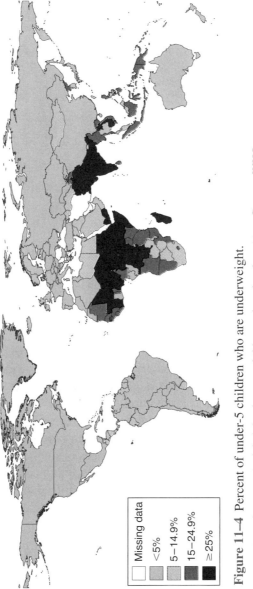

Figure 11–4 Percent of under-5 children who are underweight.

Source: Data from *WHO global database on child growth and malnutrition.* Geneva: WHO.

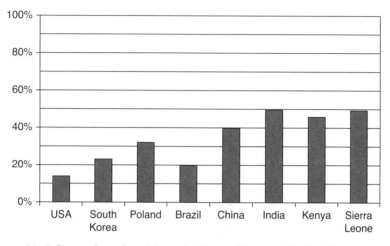

Figure 11–5 Proportion of total household spending used for food between 2006 and 2008

Source: Data from *Food security statistics by country*. Rome: FAO; 2010 October.

insecure households may report feeling hungry but not eating, worrying that their food will run out, running out of food and not having enough money to buy more, eating only a limited variety of low-cost foods, cutting the size of meals, skipping meals, and not eating for a whole day.[26]

During times of widespread hunger or **famine,** a large proportion of a population has very low food security for an extended period of time, often leading to mass migration and death. Famines are partially attributable to demographics (such as population growth) and environmental factors (such as drought), but are also due to economic and political situations. Food shortages may occur because of reduced food production, but they also happen because of increased food prices or interruptions in the food supply chain that transports food from producers to consumers. To quote Amartya Sen, a Nobel Prize–winning economist from India, "starvation is a matter of some people not *having* enough food to eat, and not a matter of there *being* not enough food to eat."[27]

As the world population increases and available croplands shrink, crop yields will have to increase to meet demand. The best way to ensure that everyone is food secure is to increase food production while also increasing environmental protection.[28] This means developing new agricultural techniques or choosing to use time-tested techniques such as crop rotation that cause as little damage to the environment as possible and also

increase yields. Food supplies can be further maximized whe
food as possible is wasted, eaten by animals, or allowed to spoil during
transportation and storage. Food distribution systems need to be strengthened so that those who are unable to produce enough food for their
families have access to surplus food produced by others. Additionally,
trade policies that make it attractive for growers to produce crops for local
consumption rather than export may also help alleviate hunger.[29]

11.7 MICRONUTRIENT DEFICIENCIES

Good nutrition requires more than just sufficient caloric intake. It also
requires a balanced diet that includes all the essential micronutrients.
Vitamin and mineral deficiencies are a common form of undernutrition in
both children and adults. A large proportion of the world's population is
at risk of iron, iodine, vitamin A, and zinc deficiencies. Most people with
severe micronutrient deficiencies live in developing countries, but there are
also pockets of micronutrient deficiencies in some high-income populations
because of dietary habits.

Some vitamin deficiencies have relatively immediate symptoms. A person with too little niacin, which is important for metabolism, will develop
pellagra and have his or her skin darken and slough off. A person with too
little riboflavin will develop rough skin and cracked lips. Thiamine deficiency causes **beriberi**, which can damage the heart and nervous system.
Too little vitamin C causes **scurvy**, which is characterized by bleeding
gums and swollen, painful joints, and decreased immune system function.

Other vitamin and mineral deficiencies have long-term consequences.
Adolescents who consume too little calcium are at risk for developing
osteoporosis as they age, and porous bones can lead to hip fractures and
other life-threatening injuries later in life. Bone strength is also reliant
upon sufficient vitamin D. Vitamin D deficiency in children whose bones
are still growing is called **rickets** (or, more informally, "knock knees").
Vitamin D deficiency in adults whose bones have stopped growing is
called **osteomalacia** and can make the bones soft and prone to breaking.
Vitamin D, the "sun vitamin," can be made in the skin if it is exposed to
sunlight for about 15 minutes daily, but deficiency is a problem in parts
of the world where women are expected to cover themselves in public, in
people who work indoors all day and avoid sun exposure, and seasonally
among people who live far from the equator and have months of darkness
each year.[30]

11.7.A Vitamin A Deficiency (VAD)

Vitamin A deficiency (VAD) is one of the most common causes of pre-ventable blindness in children.[31] Vision problems associated with VAD are related to severe dry eye (**xerophthalmia**), which can progress from night blindness and Bitot's spots (dry patches on the white of the eye) to ulcer-ation and scarring of the cornea (keratomalacia) and then complete blind-ness. Worldwide, about 190 million under-5 children (one-third of children living in countries with a per capita annual GDP less than $15,000) and 20 million pregnant women (about 15% of pregnant women in those countries) have VAD.[32] About 5 million under-5 children **(Figure 11–6)**—or nearly 1% of preschool-age children in low- and middle-income countries—and 10 million pregnant women (about 8% of pregnant women in those coun-tries) have VAD-associated night blindness.[32] Vitamin A also supports the body's immune system in fighting infections, and VAD increases the risk of dying from measles, diarrhea, and other causes.[33,34]

Yellow, orange, and dark green vegetables are the best dietary sources of vitamin A (in addition to some animal sources, such as liver). Because vitamin A is fat soluble and will only be absorbed by the body if it is eaten with fats or oils, dietary prevention of VAD requires a consistent source of both vegetables and oil. In some countries, milk, sugar, or other com-mercial products are fortified with vitamin A, but fortified foods are not

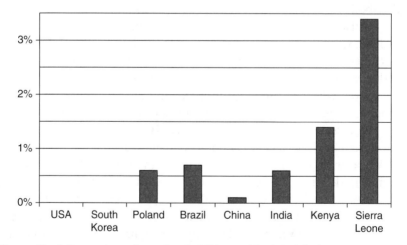

Figure 11–6 Proportion of preschool children with night blindness due to vitamin A deficiency between 1995 and 2005.

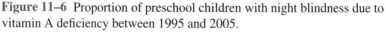

Source: Data from *Global prevalence of vitamin A deficiency in populations at risk 1995–2005: WHO global database on vitamin A deficiency*. Geneva: WHO; 2009.

available to all households that need them. Oil-filled vitamin A capsule supplements are relatively inexpensive and have prevented hundreds of thousands of child deaths and many cases of blindness,[35] but distribution can be a challenge, especially because the benefits of the capsules only last for 4 to 6 months. Some high-tech options are also available or in development. For example, "golden rice" is a genetically modified organism (GMO) that has been altered to produce the vitamin A precursor beta-carotene.[36] Golden rice is not yet widely used, in part because of concerns by some countries about allowing GMO products to be grown, but the manufacturer grants free licenses to low-income growers and humanitarian organizations.[37]

11.7.B Iodine Deficiency Disorders (IDD)

Iodine deficiency disorders (IDD) are among the most common causes of impaired cognitive function in the world.[38] The thyroid gland, located in the neck, controls body **metabolism** (the rate at which a person's body uses energy) and assists with growth. Thyroid hormones (chemical messengers that control metabolism) are made from the mineral iodine. If there is too little iodine in the diet, there is not enough iodine in the blood for the thyroid gland to function properly. In response, the thyroid gland will enlarge as it tries to collect more iodine from the blood, and it will produce a **goiter** (a swollen neck resulting from an enlarged thyroid gland). A person who cannot produce enough thyroid hormones (**hypothyroidism**) will have a low metabolism and will feel cold, tired, and apathetic. Babies born to mothers who have hypothyroidism may be stillborn or be born with a type of brain damage called **cretinism**. Adults and children who are iodine deficient often suffer from impaired mental function. About 30% of the world's population is estimated to have insufficient iodine intake.[39] Iodized salt is a cost-efficient way to reduce IDD, but only about two-thirds of the world's population is covered, and commercial salt may not reach the neediest households.[40]

11.7.C Iron Deficiency Anemia (IDA)

Red blood cells (RBCs) carry oxygen from the lungs to the rest of the cells in the body. A molecule called hemoglobin holds the oxygen inside the RBCs, and hemoglobin is made from iron. A person with too little iron is not able to make enough RBCs to efficiently transport oxygen. Symptoms of **anemia** include pale skin, fatigue, weakness, shortness of breath, headaches, an increased heart rate, and a limited ability to concentrate at work or school. When an insufficient number of RBCs is due to inadequate iron intake, this condition is called **iron deficiency anemia (IDA)**. (Other forms of anemia may be due to vitamin B12 or folic acid deficiency, blood loss, inadequate production of RBCs, or infections that destroy RBCs.)

IDA is the most common nutritional disorder in the world, affecting about 25% of the world's population (about 1.6 billion people), including about 50% of under-5 children (**Figure 11–7**), 40% of pregnant women, and 30% of nonpregnant women.[41,42] Children, pregnant women, and women who menstruate are at high risk for IDA. Children need extra iron as their body grows and their blood volume increases, pregnant women need extra iron as their blood volume expands and to reduce the risk of dying during childbirth,[43] and menstruating women and those who have recently given birth may have depleted RBCs and iron from blood loss.

IDA can be prevented and treated through increased iron intake. Iron is found in both plant and animal sources. Heme iron is found in blood and meat from animals, birds, and fish, and about 15% to 35% is absorbed by the body; nonheme iron is found in plants, eggs, and milk,

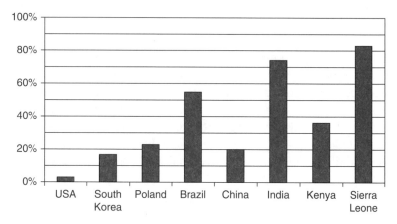

Figure 11–7 Proportion of preschool children with anemia (Hb <100 g/L) in 2006.

Source: Data from de Benoist B, McLean Erin, Egli I, Cogswell, editors. *Worldwide prevalence of anaemia 1993–2005*. Geneva: WHO; 2008.

and less than 5% is absorbed.[44] Iron can also be taken as a supplement or added to fortified foods like pastas and flours.[45] Control of infections that cause internal bleeding (like hookworm, whipworm, and schistosomiasis) or destruction of RBCs (like malaria) is also important for preventing and treating IDA.

11.7.D Zinc Deficiency

Zinc is important for immune function, growth, and child development. Any level of zinc deficiency can increase susceptibility to infection and increase the risk of death from diarrhea, malaria, and pneumonia. Several hundred thousand under-5 child deaths from these infections could potentially be prevented each year by reducing zinc deficiency in Africa and Asia.[46] Zinc is found primarily in animal sources, so people who consume a mostly plant-based diet often benefit from taking zinc supplements or eating food fortified with zinc.

11.7.E Preventing Micronutrient Deficiencies

The best way to consume micronutrients is through food. When a person's diet does not provide enough nutrients or the body is not absorbing enough of the nutrients, nonfood sources may be helpful (**Table 11–3**).[47] Micronutrient deficiencies in a population can sometimes be prevented by providing **supplements** such as multivitamin pills or by enriching or fortifying food with extra micronutrients. A food is **enriched** when some of the vitamins and minerals lost during processing are added back into the food. A **fortified** food has nutrients that are not naturally present in the ingredients added to the product. Common examples of enriched and fortified foods include vitamin A fortified sugar, folic acid and iron-enriched flours, and iodized salt. However, supplements and enriched and fortified foods may not provide vitamins and minerals in a form that has a high bioavailability. **Bioavailability** is the fraction of the vitamin or mineral consumed that is able to be absorbed and used by the body. Absorption can be increased by taking supplements with food. For example, fat-soluble vitamins must be taken with fat or oil, and iron absorption is boosted by vitamin C.

Table 11–3 Preventive and treatment interventions for maternal and child undernutrition.

Preventive Interventions (Primary Prevention)	Treatment Interventions (Secondary Prevention)
• Improved dietary intake of pregnant and lactating women	• Treatment and monitoring of severely malnourished children
• Exclusive breastfeeding for 6 months	• High-dose treatment of clinical signs of vitamin A deficiency
• Appropriate complementary child feeding for 6- to 24-month-old children	• Appropriate feeding of sick children
• Iron and folic acid supplementation for children to prevent anemia	• Oral rehydration therapy (ORT)
• Vitamin A supplementation for pregnant women and children	• Timely treatment of infectious and parasitic diseases
• Antihelminthic treatment of school-age children to prevent anemia	
• Improved hygiene and sanitation to prevent diarrhea	

Source: Information from Jamison DT, Breman JG, Measham AR, et al., editors. *Disease control priorities in developing countries*, 2nd edition. Washington DC: Oxford University Press and IBRD/World Bank; 2006.

11.8 OVERWEIGHT AND OBESITY

Overnutrition is a form of malnutrition caused by excessive intake of calories and nutrients. The average adult needs about 1800 kilocalories each day, with additional calories required for physical activity (and, if applicable, for pregnancy and lactation).[48] A person who consistently takes in more calories than the body uses will gain extra weight, become overweight, and then develop obesity (**Figures 11–8** and **11–9**). Obesity is associated with an increased risk for many diseases, including type 2 diabetes, hypertension (high blood pressure), heart disease, strokes, gallstones and other digestive disorders, back pain, arthritis of the back and hip, and several types of cancer.[49]

Overnutrition has become a concern in nearly every region of the world. Even in regions where undernutrition is still a serious problem, there are

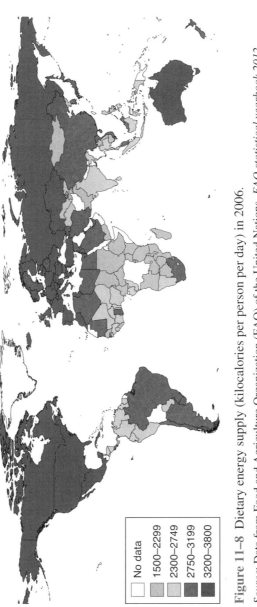

Figure 11–8 Dietary energy supply (kilocalories per person per day) in 2006.

Source: Data from Food and Agriculture Organization (FAO) of the United Nations. *FAO statistical yearbook 2012.* Rome: FAO; 2012. Table 16: Dietary energy supplies and changes in dietary composition.

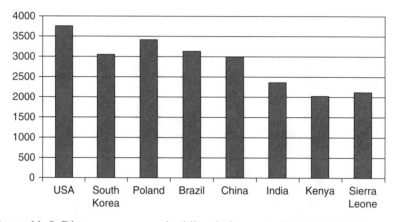

Figure 11–9 Dietary energy supply (kilocalories per person per day) between 2006 and 2008.

Source: Data from *Food security statistics by country*. Rome: FAO; 2010 October.

pockets of obesity, especially in high-income urban areas and among women.[50] In 2005, about 23% of adults worldwide were overweight or obese (**Figures 11–10** and **11–11**).[51–53] The global prevalence of adult obesity increased from about 5% of men and 8% of women in 1980 to about 10% of men and 14% of women in 2008.[54] But obesity is not just a condition of adulthood. In 2010, about 12% of under-5 children in developed countries and 6% of children in developing countries were overweight or obese.[55] The prevalence of overweight and obesity among children less than 5 years old worldwide increased from about 4% in 1990 to about 7% in 2010, and is projected to reach 9% by 2020.[55] The rate of overweight and obesity is also increasing significantly among school-aged children in nearly every region in the world.[56]

Genes influence metabolic rate, body shape (where a person carries excess weight), and the efficiency of the body at storing extra calories, but genetic change does not explain why obesity has become so much more prevalent in the past decade. It takes generations for genetic adaptation to occur, but it takes only a short time to change dietary and exercise habits. Thus, nutritional status is a function of biology and also of psychology and sociology. Nutritional science studies that use laboratory tests to quantify the amount of calories and types of nutrients in foods only explain part of the rise in obesity and other forms of malnutrition. These studies must be complemented by examinations of food preparation and eating habits and evaluations of the

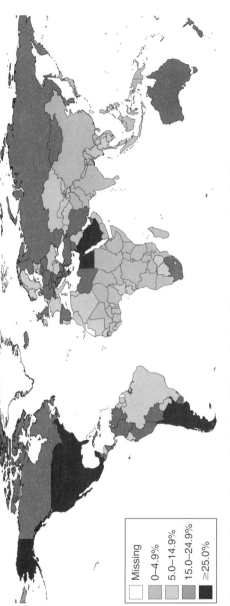

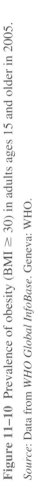

Figure 11–10 Prevalence of obesity (BMI ≥ 30) in adults ages 15 and older in 2005.

Source: Data from *WHO Global InfoBase.* Geneva: WHO.

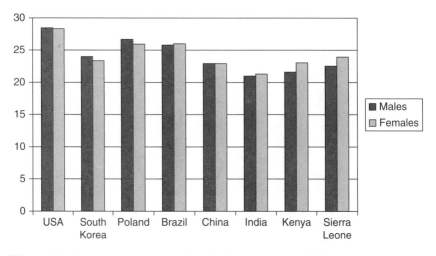

Figure 11–11 Mean age-standardized body mass index (BMI) of male and female adults ages 20 and older in 2008.

Source: Data from Global Burden of Metabolic Risk Factors of Chronic Diseases Collaborating Group. *Country trends in metabolic risk factors*. London: Imperial College London; 2011.

cultural and social aspects of eating, as these factors are significant contributors to the rising prevalence of obesity around the world.

Individuals and families who seek to reach and maintain target weights must adopt and sustain healthy behaviors. At the population level, policies that promote healthy diets and physical activity, such as health information campaigns, limits on the marketing of unhealthy food to children, taxes to increase the price of unhealthy foods, subsidies to lower the cost of healthy foods, and regulations that improve the nutrition information provided on food packages, may help prevent and reduce obesity.[57]

11.9 DISCUSSION QUESTIONS

1. What components of your diet are sources of essential nutrients like carbohydrates, proteins, fats, vitamins, and minerals? Do you get more or less than the recommended amounts in each category?
2. Design a one-day menu plan that provides healthy amounts of macronutrients, micronutrients, and energy.
3. Do you take vitamin and mineral supplements? Why or why not?

4. What governmental agencies and nongovernmental organizations in your community work to address issues of local hunger and food insecurity?
5. Do you agree that there is enough food for everyone in the world to have a healthy diet? What steps can be taken to reduce the burden caused by hunger?
6. Compare and contrast the health consequences of undernutrition and overnutrition.

REFERENCES

1. Institute of Medicine. *Dietary reference intakes for energy, carbohydrate, fiber, fat, fatty acids, cholesterol, protein, and amino acids.* Washington DC: The National Academies Press; 2005.
2. Food and Agriculture Organization (FAO) of the United Nations. *FAO statistical yearbook 2012.* Rome: FAO; 2012. Table 16: Dietary energy supplies and changes in dietary composition.
3. Hu FB, Willett WC. Optimal diets for prevention of coronary heart disease. *JAMA.* 2002;288:2569–2578.
4. Mensink RP, Zock PL, Kester AD, Katan MB. Effects of dietary fatty acids and carbohydrates on the ratio of serum total to HDL cholesterol and on serum lipids and apolipoproteins: a meta-analysis of 60 controlled trials. *Am J Clin Nutr.* 2003;77:1146–1155.
5. Klein S, Allison DB, Heymsfield SB, et al. Waist circumference and cardiometabolic risk: a consensus statement from Shaping America's Health: Association for Weight Management and Obesity Prevention; NAASO, The Obesity Society; the American Society for Nutrition; and the American Diabetes Association. *Am J Clin Nutr.* 2007;85:1197–1202.
6. *Obesity: preventing and managing the global epidemic.* Geneva: WHO; 2000.
7. *WHO Child Growth Standards. Methods and development: head circumference-for-age, arm circumference-for-age, triceps skinfold-for-age and subscapular skinfold-for-age.* Geneva: WHO; 2007.
8. *WHO Child Growth Standards. Length/height-for-age, weight-for-age, weight-for-length, weight-for-height and body mass index-for-age: methods and development.* Geneva: WHO; 2006.
9. Onyango AW, de Onis M, Caroli M, et al. Field-testing the WHO Child Growth Standards in four countries. *J Nutr.* 2007;137:149–152.
10. Kramer MS. Determinants of low birth weight: methodological assessment and meta-analysis. *Bull World Health Organ.* 1987;65:663–737.
11. Saigal S, Doyle LW. An overview of mortality and sequelae of preterm birth from infancy to adulthood. *Lancet.* 2008;371:261–269.
12. Waterlow JC. Classification and definition of protein-calorie malnutrition. *Br Med J.* 1972;3:566–569.
13. Caulfield LE, de Onis M, Blössner M, Black RE. Undernutrition as an underlying cause of child deaths associated with diarrhea, pneumonia, malaria, and measles. *Am J Clin Nut.* 2004;80:193–198.

14. Black RE, Allen LH, Bhutta ZA, et al.; Maternal and Child Undernutrition Study Group. Maternal and child undernutrition: global and regional exposures and health consequences. *Lancet.* 2008;371:243–260.

15. Collins S, Dent N, Binns P, Bahwere P, Sadler K, Hallam A. Management of severe acute malnutrition in children. *Lancet.* 2006;368:1992–2000.

16. *State of the world's children 2012.* New York: UNICEF; 2012.

17. *WHO global database on child growth and malnutrition.* Geneva: WHO.

18. Victora CG, Adair L, Fall C, et al.; Maternal and Child Undernutrition Study Group. Maternal and child undernutrition: consequences for adult health and human capital. *Lancet.* 2008;371:340–357.

19. Chilima D. Assessing nutritional status and functional ability of older adults in developing countries. *Dev Pract.* 2000;10:108–113.

20. Barrett CB. Measuring food insecurity. *Science.* 2010;327:825–828.

21. *Food security statistics by country.* Rome: FAO; 2010.

22. Kaufman PR, MacDonald JM, Lutz SM, Smallwood DM. *Do the poor pay more for food? Item selection and price differences affect low-income household food costs* (Agricultural Economic Report No. 759). Washington DC: U.S. Department of Agriculture (USDA); 1997.

23. Melgar-Quinonez HR, Zubieta AC, MkNelly B, Nteziyaremye A, Gerardo MFD, Dunford C. Household food insecurity and food expenditure in Bolivia, Burkina Faso, and the Philippines. *J Nutr.* 2006;136:1431S–1437S.

24. Coleman-Jensen A, Nord M, Andrews M, Carlson S. *Household Food Security in the United States in 2010* (ERR-125). Washington DC: USDA; 2011.

25. Beaulac J, Kristjansson E, Cummins S. A systematic review of food deserts, 1966–2007. *Prev Chronic Dis.* 2009;6:A105.

26. Bickel G, Nord M, Price C, Hamilton W, Cook J. *Guide to measuring household food security.* Alexandria VA: USDA; 2000.

27. Sen A. Ingredients of famine analysis: availability and entitlements. *Q J Econ.* 1981;96:433–464.

28. Godfray HCJ, Beddington JR, Crute IR, et al. Food security: the challenge of feeding 9 billion people. *Science.* 2010;327:812–818.

29. Maxwell S, Slater R. Food policy old and new. *Dev Policy Rev.* 2003;21:531–553.

30. Holick MF. Vitamin D deficiency. *New Engl J Med.* 2007;357:266–281.

31. Gilbert C, Muhit M. Twenty years of childhood blindness: what have we learnt? *Community Eye Health.* 2008;21:46–47.

32. *Global prevalence of vitamin A deficiency in populations at risk 1995–2005: WHO global database on vitamin A deficiency.* Geneva: WHO; 2009.

33. Fawzi WW, Chalmers TC, Herrera MG, Mosteller F. Vitamin A supplementation and child mortality: a meta-analysis. *JAMA.* 1993;269:898–903.

34. Glasziou PP, Mackerras DE. Vitamin A supplementation in infectious diseases: a meta-analysis. *BMJ.* 1993;306:366–370.

35. Mayo-Wilson E, Imdad A, Herzer K, Yakoob MY, Bhutta ZA. Vitamin A supplements for preventing mortality, illness, and blindness in children aged under 5: systematic review and meta-analysis. *BMJ.* 2011;343:d5094.

36. Tang G, Qin J, Dolnikowski GG, Russell RM, Grusak MA. Golden rice is an effective source of vitamin A. *Am J Clin Nutr.* 2009;89:1176–1783.

37. Enserink M. Tough lessons from golden rice. *Science.* 2008;320:468–471.

38. Zimmermann MB, Jooste PL, Pandav CS. Iodine-deficiency disorders. *Lancet.* 2008;372:1251–1262.
39. Andersson M, Karumbunathan V, Zimmermann MB. Global iodine status in 2012 and trends over the past decade. *J Nutr.* 2012;142:744–750.
40. Andersson M, de Benoist B, Rogers L. Epidemiology of iodine deficiency: salt iodisation and iodine status. *Best Pract Res Clin Endocrinol Metab.* 2010;24:1–11.
41. McLean E, Cogswell M, Egli I, Wojdyla D, de Benoist B. Worldwide prevalence of anaemia, WHO Vitamin and Mineral Nutrition Information System, 1993–2005. *Public Health Nutr.* 2009;12:444–454.
42. de Benoist B, McLean Erin, Egli I, Cogswell, editors. *Worldwide prevalence of anaemia 1993–2005.* Geneva: WHO; 2008.
43. Brabin BJ, Hakimi M, Belletier D. An analysis of anemia and pregnancy-related maternal mortality. *J Nutr.* 2001;131(2S–2):604S–614S.
44. Zimmermann MB, Hurrell RF. Nutritional iron deficiency. *Lancet.* 2007;370:511–520.
45. Hurrell RF. How to ensure adequate iron absorption from iron-fortified food. *Nutr Rev.* 2002;60:S7–15.
46. Fischer Walker CL, Ezzati M, Black RE. Global and regional child mortality and burden of disease attributable to zinc deficiency. *Eur J Clin Nutr.* 2009;63:591–597.
47. Jamison DT, Breman JG, Measham AR, et al., editors. *Disease control priorities in developing countries*, 2nd edition. Washington DC: Oxford University Press and IBRD/World Bank; 2006.
48. Pellett PL. Food energy requirements in humans. *Am J Clin Nutr.* 1991;51:711–722.
49. Field AE, Coakley EH, Must A, Spadano JL, Laird N, Dietz WH, Rimm E, Colditz GA. Impact of overweight on the risk of developing common chronic diseases during a 10-year period. *Arch Intern Med.* 2001;161:1581–1586.
50. Monteiro CA, Moura EC, Conde WL, Popkin BM. Socioeconomic status and obesity in adult populations of developing countries: a review. *Bull World Health Organ.* 2004:82:940–946.
51. Kelly T, Yang W, Chen CS, Reynolds K, He J. Global burden of obesity in 2005 and projections to 2030. *Int J Obesity.* 2008;32:1431–1437.
52. *WHO Global InfoBase.* Geneva: WHO.
53. Global Burden of Metabolic Risk Factors of Chronic Diseases Collaborating Group. *Country trends in metabolic risk factors.* London: Imperial College London; 2011.
54. Finucane MM, Stevens GA, Cowan MJ, et al.; Global Burden of Metabolic Risk Factors of Chronic Diseases Collaborating Group (Body Mass Index). National, regional, and global trends in body-mass index since 1980: systematic analysis of health examination surveys and epidemiological studies with 960 country-years and 9.1 million participants. *Lancet.* 2011;377:557–567.
55. de Onis M, Blössner M, Borghi E. Global prevalence and trends of overweight and obesity among preschool children. *Am J Clin Nutr.* 2010;92:1257–1264.
56. Wang Y, Lobstein T. Worldwide trends in childhood overweight and obesity. *Int J Pediatr Obes.* 2006;1:11–25.
57. Cecchini M, Sassi F, Lauer JA, Lee YY, Guajardo-Barron V, Chisholm D. Tackling of unhealthy diets, physical inactivity, and obesity: health effects and cost-effectiveness. *Lancet.* 2010;376:1775–1784.

CHAPTER 12

Global Health Payers and Players

A variety of governmental agencies, multinational organizations, private foundations, corporations, public–private partnerships, charitable groups, and individuals pay for personal and public health and implement global health research, clinical services, relief, development, advocacy, and education programs. Numerous pathways can lead to a career in global health.

12.1 HEALTH SYSTEMS

A **health system** consists of all of the people, policies, and programs that work to promote health and prevent disease in a country. The World Health Organization (WHO) has identified six core building blocks of health systems:

1. The provision of effective personal and population-based healthcare services;
2. A well-trained and productive health workforce that is able to provide quality care to all populations;
3. Access to essential medicines, vaccines, and health technologies;
4. A strong health information system that collects data about health systems performance;
5. A health financing system that enables everyone to access affordable needed services and at the same time provides incentives not to overuse services; and
6. Effective oversight of the system to ensure safety, efficiency, and accountability.[1]

The goals of health systems include improving the health of populations being served; being responsive to the expectations patients and their families have about dignity, privacy, quality, and choice; ensuring a fair

277

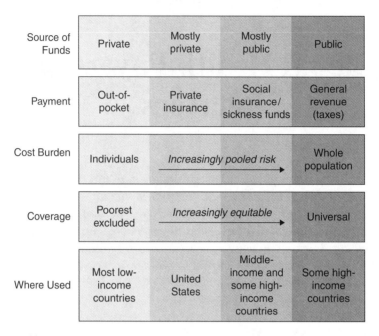

Source of Funds	Private	Mostly private	Mostly public	Public
Payment	Out-of-pocket	Private insurance	Social insurance/ sickness funds	General revenue (taxes)
Cost Burden	Individuals	*Increasingly pooled risk* →		Whole population
Coverage	Poorest excluded	*Increasingly equitable* →		Universal
Where Used	Most low-income countries	United States	Middle-income and some high-income countries	Some high-income countries

Figure 12–1 Public and private approaches to healthcare funding and coverage.
Source: Adapted from *World health report 1999*. Geneva: WHO; 1999. Figure 3.5.

financial contribution from users that does not overly burden the poor; and improving the efficiency of the system.[2]

Some countries have a healthcare system in which the medical care of individuals is usually privately funded through health insurance or the personal funds of the individual and his or her family. Others sponsor a publicly funded healthcare system that is paid for with tax revenue. Some systems pay for personal health with a combination of public and private sources (**Figure 12–1**).[3]

Most high-income countries have a government-sponsored healthcare system that is paid for through general tax revenue or through a government-run social insurance system (sometimes called a sickness fund). For example, the Republic of Korea's National Health Insurance Corporation (NHIC) and Poland's National Health Fund (NFZ) pay for nearly all health care in those countries. Health services in countries with single-payer health systems may be delivered by public or private providers. In Poland most healthcare services are provided at public facilities by clinicians who are government employees,[4] but in South Korea most services are paid for by the government but provided by private hospitals, clinics, and health centers.[5]

The services covered by universal healthcare plans and the prices for these services vary for different systems. Only some systems cover dental care and vision care. Some systems require users to pay a small fee at the time of service or a small amount for prescription medications; some do not. Some pay for all the expenses of hospitalization, while others require the patient to pay part of the cost of a hospital stay. Some allow users a choice of what types of services they want to access and how much they want to pay for them. For example, South Korean patients pay a fee if they select premium care (such as a private hospital room rather than a multibed ward) or want medical services not covered as part of the NHIC benefits package.[5] Supplemental private insurance can be purchased to pay for services not covered by the national health plan. In Brazil, everyone is entitled to free basic and advanced health care, but about one-quarter of people supplement the government health plan with private health insurance that enables them to access specialized and elective services.[6]

Common complaints about publicly funded health care include the overuse of health resources by consumers (because they do not pay directly for services) and long waiting times for access to specialists and advanced procedures.[7] However, universal healthcare systems increase equity in access to health services and improve the efficiency of the health system by reducing the underuse of health services by the poor, which in the long term saves on overall healthcare costs.[8] Single-payer systems also benefit from the streamlining of administrative and billing processes.[8]

The United States is one of the few developed countries that does not have a universal public healthcare system. The United States relies primarily on private health insurance and private healthcare providers. However, the government sponsors Medicare for the elderly and disabled and Medicaid for the country's poorest citizens, provides care to injured veterans through the Veterans Administration (VA) hospital system, and provides health care to indigenous Americans through the Indian Health Service (IHS).

Health insurance systems, whether private or public, are funded based on the principle of pooled risk. **Pooled risk** assumes that if many low-risk people and a few high-risk people all pay premiums to the insurance system over many years, then there will be a pot of money that can be used to pay for major illnesses when they occur. Only a few people will suffer a catastrophic injury or develop a very serious chronic condition, but because everyone is at risk for serious illness most people are willing to pay additional taxes or purchase insurance that protects them against the possibility of incurring an overwhelming amount of debt due to medical bills. (Pooled risk is at the core of the U.S. Patient Protection and Affordable Care Act of 2010, which makes participation in an insurance plan mandatory for those who can afford it and supplements the purchase of a private plan by those with lower incomes who do not quality for government-sponsored plans.[9])

The services provided by private health insurance companies vary greatly, just as the services provided by government plans do. Some low-cost insurance plans only cover conditions serious enough to require hospitalization. Higher-cost insurance plans may cover clinic visits, preventive care, and medications in addition to paying for hospitalizations and surgeries. In some countries, private insurance companies charge higher premiums to people with preexisting conditions, older people, and people who are in high-risk groups, and the companies have the option of denying coverage to people who have applied to be insured. These practices can prevent lower-income individuals and families from accessing health insurance, and that may put them at risk of bankruptcy if a serious illness or injury occurs.

In most low-income countries, a mix of public, not-for-profit private, and for-profit formal and informal healthcare providers are available in urban areas,[10] but there may be very few services in rural areas. Most healthcare services are paid for out-of-pocket on a pay-as-you-go basis. This means that many people who would like to access health care cannot do so because of the cost. For example, in India and Kenya the user fees that are assessed by both public and private providers at the time of service are costly for low-income households.[11,12] In Sierra Leone, free care at government facilities was introduced, in 2011, for pregnant women, breastfeeding mothers, and children younger than 5 years old.[13] However, access to health care is still limited for older children, men, and women who are not childbearing. Increasing access to affordable health services for the most vulnerable populations is one of the goals for healthcare systems in most low-income countries.

12.2 PERSONAL HEALTHCARE COSTS

Countries vary both by the type of health financing system they use and by the amount of money that is spent on health care (**Table 12–1**). High-income countries generally spend more on health care per person and more on health

Table 12–1 Health expenditures in 2009.

Country	USA	South Korea	Poland	Brazil	China	India	Kenya	Sierra Leone
Per capital total expenditure on health (PPP international $)	7960	1879	1391	921	347	124	75	110
Per capita government expenditure on health (PPP international $)	3795	1093	1006	401	182	38	33	12
Government expenditure on health as a % of total expenditure on health	47.7	58.2	72.3	43.6	52.5	30.3	43.3	10.5
Total spending on health care (in $U.S. billions) (in 2010)	2584	70	35	193	298	66	1.5	0.25
Total (public and private) expenditure on health as % of gross domestic product (GDP)	17.6	6.9	7.4	8.8	5.1	4.2	4.8	13.9
Government expenditure on health as % of total government expenditure	19.6	12.2	11.9	5.9	12.1	3.7	7.3	6.4

Source: Data from *Health system financing profile by country.* Geneva: WHO Global Health Expenditure Database; 2010; and World health statistics 2012. Geneva: WHO; 2012.

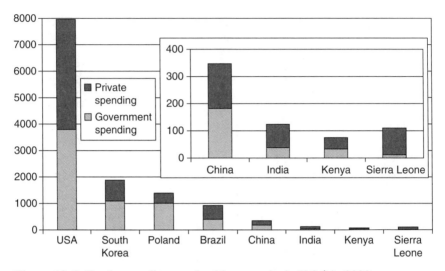

Figure 12–2 Total expenditure on health per capita in U.S.$ in 2009.
Source: Data from *World health statistics 2012*. Geneva: WHO; 2012.

care as a percentage of gross domestic product (GDP) than low-income countries. Additionally, the governments of high-income countries tend to pay for a higher percentage of healthcare costs than lower-income countries pay (**Figure 12–2**).[14,15] However, just as the types of health systems vary within one geographic region or one income group, there are variations in which entities pay for health care in different countries within regions and income brackets.

The countries with the least total spending on health generally require the greatest amount of personal health spending, both as a proportion of the healthcare bill and as a proportion of household income.[16] People who live in low-income countries must often pay for the majority of their health care themselves out-of-pocket at the time of service (**Figure 12–3**).[15] Because many residents of low-income countries have very little income, many households have a very limited ability to purchase healthcare services. An illness can quickly bankrupt a family. The poorest people might not have access to any health care at all because they cannot pay for it.

Even though access to health care is limited for many people around the world, health care is a huge part of the global economy. Worldwide, more than $4 trillion is spent on health each year, and those costs are rising.[14]

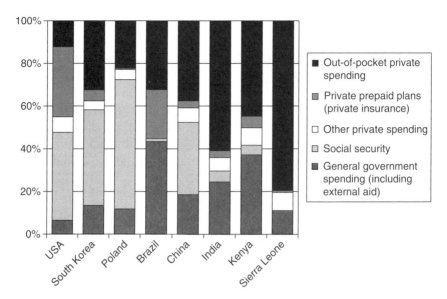

Figure 12–3 Expenditure on health by governmental (including external aid) and private sources (out-of-pocket spending and private insurance) in 2009.

Source: Data from *World health statistics 2012*. Geneva: WHO; 2012.

12.3 PAYING FOR GLOBAL PUBLIC HEALTH

Payment for health can be divided into two categories: money spent on personal health and money spent on public health. Personal health expenses relate to the health of one individual or family, such as the cost of purchasing chloroquine to treat a case of malaria, buying test strips for self-monitoring of blood glucose levels by those with diabetes, or paying for a midwife to help deliver a baby. Public health expenses relate to shared activities that protect a community or a country or the global population at large, such as the marketing of mass polio vaccination days, the use of molluscicides to kill the snails in a schistosomiasis-infected lake, or the development and testing of a new antibiotic. The money spent on local and global public health initiatives comes from somewhat different sources than the money that pays for individual health care. In addition to local and national governmental spending, global public health is funded by a combination of grants from one country to another, loans from intergovernmental agencies, and gifts from private-sector foundations, businesses, and individuals.

Donors have a variety of motivations for giving.[17] The governments of high-income countries may see providing health funding for lower-income countries as a foreign policy strategy that helps build trade alliances or as a security measure that helps protect the homeland.[18,19] Lending agencies may consider global health to be a financial investment. Philanthropic organizations may view global health as a tool for reducing poverty. Disease-specific charities may be able to increase their effectiveness by addressing concerns worldwide instead of limiting their work to a single country or region. Most of these rationales for funding global health involve benefits for the donors, the recipients, and the global population. Global health funding is about more than the global rich aiding the global poor. Global health funding is about using resources to address shared health concerns and achieve mutual goals.

12.3.A Local and National Government Funds

The majority of local and national public health initiatives around the world are paid for by taxes collected by the governments providing those services (**Figure 12–4**).[14] This is true for both developed and developing countries. Domestic spending on health significantly increased even in low- and middle-income countries between the 1990s and the 2010s.[20,21] In general, this increase has been attributed to an increasing GDP, which has increased tax revenue.

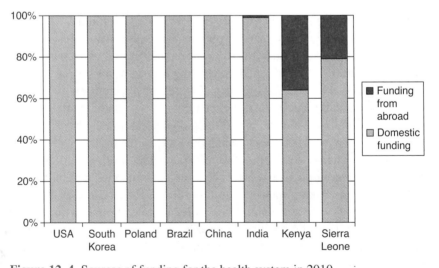

Figure 12–4 Sources of funding for the health system in 2010.

Source: Data from *Health system financing profile by country*. Geneva: WHO Global Health Expenditure Database; 2010.

12.3.B Bilateral Aid

Bilateral aid is money given directly from one country to another. For example, the United States gives more than $10 billion each year as bilateral aid, which accounts for about one-third of total U.S. foreign aid appropriations (**Figure 12–5**).[22] (Foreign aid is about 1% of the U.S. national budget. Most military assistance is provided from a separate budget line.) About 21% of total U.S. foreign aid in 2010 was devoted to health activities, up from about 5% in the late 1990s.[22] In 2010, the recipients of the most U.S. bilateral aid were Afghanistan, Israel, Pakistan, Egypt, Haiti, and Iraq (**Figure 12–6**).[22] Aid may be given in the form of equipment and commodities (such as food and computers), training (such as the education provided by Peace Corps volunteers) and expert advice, cash transfers, or economic infrastructure development (such as building schools and health clinics in postconflict areas).[22]

Most international aid is donated to lower-income countries by high-income countries that are members of the Development Assistance Committee (DAC) of the Organisation for Economic Co-operation and Development (OECD). More than $20 billion in direct aid specifically for health and health-related activities is donated by high-income countries to low- and middle-income countries each year, via bilateral aid or donations made through United Nations (UN)

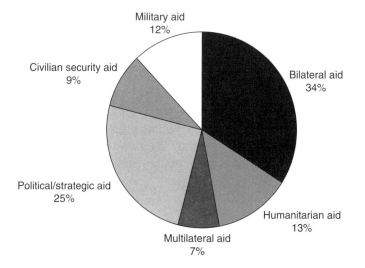

Figure 12–5 Types of U.S. foreign aid, fiscal year 2010.

Source: Data from Tarnoff C, Lawson ML. *Foreign aid: an introduction to U.S. programs and policy.* Washington DC: Congressional Research Service; 2011.

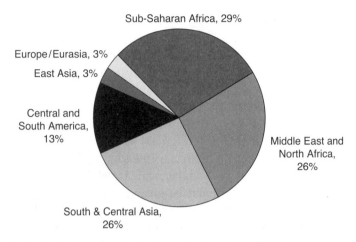

Figure 12–6 Recipients of U.S. foreign aid, fiscal year 2010.

Source: Data from Tarnoff C, Lawson ML. *Foreign aid: an introduction to U.S. programs and policy.* Washington DC: Congressional Research Service; 2011.

agencies, international health partnerships, and donations to international nongovernmental organizations (**Figure 12–7**).[23,24] The five donor nations that provide the greatest amount of **official development assistance,** or "**ODA,**" are the United States, the United Kingdom, France, Germany, and Japan, which each donated more than $10 billion in 2010.[25] As a percentage of their gross national income (GNI), the largest donors are Norway, Luxembourg, Sweden, Denmark, and the Netherlands, each of which donates more than 0.8% of its GNI.[25] (The United States donates about 0.2% of its GNI.)

Although some aid is given simply to fight poverty, aid is often tied to the political and economic interests of the donor country. For example, bilateral food aid agreements may require food to be purchased in the donor country and shipped by donor carriers to the recipient (as is the case for U.S. food assistance[22]). These kinds of bilateral aid agreements sometimes pay more attention to the business interests of donor nations than to the needs of the recipient country. However, the end result is a donation of a good or service to a less-developed country.

12.3.C The World Bank and IMF

Multilateral aid is money pooled from many donors. The World Bank, International Monetary Fund, and other UN agencies are the largest multilateral development funding institutions. Multilateral aid is often in the form of loans rather than gifts.

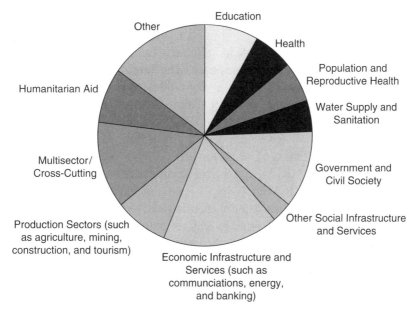

Figure 12–7 Distribution of total official development assistance (ODA) from OECD countries in 2010.

Source: Data from *DAC5 official bilateral commitments by sector*. Paris: OECD StatExtracts; 2012.

The two multilateral agencies most involved in offering **loans** (money that needs to be repaid and usually requires payment of interest on the money that has been loaned) and **grants** (money that does not have to be repaid) are the World Bank and the International Monetary Fund (IMF). Both the World Bank and the IMF were founded in 1944 during a summit held at Bretton Woods, New Hampshire, are headquartered in Washington, DC, and are "owned" by their nearly 180 member nations. But the two have distinct functions and modes of operating.[26]

The World Bank is an investment bank that makes loans to developing countries. Its board of governors is composed of representatives from each member country, who are usually member countries' ministers of finance (or the equivalent, such as the Secretary of the Treasury of the United States), and its president has always been a U.S. citizen. Because World Bank loans must be repaid with interest, lending nations can make a profit by lending money to poorer countries, assuming that the principal is repaid with interest.

The World Bank's primary lending institute is the International Bank for Reconstruction and Development (IBRD), which issues bonds in order to be able to make loans to middle-income member countries. These loans carry an interest rate that is slightly above the market rate, and they are usually supposed to be repaid within 15 years. The majority of loans are for specific infrastructure projects, although funds can also be used for other economic development purposes. The International Development Association (IDA) makes loans (and provides some interest-free credit and grants) to low-income member nations using money that has been donated from high-income countries. IDA loans are usually supposed to be paid back over a 40-year period. The World Bank Group is also home to the International Finance Corporation (IFC), the Multilateral Investment Guarantee Agency (MIGA), and the International Centre for Settlement of Investment Disputes (ICSID).

The IMF provides a structure for international monetary policy and currency exchanges, and it also makes loans to countries of any income level that have a "balance of payment" need and would otherwise not be able to make payments on their other international loans. The goal of IMF loans is to allow countries to rebuild their monetary reserves, stabilize their currencies, continue paying for imports, and create conditions for economic growth and high employment rates. The interest rates for IMF funds are usually slightly below market rates, and money received from the IMF is usually supposed to be paid back within a few years. The IMF is funded by membership fees (called "quotas") paid by its member countries, and it operates like a credit union. The IMF's managing director has always been a European.

Both the World Bank and the IMF may require countries to adhere to a Structural Adjustment Program (SAP) as a condition for receiving a loan. (Because SAPs acquired a negative reputation, loan requirements have been softened and reformulated as Poverty Reduction Strategy Papers [PRSPs] that spell out applicant countries' plans for implementing economic reforms.) **Structural adjustment** and related programs frequently require the recipient to raise taxes, reduce government spending, devalue the country's currency, eliminate price controls and subsidies, and increase production of exports. SAPs (and similar programs) are often designed to encourage capitalism through privatization of government-owned utilities and industries and deregulation of markets. This can increase the wealth of the rich business owners and government officials who live in low- and middle-income countries and negotiate the terms of international loans, because the loans can be used to support their companies (and, if corrupt leaders redirect some funds for personal use, to increase the value of their private bank accounts). But SAPs have been criticized for creating even tougher economic situations for poor households. For example, the SAP rules may put farmers and other workers in low-income countries at a competitive disadvantage because richer nations do not have the same restrictions on farm subsidies. The short-term consequences of implementing SAPs often include falling incomes, decreased social service expenditures, rising food prices, and an increased burden on women who must shift from formal wage labor to informal, low-paid work as the unemployment rate rises.[27] Additionally, there is limited evidence to support the effectiveness of SAPs at promoting economic growth.[28]

A major criticism of the international loan system is that payments on debt divert money away from education, health, clean water, and other essential human services in low-income countries. Because interest rates may increase over time, the amount that must be paid each year may not decrease significantly even if the principal and interest for some loans is repaid. And because the amount that must be repaid grows larger if debt payments are not made, the level of resulting debt can burden a country and stifle economic growth for decades.

To alleviate this burden, lending nations have agreed to forgive some of the debts of the most burdened poor countries. The World Bank's Enhanced Heavily Indebted Poor Countries (HIPC) Initiative has committed to forgiving billions of dollars of debt for low-income countries with unsustainable debt loads (measured by a debt-to-export ratio of more than 150%) that develop and implement PRSPs.[29] The HIPC cancellation only applies to loans from the IMF, the World Bank, and the African Development Fund; it does not apply to other bilateral and multilateral donors or private lenders. However, all of the eight large industrialized countries that make up the G8 (Canada, France, Germany, Italy, Japan, Russia, the United Kingdom, and the United States) pledged in 2005 to cancel the bilateral debts of the most indebted nations. The hope is that this will allow HIPCs to put more resources toward improving their health and educational systems, which will in turn contribute to ending the cycle of poverty and poor health.

12.3.D Private Foundations

Private foundations are making an increasingly significant contribution to spending on global public health. For example, the Bill & Melinda Gates Foundation has provided more than $1 billion each year in recent years to support projects such as the development and dissemination of vaccines and medications.[30] Major recipients of these funds include the GAVI Alliance, PATH, and the Global Fund to Fight AIDS, Tuberculosis and Malaria.[31] Groups like the Wellcome Trust (which is based in the United Kingdom), the Rockefeller Foundation, the Ford Foundation, the UN Foundation, and the Aga Khan Foundation also make multimillion-dollar international health grants every year.[32]

12.3.E Businesses

Each year, pharmaceutical companies like Abbott, Allergan, AstraZeneca, Bayer, Boehringer Ingelheim, Bristol-Myers Squibb, Eli Lilly and Company, GlaxoSmithKline, Johnson & Johnson, Novartis, Novo Nordisk, Roche, and Sanofi donate drugs and other products valued at more than $1 billion.[33] Some companies have made special investments in particular diseases. For example, Merck's Mectizan donation program has furthered progress toward onchocerciasis elimination,[34] and Pfizer's donations of Zithromax, a type of antibiotic, are helping the global effort to prevent blindness due to trachoma.[35] Most of the major drug companies have programs for donation of antiretroviral drugs for HIV/AIDS, and many of the companies also make donations in the areas of tuberculosis, malaria, tropical diseases, preventable diseases (especially with vaccine donations), maternal and child health, chronic diseases, and/or emergency relief.[36]

Other types of companies also make in-kind donations and fund global health programs through their own foundations as part of their **corporate social responsibility** plans. For example, the Coca-Cola Foundation, PepsiCo Foundation, and Unilever Foundation all sponsor portfolios of international water and sanitation, nutrition, and education projects, and the Johnson & Johnson Family of Companies Contribution Fund maintains a portfolio of maternal and child health projects.

In addition to being a form of humanitarian aid, and often a tax deduction, these donations help develop international markets and bring brand names to new potential customers. Populations with increased incomes and decreased health expenditures as a result of successful health initiatives have more money to spend on other goods and services. By helping potential consumers become healthy and maintain their health, companies are expanding their markets.

12.3.F Personal Donations

Millions of individuals also make donations each year to global health activities. This generosity is especially visible after major disasters. The American Red Cross alone received more than $200 million in donations after the Japanese earthquake and tsunami in 2011 and nearly $300 million after the earthquake in Haiti in 2010.[37] Child sponsorship organizations like

World Vision, Save the Children, and Compassion International are also popular recipients of charitable giving. Thousands of smaller charitable organizations rely exclusively on private donations.

Americans donated nearly $300 billion to charity in 2011, of which 73% was given by individuals (rather than foundations, bequests, or corporations).[38] In total, the donations represent about 2% of disposable income in the United States. The major recipients of funding were religious bodies ($96 billion); educational institutions ($39 billion); human services organizations providing food, clothing, shelter, and other essential goods and services domestically or internationally ($35 billion); health charities, including disease-specific support organizations, research-focused groups, and healthcare providers such as clinics and hospitals ($25 billion); international affairs charities working in the areas of relief, development, and public policy ($22 billion); community development organizations ($21 billion); arts and culture nonprofits ($13 billion); and environmental groups ($8 billion) (**Figure 12–8**).[38] Thus, a high proportion of donations across these categories went toward activities related to global health. Some of the major recipients of these funds in the United States are listed in **Tables 12–2** and **12–3**.[39] As a comparison, major international health-related charities in the United Kingdom include Save the Children, OxFam, and the British Red Cross.[40]

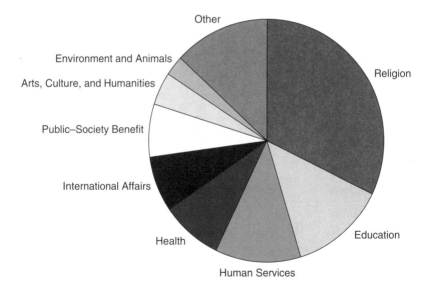

Figure 12–8 Recipients of U.S. charitable giving in 2011.

Source: Data from *Giving USA 2012: The annual report on philanthropy for the year 2011*. Executive summary. Chicago: The Giving Institute; 2012.

Table 12–2 Major international relief and development charities based in the United States.

Name	Annual Expenditures (2010–2011)	Program Expenditures (2010–2011)
Feed The Children	$1248 million	$1161 million
World Vision	$1206 million	$1066 million
Food For The Poor	$1051 million	$1018 million
Catholic Relief Services	$820 million	$774 million
AmeriCares	$665 million	$655 million
CARE	$614 million	$550 million
Operation Blessing International	$472 million	$469 million
Save the Children	$516 million	$468 million
Compassion International	$520 million	$433 million
United States Fund for UNICEF	$447 million	$405 million
MAP International	$402 million	$399 million
Direct Relief International	$309 million	$306 million
Samaritan's Purse	$336 million	$297 million
International Rescue Committee	$314 million	$287 million
Catholic Medical Mission Board	$283 million	$277 million
Brother's Brother Foundation	$274 million	$274 million
Mercy Corps	$267 million	$232 million
PATH	$257 million	$225 million
The Rotary Foundation of Rotary International	$228 million	$205 million
The Carter Center	$215 million	$201 million
CHF International	$219 million	$198 million
Project HOPE	$202 million	$190 million
Food for the Hungry	$193 million	$183 million
Doctors Without Borders, USA	$202 million	$181 million

Annual expenditures include program, administrative, and fundraising expenses.
Source: Data from *Charity directory*. Glen Rock, NJ: Charity Navigator; 2012.

Table 12–3 Major multipurpose human services and disease-specific charities based in the United States.

Name	Annual Expenditures (2010–2011)	Program Expenditures (2010–2011)
American Red Cross	$3422 million	$3157 million
Feeding America	$1180 million	$1185 million
Volunteers of America	$929 million	$831 million
American Cancer Society	$948 million	$679 million
American Heart Association	$598 million	$468 million
Susan G. Komen for the Cure	$343 million	$283 million
The Leukemia & Lymphoma Society	$281 million	$215 million
American Kidney Fund	$224 million	$219 million
National Cancer Coalition	$181 million	$175 million
Alzheimer's Association	$225 million	$169 million
Juvenile Diabetes Research Foundation International	$204 million	$168 million
March of Dimes	$206 million	$155 million
Muscular Dystrophy Association	$178 million	$139 million
American Diabetes Association	$190 million	$137 million
Elizabeth Glaser Pediatric AIDS Foundation	$144 million	$128 million
Cystic Fibrosis Foundation	$134 million	$109 million

Annual expenditures include program, administrative, and fundraising expenses.

Source: Data from *Charity directory.* Glen Rock, NJ: Charity Navigator; 2012.

12.4 TYPES OF GLOBAL HEALTH PROGRAMS

A variety of different activities can fall under the umbrella of global health services and programs. Many global health organizations and agencies work in several of these areas, while some specialize in just one domain. These areas include:

- Research and education activities that seek to understand global health concerns, identify effective solutions, and disseminate critical information to targeted audiences such as patients and families, healthcare providers, community health workers, public health professionals, policymakers, affected communities, or the general public. This is the focus of many disease-specific charities like the American Cancer Society and the American Heart Association.
- Clinical services provided by hospitals, clinics, health centers, and other direct patient care providers.
- **Relief** aid that meets the immediate needs of people who might otherwise not have access to water, food, shelter, emergency medical care, and other urgent necessities. Relief services are often required after major natural disasters and during wars.
- **Community development** programs that work with local communities to improve living conditions. One type of development program focuses on **microcredit**, very small loans (**microloans**) to novice entrepreneurs who are unable to get a loan through a conventional bank because they do not have collateral, steady employment, or a credit history, or because they are women. The interest rates are typically much lower than those offered by conventional banks, and most microcredit programs also provide some form of financial education and community support. The Grameen Foundation and other organizations help establish and support microfinance institutions. Other community development organizations may specialize in health, education, agriculture, water and sanitation, or other sectors.
- **Advocacy** initiatives that aim to increase awareness of a specific cause and to influence policy and resource allocation decisions related to that cause. For example, Amnesty International and Human Rights Watch work to bring global attention to human rights violations.
- **Logistics** efforts that deliver food, medications, medical equipment and supplies, and other goods and services to people and

communities in need. Many of the global partnerships that are working to increase vaccination coverage for children in low-income countries or to expand access to affordable medication for HIV/AIDS have expertise in the entire logistics pathway from procurement, production, and packaging to transportation, storage, and distribution.

The diversity of payers and players in global health highlight the wide variety of career paths that can lead to work in the global health arena.

12.5 IMPLEMENTING HEALTH PROGRAMS

Thousands of governmental, corporate, and nonprofit groups implement the various research and education, clinical, relief, development, advocacy, and logistics projects and programs that facilitate global health.[41,42] (**Projects** usually have clear goals and defined end dates. **Programs** are usually ongoing groups of related projects.) The agencies and organizations that manage these functions—the ones that spend global health money—are not necessarily the same ones that provide the funds for these activities.[32] Some groups specialize in fundraising; others in implementation.

The majority of clinical health services and health education programs are implemented by, or with the approval and assistance of, national ministries of health and their state or provincial and district health offices. Major relief and development efforts are also usually conducted with the approval of the national government. Supplies, technical assistance, and management oversight may be provided by UN agencies (such as the WHO, UNICEF, and other specialized programs), foreign governments (through their international development or international cooperation agencies), public–private partnerships, nongovernmental organizations, universities and colleges, businesses, and individual professionals and volunteers. Although sometimes the coordination between various groups is poor, resulting in duplication of efforts in one area, the goal is for the various players to work together to promote health, often by letting each contributor focus on its own area of expertise, whether that is water and sanitation or childhood vaccination or agricultural development or something else. The various participants in global health initiatives tend to take on different roles that are consistent with their goals or mandates and are in line with their particular capabilities.

12.5.A National and Local Governments

National governments provide the bulk of health services and payment for health systems. They decide, at least in part, who gets to use the health-care system, the choice (if any) that people have about where to seek care, the kinds of services that are covered by social security or health insurance, the level of training required for healthcare practitioners, and the types of facilities available. Even when the healthcare system is not nationalized, the government can still dictate, for example, what services must be covered by insurance and what educational and testing requirements must be fulfilled before people are licensed as doctors, nurses, dentists, and therapists.

The national government is also responsible for the public health system. It can set guidelines for nutrition, vaccination schedules, screening, and other preventive measures, and it can regulate the production and sale of health supplies, medications, and food products. It can also form public health partnerships with other nations and agencies that allow it to share information and quickly respond to infectious disease threats that require an international response. And it can negotiate with companies, for example, to secure cheaper prices on medications.

Another function of national governments is sponsoring health research. In the United States, the National Institutes of Health (NIH) is the federal focal point for medical research. The NIH is divided into more than 20 separate institutes, and research funded by nearly any of the divisions can be conducted internationally, provided that the research protocol meets rigorous standards for ethical human subjects research. The U.S. Centers for Disease Control and Prevention (CDC) is also involved in health research, and it plays a unique role in responding to international public health crises. The CDC responds to international health emergencies, including outbreaks, when invited to do so by the country or countries affected, and works with researchers in other nations to conduct field research, to set up monitoring and surveillance systems, and to train public health workers.[43] The United Kingdom's Medical Research Council (MRC), the Canadian Institutes of Health Research (CIHR), Brazil's Fundação Oswaldo Cruz (Fiocruz), the Indian Council of Medical Research (ICMR), and the Kenya Medical Research Institute (KEMRI) are other examples of nationally sponsored health research agencies.

Additionally, governments have the ability to shape public policies in ways that enhance health and reduce health disparities. The "Health in All Policies" approach recognizes that health is dependent on other critical public sectors—including agriculture, urban development, energy,

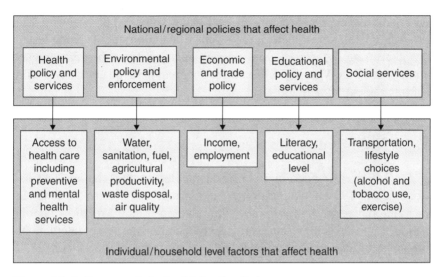

Figure 12–9 Framework for health in all policies.

commerce, education, and transportation, among others **(Figure 12–9)** — and that, conversely, a healthy population makes it possible for those other sectors to thrive.[44]

For international health initiatives, national and local governments can serve as a point of interface between local populations and international visitors. The implementation of a sponsored public health program is usually smoother and more successful when national or local government officials and local leaders have endorsed the plan.[45] For example, if a voluntary organization from the United States wants to distribute free insecticide-treated bednets (ITNs) in rural communities in Sierra Leone, the standard protocol is for the leaders of the organization to meet with local government, community organization, and/or religious leaders to ask for their support. If the project is deemed to be a locally beneficial one, the local leaders and other community representatives will be able to help the visiting group to set up a locally appropriate distribution system and to spread the word about the free ITNs to the community. The local leaders will also be able to tell the visitors if they do not need or want ITNs, if the visitors are scheduled to come at a bad time (say, during harvest time or on a day when there is a funeral or other special event), or if the presence of the visitors (who might need meals and a place to sleep) will place an undue burden on the community. Organizations that want to work on a bigger scale might need to get the approval of the national Ministry of Health and other national governmental offices. This is true for nearly all intervention programs, and essential for any projects that involve testing a new medical product. (When a new medication or other health product is being tested, the sponsoring organization must obtain approval from the ethics review committee of the Ministry of Health, or another approved authority, before starting the experimental trial.)

12.5.B United Nations Agencies

The UN was founded in 1945 by 51 member states, and by 2011 had expanded to 193 member nations. The goals of the UN are "to maintain international peace and security," "to develop friendly relations among nations," and "to achieve international co-operation in solving international problems of an economic, social, cultural, or humanitarian character."[46] The General Assembly, which is composed of one voting representative from each member state, is the main policy-setting group for the UN. The 15-member Security Council is responsible for peace-building, mediation, and security operations, and the International Court of Justice provides legal judgments and advisory opinions. The specialized functions of the UN are carried out by its agencies, offices, funds, programs, and subsidiary bodies, each of which has a unique mandate (**Table 12–4**).

The WHO is the primary health agency of the UN.[47,48] The WHO is governed by the World Health Assembly, composed of one representative from each UN member state, which convenes every May to approve a budget, make policy decisions, and approve conventions, agreements, and regulations. The first global health treaty negotiated by the WHO is the Framework Convention on Tobacco Control (FCTC), which details specific measures, such as increased taxation and comprehensive bans on advertising of tobacco products, that should be taken to reduce the demand for tobacco and the supply of tobacco.[49] More broadly, the WHO conducts research on health issues of international importance, monitors disease epidemics, collects health statistics, develops standards of practice (such as child growth charts and recommendations for laboratory and diagnostic procedures), and creates educational materials. The WHO also provides assistance to national governments that ask for technical assistance, and coordinates the health work of other UN agencies. For example, the WHO coordinated the smallpox eradication campaign in the 1960s and 1970s and is now coordinating the global polio eradication campaign.

Other UN agencies are also working on the ground in member states on health-related activities. For example, each year UNICEF provides

Table 12–4 Examples of the primary functions of United Nations agencies.

Agency, Program, Fund, or Office	Primary Work Area
United Nations Children's Fund (UNICEF)	Children
United Nations Environment Programme (UNEP)	Environmental health
World Health Organization (WHO)	Health
United Nations Programme on HIV/AIDS (UNAIDS)	HIV/AIDS
United Nations Office of the High Commissioner for Human Rights (OHCHR)	Human Rights
World Food Program (WFP)	Hunger
International Court of Justice	Justice
International Labour Organization (ILO)	Labor
United Nations Development Programme (UNDP)	National development
United Nations Population Fund (UNFPA)	Population and reproductive health issues
United Nations High Commissioner for Refugees (UNHCR)	Refugees
Food and Agriculture Organization (FAO)	Rural development
United Nations Human Settlements Programme (UN-HABITAT)	Urban development

humanitarian aid in nearly 100 countries, providing essential medications to children, treating malnutrition, supporting community water projects, distributing health kits to refugees, donating teaching materials to rural schools, assisting victims of violence, and engaging in other emergency care,[50] and each year the World Food Programme delivers emergency food aid to about 100 million people.[51]

12.5.C International Cooperation

National governments are often involved in sponsoring relief and development work internationally and cooperatively. For example, most developed countries have a governmental division dedicated to working with developing countries, and many of these agencies have a visible

Table 12–5 Examples of international development and cooperation agencies.

Country	Abbreviation	Agency
Australia	AusAID	Australian Agency for International Development
Belgium	DGDC	Belgian Development Cooperation
Canada	CIDA	Canadian International Development Agency
Denmark	Danida	Danish development cooperation
Finland	FINNIDA	Finnish International Development Cooperation
France	AFD	Agence Française de Développement
Germany	GTZ	Deutsche Gesellschaft für Internationale Zusammenarbeit
Japan	JICA	Japanese International Cooperation Agency
Norway	Norad	Norwegian Agency for Development Cooperation
Spain	AECID	Agencia Española de Cooperación Internacional para el Desarrollo
Sweden	SIDA	Swedish International Development Cooperation Agency
United Kingdom	DFID	U.K. Department for International Development
United States	USAID	U.S. Agency for International Development

presence on the ground in low-income countries (Table 12–5). While each of these agencies works to alleviate poverty and improve health, the goals, methods, and targeted recipient countries vary based on the political situations and historic connections of the donor nation. For example, the United Kingdom's Department for International Development (DFID) tends to work especially closely with member nations of the British Commonwealth, which are almost exclusively former British colonies or protectorates,[52] and the Japan International Cooperation Agency (JICA) works worldwide but is especially active in Asian countries with which it has economic ties.[53]

Foreign aid from the United States is administered by the U.S. Agency for International Development (USAID) and other entities within the U.S. Department of State, including the Peace Corps, and also by the U.S. Department of Defense (DOD), the U.S. Department of the Treasury (which

Table 12–6 U.S. Global Health Initiative principles.

Increase impact through strategic coordination and integration

Encourage country ownership and invest in country-led plans

Build sustainability through health systems strengthening

Strengthen and leverage key multilateral organizations, global health partnerships, and private sector engagement

Focus on women, girls, and gender equality

Improve metrics, monitoring, and evaluation

Promote research and innovation

Source: Information from *The United States Government Global Health Initiative strategy.* Washington DC: U.S. GHI; 2009.

manages all multilateral aid contributions), the Millennium Challenge Corporation (MCC), and other agencies.[22] Many of these efforts are coordinated by the U.S. Global Health Initiative (GHI), which has identified guiding principles for all of the country's global health programs (Table 12–6).[54]

The five core operational goals of USAID are: (1) supporting transformational development, especially in the areas of governance, human services, and economic growth; (2) strengthening fragile states; (3) supporting U.S. geostrategic interests, particularly in countries such as Iraq, Afghanistan, Pakistan, and Israel; (4) addressing transnational problems, including HIV/AIDS and other infectious diseases, climate change, and the illegal drug trade; and (5) providing humanitarian relief.[55] These goals are achieved through work in the areas of democracy, conflict prevention, and humanitarian assistance; economic growth, agriculture, and trade; and global health.[55] USAID also helps implement special presidential initiatives, such as the President's Emergency Plan for AIDS Relief (PEPFAR) and the President's Malaria Initiative (PMI), and oversees the U.S. contributions to global health partnerships.

12.5.D Global Health Partnerships

Dozens of nonprofit public–private partnerships are currently working to set and accomplish goals for selected global health issues (Table 12–7). The goals of these various global health partnerships include developing new products (such as new medicines, vaccines, and diagnostic tools),

Table 12-7 Examples of global public–private health partnerships.

Foundation for Innovative New Diagnostics (FIND)

Global Alliance for Improved Nutrition (GAIN)

Global Alliance for Vaccines and Immunisations (GAVI)

Global Fund to Fight AIDS, Malaria, and Tuberculosis (GFATM)

Health Metrics Network (HMN)

International AIDS Vaccine Initiative (IAVI)

Medicines for Malaria Venture (MMV)

Roll Back Malaria (RBM)

Stop TB Partnership (Stop TB)

UNITAID

---

distributing donated or subsidized health products, strengthening health services and health informatics systems, educating the public about particular health issues, improving the quality or regulation of products, and coordinating complex global health efforts.[56]

When these partnerships are successful, all of the involved parties benefit. The corporate sector and other private entities see a return on their investment because the collaboration pays for research and development activities, the distribution of a subsidized health product may open up new markets to donor companies, and nonprofit work boosts participating companies' public profiles. The public sector and governmental agencies attain an effective mechanism for achieving the scientific, foreign relations, and humanitarian goals of the donor countries. And global public health is advanced when these partnerships increase the visibility of specific health issues, raise funds to address these issues, stimulate research and development, establish international treatment protocols and technical standards, and improve access to health care.[57]

12.5.E Nongovernmental Organizations (NGOs)

Nongovernmental organizations (NGOs), sometime called **private voluntary organizations (PVOs)**, are nonprofit organizations that are privately managed and receive at least some of their funding from private sources. NGOs may focus on one particular issue, like cultural awareness or environmental preservation, or may address multiple issues in a particular town or region or country. NGOs may be involved in direct action like distributing food aid or may focus entirely on lobbying and advocacy. Some NGOs are **faith-based organizations (FBOs)** sponsored by religious or religiously affiliated organizations, and although they rarely require that aid recipients adhere to a particular faith or listen to an evangelistic message, they are representing a particular religious tradition. Examples of FBOs include the American Jewish World Service, Catholic Relief Services, Church World Service, Islamic Relief, and World Vision. Many **international NGOs (INGOs)** are involved in a spectrum of relief aid, development work, advocacy, and logistics; some also engage in clinical care and research.

Most large global health NGOs raise funds from individuals, private foundations, and governmental sources. One challenge for many NGOs is balancing the goals of donors and the desires of recipients. Directed donations occur when a donor gives money and stipulates that it must go to a particular cause. Sometimes this works well, but other times donors may not be aware of conditions in the recipient community. A community that wants to upgrade its local health clinic by adding a solar panel to provide electricity to the building may instead receive a microscope that they cannot use without electricity. A school may receive a donation of textbooks written in a language not spoken by any of the students. Or a donor may send old medical equipment that cannot be maintained by the community or a water pump that cannot be locally repaired. A related concern is that not all "nongovernmental" organizations are completely independent from governments, as several of the largest U.S.-based international NGOs receive a large portion of their budgets from the U.S. government. These NGOs must sometimes navigate complex political terrains.

Another challenge for NGOs operating internationally is deciding which aspects of budgeting and operations should be handled by recipient country staff and which should be managed by representatives of the donors. Some INGOs hire primarily local workers from the recipient country while others prefer to hire expatriates to be managers, accountants, and field staff. (**Expatriates**, or "expats," are people working in a foreign country for their home government, a business, the press corps, an NGO, or another organization, and who intend to move back to their home countries when their job is completed.) INGOs must also decide how closely they will work with officials from host countries and how to address potential problems with corruption and mismanagement. Some humanitarian groups feel that it is important to remain publicly neutral about political matters, and others feel compelled to speak openly about any injustices they witness. Cross-cultural communication skills are a necessity for all people working for an INGO, because they must be able to relate to both the funding agency and the host community.

NGOs also have to consider the social and political impact of their actions. The goal of most NGOs is to improve the well-being of individuals and communities, but well-intentioned efforts can sometimes have harmful side effects. The presence of a relief NGO may exacerbate conflicts by providing supplies that allow violence and instability to continue or by encouraging displaced persons to congregate in one area that could be targeted for attack. The long-term presence of a community development NGO may promote a "culture of dependency" and prevent the development of government or commercial service providers.

However, NGOs that successfully navigate these complex situations play a very important role in global health. Because most NGOs are not political, they can reach populations that might otherwise be underserved. Because NGOs often work for decades in the same communities, they build relationships and trust that allow for quick responses to emergencies, and their long-term commitments result in sustainable development. NGOs can also serve as points of connection between communities and international payers and players, using their networks to help new projects and programs quickly reach their target audiences. For example, Rotary International members all over the world have worked together on the polio eradication campaign, with local Rotary clubs in endemic areas facilitating vaccination campaigns in their communities.[58] Thus, NGOs are often the organizations that actually deliver aid to the people who need it most.

12.5.F International Committee of the Red Cross

The International Committee of the Red Cross (ICRC) works with national Red Cross and Red Crescent Societies and the International Federation of Red Cross and Red Crescent Societies to provide humanitarian aid to people in areas affected by war and other armed conflicts. The ICRC is unique among private organizations because it is an independent organization guided by its own set of rules and principles (humanity, impartiality, neutrality, independence, voluntary service, unity, and universality) but it is officially sanctioned by the Geneva Convention and international law to provide specific humanitarian services.[59] ICRC is funded through governmental support, contributions from national Red Cross and Red Crescent societies, and private donations.

The ICRC aids both civilian and military victims of conflicts by visiting prisoners of war, searching for missing persons, transmitting messages between separated family members, reunifying dispersed families, monitoring compliance with the international laws that pertain to armed conflict, and providing basic services to civilians such as food, water, and medical assistance.

National Red Cross and Red Crescent societies are autonomous from the ICRC, and provide a variety of services that meet needs in their communities. Examples of local Red Cross activities include maintaining blood banks, providing first aid training, and offering assistance to those who have been affected by natural disasters.

12.5.G International Businesses

A growing number of businesses are contractors that receive government and foundation funds to implement global health projects. For example, Chemonics International Inc., John Snow Inc., Abt Associates Inc., and Family Health International (FHI) are among the companies that received more than $100 million in 2011 to run international programs on behalf of USAID.[60]

Transnational corporations and other businesses not specializing in international development can also contribute to international health efforts by donating money and products and by helping their own workforce to be healthy—creating healthy work environments, ensuring that safety protocols are followed, covering the health expenses of workers and their families, and educating workers about health, nutrition, and injury prevention. Thus, nearly all workers have roles to play in furthering their own health, the health of their families and communities, and the health of the global public at large.

12.6 DISCUSSION QUESTIONS

1. How much do you spend out-of-pocket on health care and health-related expenses each year? What proportion of your income do you spend on health? Does this seem like a reasonable amount?
2. Do you have health insurance? If so, how much does it cost? Does it adequately cover your needs?
3. How much are you willing to pay out-of-pocket each month to have health insurance? What services would you expect to receive for that payment?

4. Have you ever made a decision not to see a doctor when sick or injured, not to fill a prescription, not to have a test your doctor recommended, or otherwise not received medical care because you were worried about your ability to pay for it? How did that make you feel?

5. Would you prefer to live in a country with a public (tax-funded) healthcare system or in a country with a privately funded healthcare system? Why?

6. Do you think your country spends too much, too little, or the right amount on international assistance?

7. If you had $100 to donate to an organization involved in global health, which one would you give to? Why?

8. If you were going to spend one month in a low-income country doing global health volunteerism, which organization would you choose to work with? Why?

9. If you were going to found a global health NGO, what specific area would you want the NGO to focus on?

10. How does your intended career path overlap with the work of global health?

REFERENCES

1. *Everybody's business: strengthening health systems to improve health outcomes: WHO's framework for action*. Geneva: WHO; 2007.

2. Murray CJL, Frenk J. A framework for assessing the performance of health systems. *Bull World Health Organ*. 2000;78:717–731.

3. *World health report 1999*. Geneva: WHO; 1999.

4. Sagan A, Panteli D, Borkowski W, et al. Poland: health system review. *Health Systems in Transition*. Copenhagen: WHO European Observatory on Health Systems and Policies; 2011.

5. Chun CB, Kim SY, Lee JY, Lee SY. Republic of Korea: health system review. *Health Systems in Transition*. Copenhagen: WHO European Observatory on Health Systems and Policies; 2009.

6. Victora CG, Barreto ML, do Carmo Leal M, et al. Health conditions and health-policy innovations in Brazil: the way forward. *Lancet*. 2011;377:2042–2053.

7. Hurst J. Challenges for health systems in member countries of the Organisation for Economic Co-operation and Development. *Bull World Health Organ*. 2000;78:751–760.

8. *World health report 2010*. Geneva: WHO; 2010.

9. Connors EE, Gostin LO. Health care reform—a historic moment in U.S. social policy. *JAMA*. 2010;303:2521–2522.

10. Basu S, Andrews J, Kishore S, Panjabi R, Stuckler D. Comparative performance of private and public healthcare systems in low- and middle-income countries. *PLoS Med*. 2012;9:e1001244.

11. Wamai RG. The Kenya health system—analysis of the situation and enduring challenges. *Japan Med Assoc J*. 2009;52:134–140.

12. Balarajan Y, Selvaraj S, Subramanian SV. Health care and equity in India. *Lancet.* 2011;377:505–515.
13. Donnelly J. How did Sierra Leone provide free health care? *Lancet.* 2011;377:1393–1396.
14. *Health system financing profile by country.* Geneva: WHO Global Health Expenditure Database; 2010.
15. *World health statistics 2012.* Geneva: WHO; 2012.
16. McIntyre D, Thiede M, Dahlgren G, Whitehead M. What are the economic consequences for households of illness and of paying for health care in low- and middle-income country contexts? *Soc Sci Med.* 2006;62:858–865.
17. Stuckler D, McKee M. Five metaphors about global-health policy. *Lancet.* 2008;372:95–97.
18. Yach D, Bettcher D. The globalization of public health, II: the convergence of self-interest and altruism. *Am J Public Health.* 1998;88:738–741.
19. Feldbaum H, Lee K, Michaud J. Global health and health policy. *Epidemiol Rev.* 2010;32:82–92.
20. Lu C, Schneider MT, Gubbins P, Leach-Kemon K, Jamison D, Murray CJL. Public financing of health in developing countries: a cross-national systematic analysis. *Lancet.* 2010;375:1375–1387.
21. *The Abuja Declaration: ten years on.* Geneva: WHO; 2011.
22. Tarnoff C, Lawson ML. *Foreign aid: an introduction to U.S. programs and policy.* Washington DC: Congressional Research Service; 2011.
23. Ravishankar N, Gubbins P, Cooley RJ, et al. Financing of global health: tracking development assistance for health from 1990 to 2007. *Lancet.* 2009;373:2113–2124.
24. *DAC5 official bilateral commitments by sector.* Paris: OECD StatExtracts; 2012.
25. *OECD factbook 2012.* Paris: OECD; 2012.
26. Driscoll DD. *The IMF and the World Bank: how do they differ?* Washington, DC: IMF; 1996.
27. Loewenson R. Structural adjustment and health policy in Africa. *Int J Health Serv.* 1993;23:717–730.
28. Easterly W. What did structural adjustment adjust? The association of politics and growth with repeated IMF and World Bank adjustment loans. *J Dev Econ.* 2005;76:1–22.
29. *Highly Indebted Poor Countries (HIPC) Initiative and Multilateral Debt Relief Initiative (MDRI)—status of implementation and proposals for the future of the HIPC Initiative.* Washington DC: IDA and IMF; 2011 Nov 8.
30. *2010 annual report.* Seattle: The Bill & Melinda Gates Foundation; 2010.
31. McCoy D, Kembhavi G, Patel J, Luintel A. The Bill & Melinda Gates Foundation's grant-making programme for global health. *Lancet.* 2009;373:1645–1653.
32. McCoy D, Chand S, Sridhar D. Global health funding: how much, where it comes from and where it goes. *Health Policy Plan.* 2009;24:407–417.
33. *Global partnerships: humanitarian programs of the pharmaceutical industry in developing nations.* Washington DC: PhRMA; 2004.
34. Thylefors B. Eliminating onchocerciasis as a public health problem. *Trop Med Int Health.* 2004;9(4 suppl):A1–A3.
35. *The end in sight: 2020 INSight.* Decatur GA: International Coalition for Trachoma Control; 2011.
36. *Developing world health partnerships directory 2010.* Geneva: International Federation of Pharmaceutical Manufacturers & Associations (IFPMA); 2010.

37. *Global impact report 2011*. Washington DC: American Red Cross; 2011.
38. *Giving USA 2012: The annual report on philanthropy for the year 2011. Executive summary*. Chicago: The Giving Institute; 2012.
39. *Charity directory*. Glen Rock, NJ: Charity Navigator; 2012.
40. *Charity trends*. Kent, UK: Charities Aid Foundation (CAF); 2012.
41. Gostin LO. A Framework Convention on Global Health: health for all, justice for all. *JAMA*. 2012;307:2087–2092.
42. Cohen J. The new world of global health. *Science*. 2006;311:162–167.
43. *Protecting the nation's health in an era of globalization: CDC's global infectious disease strategy*. Atlanta: CDC; 2002.
44. *Adelaide Statement on Health in All Policies: moving towards a shared governance for health and well-being*. Geneva: WHO; 2010.
45. Macfarlane S, Racelis M, Muli-Musiime F. Public health in developing countries. *Lancet*. 2000;356:841–846.
46. *Charter of the United Nations*. San Francisco: UN; 1945.
47. Koplan JP, Bond TC, Merson MH, et al.; Consortium of Universities for Global Health Executive Board. Towards a common definition of global health. *Lancet*. 2009;373:1993–1995.
48. Brown TM, Cueto M, Fee E. The World Health Organization and the transition from "international" to "global" public health. *Am J Public Health*. 2006;96:62–72.
49. Shibuya K, Ciecierski C, Guindon E, Bettcher DW, Evans DB, Murray CJL. WHO Framework Convention on Tobacco Control: development of an evidence based global public health treaty. *BMJ*. 2003;327:4–157.
50. *2011 UNICEF humanitarian action for children: building resilience*. New York: UNICEF; 2011.
51. *Fighting hunger worldwide: the World Food Programme's year in review, 2010*. Rome: WFP; 2011.
52. *DFID annual report and accounts 2011–2012*. London: DFID; 2012.
53. *Japan International Cooperation Agency annual report 2011*. Tokyo: JICA; 2011.
54. *The United States Government Global Health Initiative strategy*. Washington DC: U.S. GHI; 2009.
55. *USAID primer: what we do and how we do it*. Washington DC: USAID; 2006.
56. Widdus R. Public-private partnerships for health: their main targets, their diversity and their future directions. *Bull World Health Organ*. 2001;79:713–720.
57. Buse K, Harmer AM. Seven habits of highly effective global public-private health partnerships: practice and potential. *Soc Sci Med*. 2007;64:259–271.
58. Majiyagbe J. The volunteers' contribution to polio eradication. *Bull World Health Organ*. 2004;82:2.
59. *Annual report 2011*. Geneva: ICRC; 2012.
60. *USAID implementing partners (fiscal year 2011)*. Washington DC: USAID; 2012.

CHAPTER 13

Globalization and Health

Globalization contributes to the health transitions that are occurring in many parts of the world by mixing diverse populations in rapidly growing cities, transporting infections across the globe, altering dietary practices, and accelerating environmental changes.

13.1 GLOBALIZATION AND GLOBAL HEALTH

One of the key components of global health as a field new and distinct from international health is its focus on issues common to all countries in the world. Globalization is making many of these concerns more prominent, including urbanization and health, emerging infectious diseases, food safety, security, and the health impacts of global environmental change.

Globalization has many definitions, most of which are very specific to a particular discipline. For example, economists use globalization to refer to the expansion and integration of economic activity and policies between nations.[1] Globalization is seen in the increasing number of global governmental and nongovernmental organizations, the proliferation of multilateral trade agreements, increases in foreign direct investment, the rise of global supply chains, increased population mobility (including tourism, urban migration, and forced displacements), and increased cultural diffusion. The globalization of the world economy is very evident in the items people use on a daily basis. For example, many of the telecommunications devices, clothes, appliances, and other consumer goods purchased in the United States are imported from other countries.[2]

Globalization is not new to the field of public health. Infectious diseases like plague and smallpox spread across Europe and Asia more than a thousand years ago when sea and land trade routes, like the Silk Road, linked China, India, and the Mediterranean. The infectious diseases carried by the Europeans who explored the Americas in the 15th century caused the decimation of many indigenous American populations, and some infections indigenous to the Western hemisphere (such as syphilis) made their way back to Europe and sparked mass epidemics.[3] Early European explorers to the New World also brought tobacco from the Americas to Europe, increasing the prevalence of chronic diseases. (And, more recently, as tobacco use declines in the United States and some other high-income world regions, tobacco marketing and sales in Asia, Latin America, Africa, and Eastern Europe are increasing.[4])

Infectious diseases have never stopped at national boundaries, and modern transportation allows for a new infectious disease that emerges in any part of the world to be transported by aircraft to any other part of the world within hours rather than weeks or months. The original cases of SARS (severe acute respiratory syndrome) occurred in Guangdong, in southern China, in November 2002; in March 2003, SARS spread to Hong Kong and then, days later, a secondary outbreak occurred in Toronto, Canada, with additional cases in more than two dozen countries.[5] If a strain of highly pathogenic avian influenza develops the ability to spread easily from human to human, an even faster and more widespread dissemination of the infection across the globe is expected.[6] Globalization means that humans are tied together, and a problem in one part of the world can quickly become a global issue.[7]

New concerns about globalization and health move beyond infectious disease outbreaks (which remain a worry) to encompass drug resistance, noncommunicable diseases (NCDs), nutrition, the safety of imported goods (including, for example, toys coated in lead paint as well as foods with microbial or chemical contaminants), peace and conflict, bioterrorism, global climate change, and a host of other issues.

13.2 URBANIZATION AND HEALTH

On average, urban residents have greater access than rural residents to water and sanitation, to a relatively reliable public transportation system, and to healthcare providers and health technologies. Electricity in cities reduces cooking time and makes it easier to store food safely. Communications systems, such as radio and television, broadcast news and entertainment shows as well as emergency warnings and health messages. Urban women have more opportunities to pursue additional education and to find employment outside the home. Pregnancy in cities is safer because of greater access to antenatal care and assistance by medical professionals during delivery.

However, the benefits of **urbanicity** are not available to all urban residents.[8,9] **Table 13–1** compares rural, unplanned urban, and planned urban communities. Many people who move to cities end up living in unplanned settlements (sometimes called shantytowns, slums, or squatter camps) where

Table 13–1 Comparison of health risks associated with rural living, unplanned urban living, and planned urban living.

Sector	Rural	Unplanned Urban	Planned Urban
Water	• May have minimal access to improved water sources • Risk of microbial contamination	• May have minimal access to affordable clean water • Risk of microbial and industrial/agricultural chemical contamination	• Reliable access to safe, clean drinking water
Sanitation	• May have inadequate sanitation facilities • Open defecation in a field away from the house may be common	• May have inadequate sanitation facilities • Open defecation in the street may be common	• Sewage system
Trash disposal	• Solid waste is burned or buried	• No collection of solid waste • Trash heaps create a habitat for insect and rodent vectors	• Solid waste is collected and removed
Fuel	• Solid fuels, which may be able to be collected locally	• Solid fuels, which may be expensive	• Electricity
Nutrition	• May have limited ability to purchase food • Can usually grow, gather, or hunt for food	• May have limited access to affordable, healthy foods • May not have space for a garden	• Adequate access to healthy and safe dietary choices
Health facilities	• Facilities may be far from home and may provide only basic care	• Facilities may be crowded and understaffed	• Basic, emergency, and specialty healthcare (including mental health and rehabilitation) facilities are available

(Continues)

Table 13–1   *(Continued)*

Sector	Rural	Unplanned Urban	Planned Urban
Air quality	• Indoor air pollution from burning biomass	• Both indoor and outdoor air pollution • Noise pollution	• Some outdoor air pollution • Some indoor air pollution from building materials
Chemical Hazards	• Potential exposure to agrochemicals like fertilizer and pesticides	• Potential exposure to industrial waste	• Little exposure to industrial or agricultural hazards

the quality of life is generally worse than rural life. Poorly constructed homes, often made from cardboard, scraps of metal and wood, or other found items, provide little comfort or privacy. Residents may not have access to toilets, and trash and human waste may collect near the home and attract rodents and insects. Living in close proximity to large numbers of people and their animals increases the risk of insect borne and animal borne diseases. Violence and road-traffic accidents (often of the motor vehicle versus pedestrian variety) may be common. Urban workers may face new occupational hazards, and may not have access to affordable emergency healthcare services. It may be difficult to grow or to purchase nutritious foods, and there may be little time or space for exercising. Unplanned communities in urbanizing cities often form in undesirable locations near noisy and polluted highways or industrial centers that exacerbate asthma and cardiovascular conditions. Informal dwellings are often built in floodplains or on other vulnerable lands, and lack of drainage systems means that floods carry feces and other waste into homes.

Each day, thousands of people move from rural areas to cities in search of better jobs, higher incomes, more social opportunities, and greater conveniences. This process of **urbanization** affects both urban and rural residents. Rural women, for example, may bear a particularly heavy burden when their husbands move to cities to find wage employment, leaving the women with the responsibility of completing all of the household chores. Or parents who move to the city may have to leave their children in the care of grandparents, which puts a strain on three generations.

Although urbanization is occurring in nearly every part of the world (**Figures 13–1 and 13–2**),[10,11] the rates are particularly high in developing countries, which are now home to many of the world's largest metropolitan

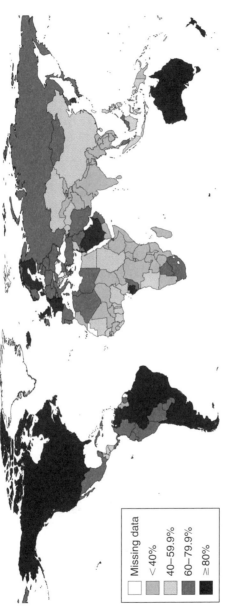

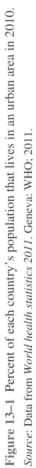

Figure 13–1 Percent of each country's population that lives in an urban area in 2010.
Source: Data from *World health statistics 2011.* Geneva: WHO; 2011.

areas (**Table 13–2**).[12] **Figure 13–3** highlights the trend in low-income countries toward rapid urbanization. In these areas, the birth rates remain high in both rural and urban areas, but rural-to-urban migration causes cities to grow at an especially rapid rate. In many high- and middle-income regions, birth rates are low and rural-to-urban migration is causing rural populations to shrink.[12]

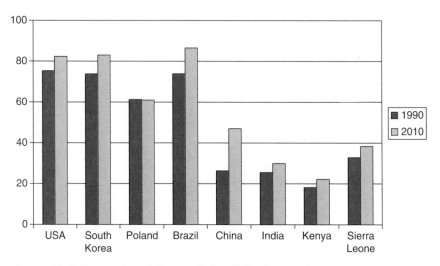

Figure 13–2 Proportion of the population living in an urban area.
Source: Data from *Human development report 2010*. New York: UNDP; 2010.

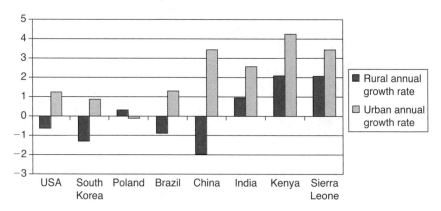

Figure 13–3 Rural and urban population growth rates between 2005 and 2010.
Source: Data from *World urbanization prospects, the 2011 revision*. New York: Department of Economic and Social Affairs, United Nations; 2012.

Table 13–2 The world's megacities (urban areas of 10 million or more inhabitants) in 2011. Cities in low- and middle-income countries are shaded in grey.

Rank	Metropolitan Area	Population
1	Tokyo, Japan	37.2 million
2	Delhi, India	22.7 million
3	Mexico City, Mexico	20.4 million
4	New York City, USA	20.4 million
5	Shanghai, China	20.2 million
6	São Paulo, Brazil	19.9 million
7	Mumbai, India	19.7 million
8	Beijing, China	15.6 million
9	Dhaka, Bangladesh	15.4 million
10	Kolkata, India	14.4 million
11	Karachi, Pakistan	13.9 million
12	Buenos Aires, Argentina	13.5 million
13	Los Angeles, USA	13.4 million
14	Rio de Janeiro, Brazil	12.0 million
15	Manila, Philippines	11.9 million
16	Moscow, Russia	11.6 million
17	Osaka, Japan	11.5 million
18	Istanbul, Turkey	11.3 million
19	Lagos, Nigeria	11.2 million
20	Cairo, Egypt	11.2 million
21	Guangzhou, China	10.8 million
22	Shenzhen, China	10.6 million
23	Paris, France	10.6 million

Source: Data from *World urbanization prospects, the 2011 revision*. New York: Department of Economic and Social Affairs, United Nations; 2012.

13.3 EMERGING INFECTIOUS DISEASES

Even as modern science has allowed the control and even eradication of some diseases, other diseases previously not found in humans are appearing. **Emerging infectious diseases (EIDs)** occur when a new pathogen begins to affect human populations or an existing pathogen changes the kind of disease it causes. The agent might evolve in a way that makes it easier to transmit to a susceptible person (increased **transmissibility**) and, therefore, more common (increased incidence). It might change so that it causes a new set of symptoms or more severe symptoms (increased virulence). In some cases, an infectious agent that usually affects only nonhuman hosts may adapt in a way that makes it infectious to humans. Sometimes an infectious agent may change in a way that allows for a different portal of entry, perhaps developing the ability to spread through airborne transmission. Other infections, called **reemerging infections**, were controlled at some point in the past but are becoming problematic again.[13–15] Consider just a few of the many EIDs identified in recent decades:

- Within months of methicillin being released for use as an antibiotic in 1960, cases of methicillin-resistant *Staphylococcus aureus* (MRSA) were reported.[16] MRSA is very difficult to treat, and it can cause severe "flesh-eating" infections (necrotizing fasciitis) and bloodstream infections. MRSA is now common in hospitals (where it is called hospital-acquired or HA-MRSA), but the infection can also be transmitted by unsterilized sports equipment and other everyday items that cause community-acquired or CA-MRSA. Drug-resistant strains of bacteria are often hardier than drug-sensitive strains, so inappropriate access to drugs in one nation (such as infected persons taking an inappropriate type of antibiotic or too few doses of an appropriate one) can rapidly cause a global antimicrobial resistance problem.[17]
- Legionnaires' disease is a severe type of pneumonia that was first identified in 1976 following a conference of the American Legion in Philadelphia.[18] (The mild form is called Pontiac fever.) The bacteria that cause Legionnaires' disease live in water. When modern water distribution systems like air cooling units, spas, and humidifiers aerosolize the bacteria, they can be inhaled and lung infections can occur.[19]
- An outbreak of Ebola virus, a tropical hemorrhagic fever, was first reported in 1976.[20] Outbreaks are rare, but still occur in central Africa,

and the case fatality rate is high.[21] The reservoir for the infection remains unconfirmed, even though international research teams have been searching for years for proof of an animal host.[22]

- Although hantaviruses have caused human disease in many parts of the world for a long time, hantavirus pulmonary syndrome (HPS) was first seen in 1993 in the isolated Four Corners region of the southwest United States. Several young adults developed severe pneumonia after they inhaled aerosolized rat urine or feces while doing a spring cleaning of rural summer homes.[23] HPS outbreaks have since been reported in Central America and South America.[24]

- The first cases of acquired immunodeficiency syndrome (AIDS) were diagnosed in 1981 in the United States.[25] The human immunodeficiency virus (HIV) was not identified until several years later.[26] By the mid-1990s, cases had been reported from nearly every country in the world, and more than 5 million people had died of AIDS.[27]

- Cholera, a waterborne bacterial infection that can travel in ocean waters from one nation's shores to another, appeared in South America for the first time in nearly 100 years in 1991. It was first identified in Peru but quickly spread to Ecuador and Colombia, and in less than a year it had spread throughout South America and Central America, including to Mexico and several Caribbean countries.[28,29]

- Although cases have occurred in Egypt, Sudan, and Uganda for decades, an outbreak of encephalitis due to West Nile Virus happened in the United States for the first time in 1999.[30] The virus cycles between mosquitos and vertebrates (usually birds, but sometimes humans or other animals). A small proportion of infected humans develop severe nervous system complications.[31] Just a few years after the first cases were identified in New York, cases had been reported from nearly all of the contiguous states.[32]

The U.S. Institute of Medicine reports that these new health threats derive from a complex interaction of genetic and biological factors; physical environmental factors; ecological factors; and social, political, and economic factors (**Table 13–3**).[33] As the world population increases (#6), humans and domestic animals move into previously uninhabited natural environments (#5) and are exposed to new plants, animals, and microbes. Alteration of the environment (#4), such as deforestation, dam building, and manipulation of wetlands, creates new environmental reservoirs for infectious agents and their hosts, and natural disasters (#3) like floods

Table 13–3 Risk factors for emerging infections.

1	Microbial adaptation and change
2	Human susceptibility to infection
3	Climate and weather
4	Changing ecosystems
5	Economic development and land use
6	Human demographics and behavior
7	Technology and industry
8	International travel and commerce
9	Breakdown of public health measures
10	Poverty and social inequality
11	War and famine
12	Lack of political will
13	Intent to harm

Source: Information from Smolinski, MS, Hamburg MA, Lederberg J, editors. Committee on Emerging Microbial Threats to Health in the 21st Century. Institute of Medicine. *Microbial threats to health: emergence, detection, and response.* Washington DC: The National Academics Press; 2003.

and droughts can alter the landscape and introduce new infectious agents to a region. Changes in dietary and other behaviors (#6) that become trendy and spread globally may also facilitate transmission. Urbanization facilitates emergence as people with different strains of infections interact with one another (#2) and create new habitats for vectors (#5). Technology is also speeding up the rate of emergence. Modern transportation (#8) has made it possible for an infectious person to travel nearly anywhere in the world within hours. Healthcare innovations (#7) have created new risks and risk groups. Advanced medical therapies like the immunosuppressive drugs used by people who have had organ transplants and the technology for keeping premature infants alive have created new populations of highly susceptible people (#2). **Nosocomial infections** (also called **hospital-acquired infections**, or **HAIs**) may be very hardy and difficult to treat, and antimicrobial resistance is increasing (#1). Other technological advances have created new places for infectious agents to grow and new methods of dispersion. New infectious diseases can emerge anywhere in the world and spread quickly, so the distinction between local public health problems and global ones is increasingly limited.

13.4 NUTRITION AND FOOD SAFETY

Nutrition globalization is seen in changing eating habits, the increasing variety of foods on grocery store shelves, the growing number of international restaurant chains, and the global marketing of food products. International food markets have grown significantly in recent decades. For example, the proportion of food consumed in the United States that is imported increased from 12% in 1990 to 14% in 2000 to 17% in 2009 (**Figure 13–4**).[34] This cross-border trade in foods has created a new set of concerns about food safety.

A wide variety of foods have been implicated in outbreaks, including fruits and vegetables, meats and poultry, eggs, seafood, dairy products, bakery items, and unpasteurized fruit juices.[35] The causative agents in foodborne outbreaks include a diversity of bacteria (*Campylobacter, E. coli, Listeria, Salmonella, Shigella*, and others), parasites (such as *Cryptosporidium, Giardia*, and *Toxoplasma gondii*), and viruses (including noroviruses, rotaviruses, astroviruses, and hepatitis A virus, among others).[36] In addition to microbial contamination, chemical contaminants are increasing threats to health. Concerns have been raised

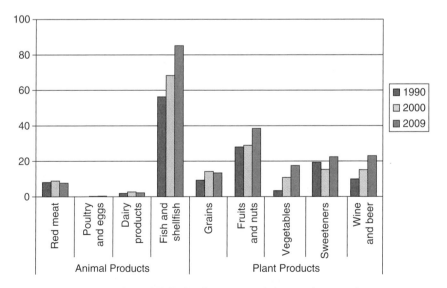

Figure 13–4 Proportion of U.S. foods consumed that are imported.

Source: Data from *Import share of consumption*. Washington DC: Economic Research Service, United States Department of Agriculture; 2012 May 30.

about heavy metal poisoning from mercury in fish, pesticide residues, chemical additives and preservatives, and other issues.[37] (These complex considerations have contributed to the development of the One Health concept that promotes the integration of human, animal, and environmental health initiatives.[38])

While most outbreaks are caused by locally grown and processed foods,[39] an increasing number of large multinational foodborne outbreaks are being reported.[40] The *Codex Alimentarius* International Food Standards, which are compiled by scientific panels hosted by the United Nations, provide guidelines about food safety, but these are not binding on countries or food producers, and they can be difficult to enforce.[41] Additionally, labeling requirements are not standardized across markets, and countries have different expectations about the use of additives and preservatives, fortification and enrichment with vitamins and minerals, and the use and labeling of genetically modified organisms (GMOs). As the food industry becomes increasingly global, it may become more difficult for governments and consumers to have confidence that their food supply is safe. However, several simple food safety practices can help protect consumers at home (**Table 13–4**).[42]

Globalization is also having an impact on social and cultural eating behaviors, breastfeeding practices and attitudes, and perceptions of physical beauty. Some anthropologists have used the terms New World Syndrome, "Coca-colonization," and "McDonaldization" to refer to the diseases of affluence (such as obesity, diabetes, heart disease, and hypertension) that occur after a population replaces its traditional diet with processed foods.[43,44] Dietary changes may include increased portion sizes, more snacking, more meals eaten outside the home, replacing water with sweetened beverages,

Table 13–4 Key food safety practices.

Clean	Wash hands and surfaces often
Separate	Avoid cross-contamination between uncooked and ready-to-eat foods
Cook	Cook meats, eggs, and dairy products to a proper temperature
Chill	Refrigerate foods promptly to keep them at a safe temperature

Source: Information from Medeiros LC, Hillers VN, Kendall PA, Mason A. Food safety education: what should we be teaching to consumers? *J Nutr Educ*. 2001; 33:108–113.

eating more animal protein, cooking with more oil, adding more sweeteners to the diet, and shifting from consuming whole grains to refined grains.[45] This nutrition transition can result from a variety of globalization processes, including urbanization, new technologies, global media, and international transportation and trade.

A related change includes adaptations in cultural perceptions of beauty. When the painters of the European Renaissance wanted to show beautiful, powerful women, they portrayed women with rolls of fat and rounded curves. In some cultures today, larger women are still seen as having ideal body shapes and greater weight is associated with perceived fertility. When resources are scarce, having greater weight is often a sign of wealth because it shows that the household has more than enough calories and does not have to expend so many of them in physical labor. On the other hand, the women who model on the fashion runways in Paris and Milan and those who are Hollywood stars tend to be extremely skinny. In industrialized societies, being underweight is often an indication of wealth because richer households have the time and money to prepare healthy foods and exercise whereas working-class households rely on cheap fast foods and work long hours at jobs that are often sedentary.

However, globalization is influencing attitudes toward food and body image. Although eating disorders like anorexia nervosa and bulimia nervosa are still relatively rare in non-Western cultures, there are reports from many countries of cases being identified.[46] (Anorexia nervosa is a condition in which a person has a distorted body image and feels fat even when emaciated. A person with anorexia nervosa follows a very restricted diet, exercises excessively, and may use laxatives and other methods of losing weight. Bulimia nervosa is when a person engages in frequent binge-purge cycles, eating thousands of calories at one sitting then inducing vomiting and using laxatives to get rid of the calories ingested.) More importantly, dissatisfaction with body shape is becoming more common, especially as the idealized bodies of movie stars and the touched-up bodies of magazine cover models are broadcast to larger audiences. For example, recent studies of ideal body size in Pacific Island nations like Fiji, Tonga, and Samoa, which have some of the highest rates of obesity in the world, have found growing dissatisfaction with body size, a trend toward thin bodies being seen as ideal, and the beginnings of unhealthy weight loss behaviors like purging.[47–50] Thus, attitudes toward food and perceptions about body shape are being imported and exported globally along with foods and food products.

13.5 BIOTERRORISM AND SECURITY

Bioterrorism is the deliberate release of pathogens, chemicals, or other agents that can cause illness and possibly death of people, animals, or plants. Chemical and biological warfare are not new.[51] During the Tartar siege of the city of Kaffa (now in the Ukraine) in the 14th century, the bodies of plague victims were catapulted over city walls to spark an epidemic. During the French and Indian War in the 1760s, the British army sent smallpox-infected blankets to American Indians who supported the French. During World War I, several European nations used biological agents against the livestock of enemies. What is new is that there are now more tools available for creating and spreading bioterror agents and the scale on which such acts can occur is much larger.

A bioweapon may be selected because it produces severe disease or death, the target population is susceptible to the agent, and the target population has limited or no access to immunization or treatment. Additionally, a particular agent may be selected for use because it can be produced relatively easily and rapidly, is relatively inexpensive, is environmentally stable, has a low infectious dose, has a simple delivery mechanism (such as through air, water, or food), is highly infectious, has a desirable incubation period (either short so immediate disease is produced or somewhat longer so that the asymptomatic contagious stage is lengthy), and/or causes disease that is difficult to diagnose.[52] While the goal of some bioterrorists is to kill or seriously injure masses of people, the most common goal is to cause widespread fear, panic, and social disruption.

In the United States, potential bioterror agents are classified into three categories (**Table 13–5**).[53] Category A represents high-priority agents that pose a significant risk because they can be easily transmitted from one person to another or have high mortality rates. Category A agents include anthrax, smallpox, plague, botulism, tularemia, and viral hemorrhagic fevers like Ebola and Marburg virus. Anthrax is of particular concern because it was used in a postal bioterrorism attack in the United States in 2001.[54,55] Naturally occurring cases of anthrax (*Bacillus anthracis*) are diagnosed every year in people who work with sheep and livestock because anthrax forms spores (dormant bacteria) that can survive in the environment for years. These cases are usually skin (cutaneous) infections. In the laboratory, anthrax can be made into a fine powder, creating an inhalational anthrax that affects the lungs. Anthrax is not passed from person to person, but the weaponized form can be aerosolized and breathed in. The disease

Table 13–5 U.S. classifications of potential bioterrorism agents.

Category	Agents
Category A	• Anthrax (*Bacillus anthracis*)
	• Botulism (*Clostridium botulinum* toxin)
	• Plague (*Yersinia pestis*)
	• Smallpox (variola major)
	• Tularemia (*Francisella tularensis*)
	• Viral hemorrhagic fevers (such as Ebola, Marburg, Lassa, and Machupo viruses)
Category B	• Brucellosis
	• Glanders (*Burkholderia mallei*)
	• Melioidosis (*Burkholderia psudomallei*)
	• Psittacosis (*Chlamydia psittaci*)
	• Q fever (*Coxiella burnetii*)
	• Typhus fever (*Rickettsia prowazekii*)
	• Alphaviruses that cause encephalitis (such as Venezuelan equine encephalitis [VEE], eastern equine encephalitis [EEE], and western equine encephalitis [WEE])
	• Toxins (such as ricin, Staphylococcal enterotoxin B, and the epsilon toxin of *Clostridium perfringens*)
	• Food safety threats (such as *Salmonella*, *Escherichia coli* O157:H7, and *Shigella*)
	• Water safety threats (such as *Vibrio cholerae* and *Cryptosporidium parvum*)
Category C	• Emerging infectious diseases (such as hantavirus and Nipah virus)

Source: Adapted from Rotz LD, Khan AS, Lillibridge SR, Ostroff SM, Hughes JM. Public health assessment of potential biological terrorism agents. *Emerg Infect Dis.* 2002;8:225–230.

can be easily cured with antibiotics if is detected early, but advanced cases are often fatal.

Category B agents are moderately easy to spread, have a moderate illness rate, and usually cause relatively few deaths. Examples of Category B agents include brucellosis, ricin (a toxin from *Ricinus communis*, which is found in castor beans), Q fever, typhus fever, and viral encephalitis infections. This category also includes food safety threats such as *Salmonella, Shilgella,* and *E. coli O157:H7* and water supply threats such as cholera and cryptosporidiosis. Category C agents are emerging infectious diseases like hantavirus that are potential threats in part because they are not well understood. Chemical agents may also pose a threat (**Table 13–6**).[56]

The best defense against a bioterrorist attack is early detection so that an outbreak can be contained and exposed or at risk people can receive immunization, postexposure prophylaxis, and/or medical treatment. This requires a strong laboratory network, trained public health departments that are prepared to coordinate response activities, the cooperation of healthcare providers and emergency responders, and an adequate stockpile

Table 13–6 Possible chemical bioweapons.

Category	Examples
Nerve agents	tabun, sarin, soman, GF, VX
Blood agents	hydrogen cyanide, cyanogen chloride
Blister agents	lewisite, nitrogen and sulfur mustards, phosgene oxime
Heavy metals	arsenic, lead, mercury
Volatile toxins	benzene, chloroform, trihalomethanes
Pulmonary agents	phosgene, chlorine, vinyl chloride
Incapacitating agents	BZ
Explosive nitro compounds and oxidizers	ammonium nitrate combined with fuel oil
Flammable industrial gases and liquids	gasoline, propane
Poisonous industrial gases, liquids, and solids	cyanides, nitriles
Corrosive industrial acids and bases	nitric acid, sulfuric acid
Other agents	esticides, dioxins, furans, polychlorinated biphenyls (PCBs)

Source: Adapted from Biological and chemical terrorism: strategic plan for preparedness and response. Recommendations of the CDC Strategic Planning Workgroup. *MMWR Recomm Rep*. 2000;49(RR-1):1–14.

of essential vaccines and medications.[53] Strong communication systems are also necessary for keeping the public informed of developments and encouraging appropriate personal responses. Global communication may also play a key role in preventing some acts of terrorism and responding to attacks that do occur.

13.6 GLOBAL ENVIRONMENTAL CHANGE AND HEALTH

A recent study estimated that about 24% of the global disease burden can be attributed to environmental factors such as water, sanitation, indoor and outdoor air pollution, noise, housing risks, chemicals, the recreational environment, water resources management, land use and the built environment, radiation, and occupational exposures (**Table 13–7**).[57] Many of these diseases could be prevented with modest environmental interventions. For example, digging pit latrines reduces the incidence of diarrhea and also keeps feces from contaminating water supplies. And vector control, such as spraying insecticide to reduce the mosquito population and the incidence of malaria, can be minimally damaging to the environment if the chemicals are applied correctly.

Infrastructural development—building permanent structures, terracing slopes for agricultural use, converting forests to farms, paving streets, installing electric lines and sewers, building dams, extracting fossil fuels to make oil and other petroleum products, and a host of other activities—has increased the quality of life for billions of people. Many of these environmental changes are beneficial for health and have minimal impact on the environment. However, any environmental change may also create a new set of health concerns (**Table 13–8**).[58–60]

The immediate effects of most human activities are local, but the distinction between local and global environmental change is getting blurrier. The air pollution created by millions of commuters driving to work each day in one city does not just damage their airspace, but that of their neighbors. The solid waste products, including hazardous materials, that are produced in one country may be transported across national boundaries as rich countries pay others to take on the long-term environmental risk of storing potentially toxic waste.[61] Deforestation and habitat destruction, soil erosion and salinization, water management problems, overhunting and overfishing, invasive species (which may crowd out local flora and fauna), human population growth, and increasing use of resources per capita can all have local and global impacts.[62]

Table 13–7 Percent of disease attributable to environmental risk factors.

Disease	% of Cases Attributable to the Environment	Primary Environmental Risk Factor (>25% of Cases Attributable to the Risk Factor)
Intestinal nematode infections	100%	Water, sanitation, and hygiene
Trachoma	100%	Water, sanitation, and hygiene
Schistosomiasis	100%	Water, sanitation, and hygiene
Japanese encephalitis	95%	Water resources management
Dengue	95%	Housing risks
Diarrheal diseases	94%	Water, sanitation, and hygiene
Drowning	72%	Recreational environment
Unintentional poisonings	71%	Chemicals
Lymphatic filariasis	66%	Water, sanitation, and hygiene
Chagas disease	56%	Housing risks
Malnutrition	50%	Water, sanitation, and hygiene
Lower respiratory infections	42%	Indoor air pollution
Malaria	42%	Water resources management
Road-traffic accidents	40%	Land use and built environment

Source: Data from Prüss-Üstün A, Corvalán C. How much disease burden can be prevented by environmental interventions? Epidemiology. 2007;18:167–178.

Globalization can also benefit environmental health by encouraging the use of sustainable practices. In a global marketplace, the choices any person makes about where to live, work, and travel, and what to purchase, can have a significant influence on others around the world. For example, the growing demand for organic foods and other organic products in high-income countries has created an incentive for farmers to minimize the use of chemicals on their crops. As a result, a growing number of farmers in countries of all income levels have adopted new growing techniques.[63]

Table 13–8 Examples of health effects of local environmental change.

Environmental Change	Possible Pathways	Possibly Increased Disease Outcomes
Dam building and irrigation	Increased snail habitat and human contact with water	Schistosomiasis
	Increased insect breeding sites	Vectorborne infections
	Increased moist soil	Helminth infections
Urbanization	Lack of access to clean drinking water and sanitation for residents in low-quality housing areas	Diarrheal diseases and helminthiases
	Increased trash that attracts rodents	Plague, hantavirus
	More *Aedes aegypti* mosquito breeding sites	Dengue
	Crowded housing	Mental illness, war/violence, tuberculosis and respiratory infections
	Immigration of susceptible people	Communicable diseases
Deforestation	Increased insect breeding sites	Vectorborne infections
	Increased contact with animal reservoirs	Zoonotic infections
Reforestation	Increased contact with tick vectors and increased outdoor exposure	Lyme disease
Agricultural intensification	Increased antibiotic and pesticide use promotes drug and insecticide resistance	Poisoning, vectorborne infections, drug-resistant infections
	Increased contact with vectors	Vectorborne infections

Source: Information from Moore M, Gould P, Keary BS. Global urbanization and impact on health. *Int J Hyg Environ Health*. 2003;206:269–278; and Wilson ML. Ecology and Infectious Disease. In: Aron JL, Patz JA, editors. *Ecosystem change and public health*. Baltimore MD: The Johns Hopkins University Press; 2001; and *Global environmental outlook year book 2004/2005*. Nairobi, Kenya: UNEP; 2005.

However, the cumulative effect of the intensified use of natural resources across the planet appears to be contributing to global climate change. The Intergovernmental Panel on Climate Change (IPCC), which reviews and synthesizes scientific data about climate and weather, has expressed certainty that global warming is occurring and will continue to occur for centuries to come. The IPCC has also concluded that the observed changes are very likely due to human activity.[64] The impacts of global climate change include land degradation, water and air quality issues, a loss of biodiversity, and temperature and precipitation extremes (**Figure 13–5**),[65] all of which can have a significant impact on human health.[66]

While cycles of climate change have occurred throughout history, there is growing concern about the pace of global warming. The IPCC predicts that climate change will mean more frequent hot days and nights and fewer cold days and nights, an increasing frequency of heat waves, an increase in the frequency of heavy precipitation events in some areas and an increase in droughts in others, an increase in tropical cyclone (hurricane) activity, and an increase in the incidence of extremely high sea levels.[64] In addition to temperature extremes and variable weather cycles, there may be continued ozone depletion and increased ultraviolet radiation. Global warming can also lead to acid precipitation (acid rain), loss of biodiversity, desertification, and resource depletion (such as the loss of potable water supplies). These changes can have direct effects on human health (**Table 13–9**).[67]

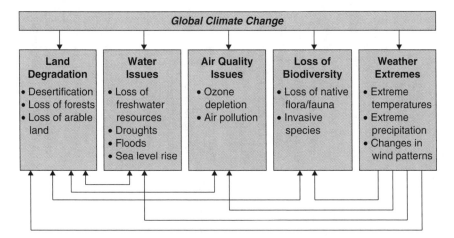

Figure 13–5 Examples of the signs of global environmental change.

Table 13–9 Examples of human health effects of global climate change.

Diseases	Mechanism
Asthma and allergies	Changes in air quality (due to increased pollen, mold, toxins, or dust) may increase the prevalence and severity of respiratory diseases
Skin cancer and cataracts	Increased exposure to ultraviolet radiation (due to a decrease in stratospheric ozone) may increase the incidence of skin cancer and cataracts
Cardiovascular disease	High temperatures and poor air quality increase the incidence of heart attacks and strokes
Nutritional diseases	Changes in temperature and precipitation can reduce crop yields and lead to undernutrition
Mental health	The stresses associated with extreme weather events could increase the incidence and severity of psychological disorders
Infectious diseases	Climate change has the potential to increase the incidence of vectorborne (insect-transmitted) and zoonotic (animal) diseases as well as waterborne diarrheal diseases

Source: Information from The Interagency Working Group on Climate Change and Health. *A human health perspective on climate change: a report outlining the research needs on the human health effects of climate change.* Research Triangle Park NC: Environmental Health Perspectives/National Institute of Environmental Health Sciences (NIEHS); 2010.

Climate change will affect every individual, community, and nation. Heat waves in the United States, Europe, India, and other regions of the world have already been responsible for the deaths of older adults and those with respiratory diseases.[68] Each year, floods cause the deaths of thousands of people and animals, destroy homes and crops, and damage infrastructure, including hospitals, roads, and sewage systems.[69] The poor bear the highest burden, because most of the deaths from extreme weather occur in low-income areas.[70]

Regardless of arguments about the precise causes of global warming, these alarming trends support the notion that humans should try to tread more lightly on the Earth. For example, alternative energy sources that harness solar, wind, or wave power may be able to produce energy that creates less pollution and less environmental damage than carbon-based fuels, hydroelectric power (which requires the building of massive dams and flooding of large swaths of land), and nuclear power (which remains dangerous because of the risk of a meltdown). The short- and long-term risks and benefits of projects that alter the environment should be carefully considered before projects are initiated, and the assessments should include health and environmental evaluations as well as economic considerations. Preventive measures should be implemented, such as using locally appropriate building materials and housing styles and not building homes in especially vulnerable locations.[71] Additionally, global monitoring and communications systems need to be strengthened so that potentially catastrophic events like widespread famines can be prevented and addressed.[66] In a globalized world, everyone has a stake in creating and sustaining a healthy environment.[72]

13.7 DISCUSSION QUESTIONS

1. How is globalization beneficial for individual and public health? How is globalization harmful?
2. If you were a poor resident of a low-income country, would you rather live in a rural area or an urban area? Why?
3. How worried should humans be about the emergence of new infectious diseases? Is there anything that we can do to reduce the risk of EIDs?
4. What are some examples of recent foodborne outbreaks? What were the food sources that spread the infection? Was global trade a factor in these outbreaks?
5. Describe the physical characteristics that make a man or woman attractive in your culture. How have your own ideals about beauty been shaped by culture?
6. What do your state/province and/or country recommend that you do to prepare for a possible act of bioterrorism? Have you taken the recommended steps? Why or why not?
7. What changes in the natural and built environments of your community have increased the health of local residents? What changes have decreased the health of the community?
8. What steps can you take to minimize your ecological footprint?

REFERENCES

1. Sachs J. International economics: unlocking the mysteries of globalization. *Foreign Policy.* 1998;110:97–111.
2. *The world factbook.* Washington DC: Central Intelligence Agency; 2012.
3. Morens DM, Folkers GK, Fauci AS. Emerging infections: a perpetual challenge. *Lancet Infect Dis.* 2008;8:710–719.
4. Glynn T, Seffrin JR, Brawley OW, Grey N, Ross H. The globalization of tobacco use: 21 challenges for the 21st century. *CA Cancer J Clin.* 2010;60:50–61.
5. Cherry JD. The chronology of the 2002–2003 SARS mini pandemic. *Pediatr Respir Rev.* 2004;5:262–269.
6. Viboud C, Bjørnstad ON, Smith DL, Simonsen L, Miller MA, Grenfell BT. Synchrony, waves, and spatial hierarchies in the spread of influenza. *Science.* 2006;312:447–451.
7. Bettcher D, Lee K. Globalisation and public health. *J Epidemiol Commun Health.* 2002;56:8–17.
8. Moore M, Gould P, Keary BS. Global urbanization and impact on health. *Int J Hyg Environ Health.* 2003;206:269–278.
9. Vlahov D, Galea S. Urbanization, urbanicity, and health. *J Urban Health.* 2002;79(suppl 4):S1–S12.
10. *World health statistics 2011.* Geneva: WHO; 2011.
11. *Human development report 2010.* New York: UNDP; 2010.
12. *World urbanization prospects, the 2011 revision.* New York: Department of Economic and Social Affairs, United Nations; 2012.
13. Morens DM, Folkers GK, Fauci AS. The challenge of emerging and re-emerging infectious diseases. *Nature.* 2004;430:242–249.
14. Fauci AS. Infectious diseases: considerations for the 21st century. *Clin Infect Dis.* 2001;32:675–685.
15. Gubler DF. Resurgent vector-borne diseases as a global health problem. *Emerg Infect Dis.* 1998;4:442–450.
16. Grundmann H, Aires-de-Sousa M, Boyce J, Tiemersma E. Emergence and resurgence of meticillin-resistant *Staphylococcus aureus* as a public-health threat. *Lancet.* 2006;368:874–885.
17. MacPherson DW, Gushulak BD, Baine WB, et al. Population mobility, globalization, and antimicrobial drug resistance. *Emerg Infect Dis.* 2009;15:1727–1731.
18. Fraser DW, Tsai TR, Orenstein W, et al. Legionnaires' disease: description of an epidemic of pneumonia. *N Engl J Med.* 1997;297:1189–1197.
19. Breiman RF, Butler JC. Legionnaires' disease: clinical, epidemiological, and public health perspectives. *Semin Respir Infect.* 1998;13:84–89.
20. Pourrut X, Kumulungui B, Wittmann T, et al. The natural history of Ebola virus in Africa. *Microbes Infect.* 2005;7:1005–1014.
21. Feldmann H, Geisbert T. Ebola haemorrhagic fever. *Lancet.* 2011;377:849–862.
22. Leroy EM, Rouquet P, Formenty P, et al. Multiple Ebola virus transmission events and rapid decline of central African wildlife. *Science.* 2004;303:387–390.
23. Hantavirus Pulmonary Syndrome—United States: updated recommendations for risk reduction. *MMWR. Recomm Rep.* 2002;51 (RR-9).
24. Jonsson BC, Moraes Figueiredo LT, Vapalahti O. A global perspective on hantavirus ecology, epidemiology, and disease. *Clin Microbiol Rev.* 2010;23:412–441.

25. Jaffe HW, Bregman DJ, Selik RM. Acquired immune deficiency syndrome in the United States: the first 1000 cases. *J Infect Dis.* 1983;148:339–345.
26. Mortimer PP. ABC of AIDS: the virus and the tests. *Br Med J (Clin Res Ed).* 1987;294:1602–1605.
27. Quinn TC. Global burden of the HIV pandemic. *Lancet.* 1996;348:99–106.
28. Update: Cholera Outbreak—Peru, Ecuador, and Colombia. *Morb Mort Wkly Rep.* 40;13:225–227.
29. Update: Cholera—Western Hemisphere, 1992. *Morb Mort Wkly Rep.* 1992; 41(36):667–668.
30. Hayes EB, Komar N, Nasci RS, Montgomery SP, O'Leary DR, Campbell GL. Epidemiology and transmission of West Nile Virus disease. *Emerg Infect Dis.* 2005;11:1167–1173.
31. Hayes EB, Gubler DJ. West Nile virus: epidemiology and clinical features of an emerging epidemic in the United States. *Annu Rev Med.* 2006;57:181–194.
32. Lindsey NP, Staples JE, Lehman JA, Fischer M; U.S. CDC. Surveillance for human West Nile Virus disease—United States, 1999–2008. *MMWR Surveill Summ.* 2010;59:1–17.
33. Smolinski, MS, Hamburg MA, Lederberg J, editors. Committee on Emerging Microbial Threats to Health in the 21st Century. Institute of Medicine. *Microbial threats to health: emergence, detection, and response.* Washington DC: The National Academics Press; 2003.
34. *Import share of consumption.* Washington DC: Economic Research Service, United States Department of Agriculture; 2012.
35. Dewaal CS, Hicks G, Barlow K, Alderton L, Vegosen L. Foods associated with foodborne illness outbreaks from 1990 through 2003. *Food Protection Trends.* 2006;26:466–473.
36. Mead PS, Slutsker L, Dietz V, et al. Food-related illness and death in the United States. *Emerg Infect Dis.* 1999;5:607–625.
37. Olson ED. Protecting food safety: more needs to be done to keep pace with scientific advances and the changing food supply. *Health Aff.* 2011;5:915–923.
38. King LJ, Anderson LR, Blackmore CG. Executive summary of the AVMA One Health Initiative Task Force report. *J Am Vet Med Assoc.* 2008;233:259–261.
39. Altekruse SF, Cohen ML, Swerdlow DL. Emerging foodborne diseases. *Emerg Infect Dis.* 1997;3:285–293.
40. Lynch MF, Tauxe RV, Hedberg CW. The growing burden of foodborne outbreaks due to contaminated fresh produce: risks and opportunities. *Epidemiol Infect.* 2009;137:307–315.
41. Livermore MA. Authority and legitimacy in global governance: deliberation, institutional differentiation, and the Codex Alimentarius. *New York University Law Rev.* 2006;81:766–801.
42. Medeiros LC, Hillers VN, Kendall PA, Mason A. Food safety education: what should we be teaching to consumers? *J Nutr Educ.* 2001;33:108–113.
43. Weiss KM, Ferrell RF, Hanis CL. A New World Syndrome of metabolic diseases with a genetic and evolutionary basis. *Am J Physical Anthropol.* 1984;27(suppl S5):153–178.
44. Diamond J. The double puzzle of diabetes. *Nature.* 2003;423:599–602.
45. Popkin BM. Global nutrition dynamics: the world is shifting rapidly toward a diet linked with noncommunicable diseases. *Am J Clin Nutr.* 2006;84:289–298.

46. Makino N, Tsuboi K, Dennerstein L. Prevalence of eating disorders: a comparison of Western and non-Western countries. *Med Gen Med*. 2004;6:49.

47. Becker AE, Gliman SE, Burwell RA. Changes in prevalence of overweight and in body image among Fijian women between 1989 and 1998. *Obes Res*. 2005;13:110–117.

48. Becker AE. Television, disordered eating, and young women in Fiji: negotiating body image and identity during rapid social change. *Cult Med Psychiatry*. 2004;28:533–559.

49. Brewis AA, McGarvey ST, Jones J, Swinburn BA. Perceptions of body size in Pacific Islanders. *Int J Obes*. 1998;22:185–189.

50. Craig P, Halavatau V, Comino E, Caterson I. Perception of body size in the Tongan community: differences from and similarities to an Australian sample. *Int J Obes*. 1999;23:1288–1294.

51. Noah DL, Huebner KD, Darling RG, Waeckerle JF. The history and threat of biological warfare and terrorism. *Emerg Med Clin N Am*. 2002;20:255–271.

52. Beeching NJ, Dance DAB, Miller ARO, Spencer RC. Biological warfare and bioterrorism. *BMJ*. 2002;324:336–339.

53. Rotz LD, Khan AS, Lillibridge SR, Ostroff SM, Hughes JM. Public health assessment of potential biological terrorism agents. *Emerg Infect Dis*. 2002;8:225–230.

54. Inglesby TV, O'Toole T, Henderson DA, et al. Anthrax as a biological weapon, 2002: updated recommendations for management. *JAMA*. 2002;287:2236–2252.

55. Jernigan DB, Raghunathan PL, Bell BP, et al. Investigation of bioterrorism-related anthrax, United States, 2001: epidemiologic findings. *Emerg Infect Dis*. 2002;8:1019–1028.

56. Biological and chemical terrorism: strategic plan for preparedness and response. Recommendations of the CDC Strategic Planning Workgroup. *MMWR Recomm Rep*. 2000;49(RR-1):1–14.

57. Prüss-Üstün A, Corvalán C. How much disease burden can be prevented by environmental interventions? *Epidemiology*. 2007;18:167–178.

58. Myers SS, Patz JA. Emerging threats to human health from global environmental change. *Annu Rev Environ Resour*. 2009;39:223–252.

59. Wilson ML. Ecology and Infectious Disease. In: Aron JL, Patz JA, editors. *Ecosystem change and public health*. Baltimore MD: The Johns Hopkins University Press; 2001.

60. *Global environmental outlook year book 2004/2005*. Nairobi, Kenya: UNEP; 2005.

61. Liddick D. The traffic in garbage and hazardous wastes: an overview. *Trends Organized Crime*. 2010;13:134–146.

62. Diamond J. *Collapse: how societies choose to fail or succeed*. New York: Viking; 2005.

63. Willer H, Kilcher L, editors. *The world of organic agriculture: statistics and emerging trends 2012*. Bonn, Germany: International Federation of Organic Agriculture Movements; 2012.

64. Intergovernmental Panel on Climate Change. *Climate change 2007: the physical science basis. Summary for policymakers*. Geneva: IPCC; 2007.

65. Rockström J, Steffen W, Noone K, et al. A safe operating space for humanity. *Nature*. 2009;461:472–475.

66. Costello A, Abbas M, Allen A, et al. Managing the health effects of climate change. *Lancet*. 2009;373:1693–1733.

67. The Interagency Working Group on Climate Change and Health. *A human health perspective on climate change: a report outlining the research needs on the human*

health effects of climate change. Research Triangle Park NC: Environmental Health Perspectives/National Institute of Environmental Health Sciences (NIEHS); 2010.

68. Kovats RS, Hajat S. Heat stress and public health: a critical review. *Annu Rev Public Health.* 2008;29:41–55.

69. Alderman K, Turner LR, Tong S. Floods and human health: a systematic review. *Environ Int.* 2012;47:37–47.

70. McMichael AJ, Friel S, Nyong A, Corvalan C. Global environmental change and health: impacts, inequalities, and the health sector. *BMJ.* 2008;336:191–194.

71. Frumkin H, Hess J, Luber G, Malilay J, McGeehin M. Climate change: the public health response. *Am J Public Health.* 2008;98:435–445.

72. McMichael AJ, Beaglehole R. The changing global context of public health. *Lancet.* 2000;356:495–499.

CHAPTER 14

Health, Human Rights, and Humanitarian Aid

Access to basic health care is considered to be a fundamental human right, but wars, civil conflicts, and natural disasters can restrict access to health services. Local and international organizations can help by responding to urgent needs, assisting with long-term recovery, and helping to prevent and prepare for future catastrophes.

14.1 HEALTH AND HUMAN RIGHTS

The preamble to the Constitution of the World Health Organization (WHO), which has been affirmed by the nearly 200 countries that have membership in the United Nations (UN), lists nine health principles (**Table 14–1**). The boldest claim is that "the enjoyment of the highest attainable *standard of health* is one of the fundamental *rights* of every human being."[1] This statement calls for the standard of health to be raised so that everyone has access to at least basic medical and psychological care (principle 7), especially people who are members of vulnerable population groups (principles 2 and 6). The preamble also notes that health is linked with peace (principles 3, 4, and 5), that areas with poor health standards put everyone at risk for outbreaks of infectious disease (principle 5), and that both the public (principle 8) and governments (principle 9) must take active responsibility for public health. Two key terms require careful definitions: human rights and standard of health.

A **human right** is an entitlement that is due to every person simply because of being human. Human rights are considered to be universal (available to everyone) and irrevocable (something that cannot be taken away). Many of these rights are spelled out in the Universal Declaration of Human Rights (UDHR), which was unanimously adopted by the member

Table 14–1 Health principles from the Preamble to the Constitution of the World Health Organization.

1	Health is a state of complete physical, mental, and social well-being and not merely the absence of disease or infirmity.
2	The enjoyment of the highest attainable standard of health is one of the fundamental rights of every human being without distinction of race, religion, political belief, economic, or social condition.
3	The health of all peoples is fundamental to the attainment of peace and security and is dependent upon the fullest cooperation of individuals and States.
4	The achievement of any State in the promotion and protection of health is of value to all.
5	Unequal development in different countries in the promotion of health and control of disease, especially communicable disease, is a common danger.
6	Healthy development of the child is of basic importance; the ability to live harmoniously in a changing total environment is essential to such development.
7	The extension to all peoples of the benefits of medical, psychological, and related knowledge is essential to the fullest attainment of health.
8	Informed opinion and active cooperation on the part of the public are of the utmost importance in the improvement of the health of the people.
9	Governments have a responsibility for the health of their peoples which can be fulfilled only by the provision of adequate health and social measures.

Source: Reproduced from the World Health Organization. The Constitution of the World Health Organization. http://whqlibdoc.who.int/hist/official_records /constitution.pdf.

states of the UN in 1948 (**Table 14–2**).[2] Articles 3 to 21 define civil and political rights that protect the foundational freedoms of humans, such as the right to privacy and the right to freedom from torture. These rights are about protections rather than provisions, and they can be granted and upheld with limited financial costs to the government. Articles 22 to 28 outline economic, social, and cultural rights that, if realized, would contribute to human flourishing. These rights, such as the right to social security, the right to education, and the right to a standard of living adequate for health and well-being, obligate governments to provide certain services to their people.[3]

Table 14–2 Human rights listed in the Universal Declaration of Human Rights.

Human Right	UDHR Articles
Right to equal dignity and human rights for all humans	1, 2, 6
Right to life, liberty, and security of person	3
Freedom from slavery and servitude	4
Freedom from torture and cruel, inhuman, or degrading treatment or punishment	5
Freedom from discrimination	7
Freedom from arbitrary arrest, detention, or exile	9
Right to a fair trial	8, 10, 11
Right to privacy	12
Freedom of movement	13
Right to asylum	14
Right to a nationality	15
Right to marry and found a family	16
Right to own property	17
Freedom of thought, conscience, and religion	18
Freedom of opinion and expression	19
Freedom of peaceful assembly and association	20
Right to participate in government	21
Right to social security	22
Right to work	23
Right to rest and leisure	24
Right to a standard of living adequate for the health and well-being of the individual and his/her family, including food, clothing, housing, medical care, and necessary social services, and the right to security in the event of unemployment, sickness, disability, widowhood, or old age	25
Right to education	26
Right to participate in the cultural life of a community	27

Source: Adapted from United Nations Human Rights. The Universal Declaration of Human Rights. http://www.ohchr.org/en/udhr/Pages/UDHRIndex.aspx.

The **standard of health** refers to targets that governments set for improving the health of their populations. The UN High Commissioner for Human Rights has clarified what is meant by the right to the "highest attainable standard of health": "The right to health does not mean the right to be *healthy*, nor does it mean that poor governments must put in place expensive services for which they have no resources. But it does require governments and public authorities to put in place policies and action plans [which] will lead to available and accessible healthcare for all in the shortest possible time. To ensure that this happens is the challenge facing both the human rights community and public health professionals."[4] In other words, no one can guarantee *health* for anyone—many diseases have no known preventable cause and no known cure—but governments can strive to increase access to preventive and therapeutic services, starting with a basic package of healthcare services (such as antenatal care, childhood vaccinations, treatment for common infectious diseases, and access to clean water) and then expanding the range of services that are available to the whole population.[5]

The goals of the field of health and human rights include exposing human rights violations, increasing accountability for governments and other organizations involved in health and human services, providing education about rights, and improving access to health and related services.[6] Achieving the highest attainable standard of health requires increasing access to health care and to the tools for health.

14.2 ACCESS TO HEALTH

Access to health is a major economic and political concern in most countries. In the United States, recent changes in healthcare policy have sparked debates about how to increase the proportion of the population with health insurance, contain rising healthcare costs, and regulate private health insurance plans, and whether to expand government healthcare coverage to include those who are not poor, old, or government employees.[7] Brazil is trying to reduce remaining health disparities by increasing revenue for its universal public healthcare system and improving the quality of services provided.[8] China is seeking to increase medical insurance coverage, to ensure access to essential medications, and to invest more resources in primary health care and preventive health services.[9] India is pursuing options for reducing the high out-of-pocket healthcare expenses that restrict access to health services for low-income households.[10]

Sierra Leone introduced free maternal and child health care at public facilities in 2011, and is now trying to figure out how to pay for the plan.[11] Every country has to make decisions about what healthcare services should be provided and who should pay for those services, and these decisions have human rights implications.

A first major access to health issue is whether health care should be seen as a basic social right or if it should be treated like a commodity that can be bought and sold.[12] Some countries have national constitutions or laws that recognize the right to health.[13] These countries, which include Brazil and Poland, typically have healthcare systems that provide universal (or nearly universal) health care that is funded through tax revenue.[14,15] Everyone in these countries has access to a package of essential health services at no cost to them beyond what they pay in taxes. Other countries have healthcare systems that are primarily private. A package of free or subsidized essential healthcare services may be provided to children and low-income adults by the government, but some critical health services may cost too much to be accessed by these households. Human rights activists say that if health is a human right it is unjust that poor people so often do not have access to even the minimum level of health care that will allow them to live healthy and productive lives, especially as most poor people are born into poverty.[12]

Given that every country has limited resources available for health, a related issue is about the package of healthcare services that should be available to everyone. The right to health does not mean the right for everyone to have access to every health resource on demand. Difficult decisions have to be made about how to prioritize distribution of health goods and services, like deciding who will be eligible for a particular surgery, which medications will be part of the health system's formulary, and which routine preventive health services and screenings will be covered. The unfortunate reality is that most health systems cannot provide a heart transplant to everyone who needs one to stay alive, high-tech and expensive cancer treatments for everyone who would benefit from them, or years of intensive rehabilitation for everyone whose quality of life would improve with more extensive therapy. Judgments about what health systems will cover have to consider the number of medical specialists and support staff available to do procedures, the types of healthcare facilities available, the cost-effectiveness of various medicines and health technologies, and the improvements in quality of life associated with various interventions.[16]

However, the general consensus is that the right to health includes the right to access at least basic healthcare services, essential medications and health technologies, and water and other foundational resources for health.

14.2.A Access to Health Care

The right to health care is one of many human rights recognized in the Universal Declaration of Human Rights. Article 25 states that "everyone has the right to a standard of living adequate for the health and well-being of himself and of his family, including food, clothing, housing, and *medical care* and necessary social services."[2]

Several key criteria are used to evaluate access to health care:[17]

- *Availability*: There should be an adequate number of medical and public health facilities that are functioning, staffed, and stocked with the necessary supplies.
- *Accessibility*: Health care should be geographically and physically accessible to everyone, regardless of residential location and physical ability.
- *Affordability*: Health care should be economically accessible. Payment for services should be commensurate with ability to pay.
- *Acceptability*: Health care should be respectful of patients from all ethnicities, sexes, ages, and other population groups. This may mean adapting to cultural expectations, such as ensuring that a female healthcare provider examines female patients in nonemergency situations if that is the cultural expectation of the patient.
- *Quality*: Health facilities should be well maintained and stocked with appropriate supplies, and healthcare staff should be appropriately skilled.

These set a minimum standard for access to health care. They do not specify what constitutes an appropriate level of access to health personnel, medical specialists, tests and procedures, medications, and health technology because access is dependent on a country's resources. Lower-income countries generally have lower standards of health because they have more limited resources. Those limits include too few healthcare workers (**Table 14–3**),[18] a situation exacerbated by "**brain drain**," the migration of healthcare professionals trained in low-income countries to higher paying jobs in high-income countries.[19] Ideally, every country should be working toward increasing access to and quality of health personnel and services.

14.2.B Access to Medication

Creating and testing new medications is a long and expensive process costing about $1 billion, on average, for each new product.[20] In exchange for their research and development (R&D) investments, pharmaceutical

Table 14-3 Healthcare personnel and services per 10,000 people in 2010.

Country	USA	South Korea	Poland	Brazil	China	India	Kenya	Sierra Leone
Physicians	24.2	20.2	21.6	17.6	14.2	6.5	--	0.2
Psychiatrists	0.8	0.5	0.5	0.3	0.1	<0.05	<0.05	<0.05
Nurses/midwives	98.2	52.9	58.0	64.2	13.8	10.0	--	1.7
Dentistry personnel	--	5.0	3.2	11.7	0.4	0.8	--	<0.05
Pharmaceutical personnel	--	12.1	6.3	5.4	2.5	5.2	--	0.3
Community health workers	--	--	--	--	8.3	0.5	--	0.2
Hospital beds	30	103	67	24	42	9	14	--
Psychiatric hospital beds	3.4	19.1	5.4	1.9	1.4	0.2	--	0.3

--: data not available

Source: Data from *World health statistics 2012.* Geneva: WHO; 2012.

companies with a new product that has been shown to be safe and effective are granted a **patent** for the drug and given exclusive rights to sell that drug for at least five years (and often much longer that that).[21] Generic versions of the patented drug cannot be sold legally until after the expiration of the exclusivity period. This provides the company with a window of opportunity in which to recoup R&D costs and possibly make a profit.

International trade agreements from the World Trade Organization (WTO), a UN agency, enforce the patents issued by member nations (Table 14–4). For example, the TRIPS (Trade-Related Aspects of Intellectual Property Rights) agreement standardized intellectual property laws. The World Intellectual Property Organization (WIPO) also protects patents, copyrights, and registered trademarks, including those for health-related products. Additionally, bilateral and multilateral trade agreements between two or more countries may include clauses that further restrict access to cheaper drugs. (These are sometimes called "TRIPS Plus" agreements because they require more protections on intellectual property than TRIPS does.) For example, trade agreements might extend the duration of a patent on a pharmaceutical agent and enforce rules that prohibit generic versions of the drug from being produced or imported. These agreements may inhibit the ability of low- and middle-income countries to take action to procure or to produce their own cheaper medications.

Table 14–4 Health aspects of international trade agreements.

Trade Agreement	Health Aspects
General Agreement on Trade in Services (GATS)	Treats human services such as health care, water, sanitation, and education as commodities subject to trade rules. Also addresses some safety regulations, handling of hazardous materials, licensing of medical practitioners, and other aspects of health.
General Agreement on Tariffs and Trade (GATT)	Allows for countries to ban certain products to protect public health, but directs more attention to protecting intellectual property rights like drug patents.
Trade-Related Aspects of Intellectual Property Rights (TRIPS)	Protects patents, copyrights, trademarks, and industrial designs across national boundaries and, therefore, limits the production of certain protected medications. Contains safeguards that are supposed to ensure access to essential medications.

Many of the concerns about access to essential medicines came to light as a result of the unmet need for low-cost antiretroviral drugs (ARVs) to combat HIV/AIDS in Africa.[22] As the HIV/AIDS pandemic expanded in the 1990s, the new ARVs that were saving lives in high-income countries were too expensive to be widely used in low-income regions. Countries like Brazil, India, and South Africa that tried to produce generic versions of patented ARVs (or to import generic drugs produced elsewhere) faced penalties for violating international intellectual property regulations. In the early 2000s, pharmaceutical companies, ministries of health, and advocacy groups worked together to make patented drugs available at a lower price to low-income countries, and the WTO clarified that the TRIPS agreement "should be interpreted and implemented in a manner supportive of WTO members' right to protect public health and, in particular, to promote access to medicines for all."[23] Countries facing a "national emergency or other circumstances of extreme urgency" could issue "compulsory licenses" for drugs to be manufactured locally. (However, restrictions still applied to imported medications, and few low-income countries had manufacturing capabilities.) By 2010, the Global Fund, PEPFAR (the U.S. President's Emergency Plan for AIDS Relief), and other programs had helped to significantly increase the proportion of people with HIV infection worldwide who were taking ARVs, and the majority of the ARVs were generics.[22]

HIV medications are not the only drugs with limited availability in low-income countries, and other initiatives are seeking to increase access to a variety of critical pharmaceutical agents. For example, the Médecins Sans Frontières (Doctors Without Borders) Campaign for Access to Essential Medicines is lobbying for lower prices, limits on patents, and the development of new diagnostic tests and medicines for common infectious diseases and neglected tropical diseases.[24]

Additionally, to avoid the issue of patent protection entirely, public–private partnerships, which are often funded by philanthropic organizations, have been formed to develop new drugs for neglected tropical diseases.[25] These partnerships usually target drugs for diseases that for-profit companies are unlikely to invest in because of the limited revenue expected from a product created solely for use in low-income regions. Drugs produced by these partnerships will be available at a low cost as soon as they are proven to be safe and effective.

However, significant inequalities in access to medications remain. The WHO's core list of essential medicines that healthcare systems should stock includes about 800 anti-infective, anti-allergic, analgesic, antipsychotic, and hormonal drugs along with medications for noncommunicable diseases such as epilepsy, migraines, heart disease, asthma, and gastrointestinal diseases.[26] The typical low- or middle-income country only includes about 400 medications on its national essential medicines list, about half of the drugs recommended by the WHO expert panel.[27] In contrast, the typical high-income country has a formulary with more than double the number of drugs on the WHO list.

As a result, people in high-income countries have much greater access to medications than people in other parts of the world (**Figure 14–1**). On average, people in high-income countries spend about $432 per year on medications (public and private spending combined), compared to $84 in upper middle-income countries, $31 in lower middle-income countries, and $8 in low-income countries (**Figure 14–2**).[28] High-income and low-income countries are home to similar proportions of the world's population (16% and 17%, respectively), but high-income countries make 78.5% of global pharmaceutical purchases, while low-income countries account for only 1% of sales.[29]

14.2.C Access to Health Technology

Breaking the cycle of disease and poverty requires increased access to health technologies—such as medications, vaccines, and bednets, and also water filters, solar cookers, and other assistive devices—but many

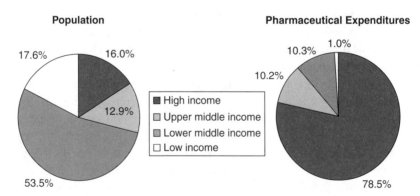

Figure 14–1 Total population and global pharmaceutical sales by country income level in 2006.

Source: Data from Lu Y, Hernandez P, Abegunde D, Edejer T. Medicine expenditures. In: *The world medicines report*. Geneva: WHO; 2011.

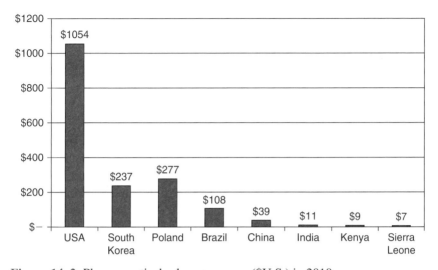

Figure 14–2 Pharmaceutical sales per person ($U.S.) in 2010.

Source: Data from *The pharmaceutical industry and global health: facts and figures.*
Geneva: International Federation of Pharmaceutical Manufacturers & Associations
(IFPMA); 2011.

of the health tools that are effective and relatively affordable remain prohibitively expensive for the poorest households. Simple interventions like insecticide-treated bednets and multivitamins could be adopted for wider use if the global community had the collective will to see that these lifesaving technologies are distributed at low or no cost to the people who need them most.

Thus, the product development cycle for technology for global health does not end when a product is completed and has been field tested. The technology must also be made available for widespread use. The Bill & Melinda Gates Foundation, which makes large donations to researchers creating new technologies for health, recognizes this progression with a four-step process of discovery, development, delivery, and advocacy (which is aimed at sustainability and public policy).[30] The "delivery" phase requires an organizational structure to be in place in the field to coordinate dissemination efforts. Additionally, the technology must be easily and reliably available to those who have chosen to use it, it must be affordable, and it must gain local acceptance and be adopted for use by the end user and not just the national government.[31] In other words, technology is necessary for improving health, but the existence of a helpful tool for health is not enough. A tool only becomes helpful for global health when the people who would benefit most from it have access to it and choose to use it. Access to new technologies requires product advocacy and buy-in from a variety of stakeholders, including donors, policymakers, and end users.[31]

14.2.D Access to Water

Because water is a basic human need—something like air that everyone requires on a daily basis just to survive—access to water is a human right.[32] This does not mean that everyone has a right to an unlimited amount of free water. It does mean that everyone has a right to an adequate quantity of clean water for consumption and hygiene (about 20 to 50 liters daily) at a reasonable cost.[33]

Increasing access to water requires investments in water system infra-structure, which usually means digging new groundwater wells and pro-tecting surface water sources, installing miles of pipelines and pumps to transport water from the source to consumers, and sometimes also con-structing facilities to store and treat the water. These improvements can be expensive, and the costs of building and maintaining the water system must usually be recouped through taxes or user fees. Additionally, user fees help promote conservation, which is important in places where freshwater resources are limited. Thus, water is now considered to be both a consumer good and an essential human need.[34] These sometimes contradictory defini-tions have at times led to significant tensions.

One concern is about the ability of poor households to afford the water they need, especially following water privatization. For example, massive protests occurred in 2000 in Cochabamba, Bolivia's third largest city, after the government leased the city's water rights to a U.S.-based corporation in order to improve services and to satisfy a condition of a World Bank loan.[35] In order to raise capital for modernizing the water system, the company significantly increased user fees. For many low-income households, the higher cost of water was a huge burden. There was no legal way to reduce the cost of the household's water, because residents were banned from using other water sources, such as personal wells and storage tanks, and were even forbidden to collect rainwater without a paid permit.[36] After several months of escalating protests, the water system was renationalized. However, other countries in Latin America, Asia, Africa, and other parts of the world are now experimenting with water privatization.[37] Concerns remain about how to ensure that the poorest residents do not suffer under new policies, and about what alternatives exist for increasing access to safe drinking water.

A related set of questions exist about ownership of various water resources, especially in areas where a growing human population and agricultural intensification have placed extreme demands on the watershed. For example, water supplies are becoming a crucial issue in the American West. In many of the western states, water rights sold (often many decades ago) to cities, farmers, ranchers, and miners define who owns various supplies of water. As was the case in Cochabamba, rainwater collection by those who do not own rights to the local watershed is illegal.[38] Thirsty cities like Los Angeles and Las Vegas that require additional water for their growing populations have to purchase water rights from increasingly remote sources, which may result in the water from distant rivers being rerouted to the city. In some cases, diversion of water or excessive use of water by upstream consumers has left those downstream with a much reduced supply of water.[39] It can be difficult for those downstream populations to make a legal case for their right to the missing water, especially if the water crosses a state or national border (such as the U.S.–Mexican border). The growing concerns about water scarcity require conservation of precious water resources (including the reduction of water loss during transport), clarification of the laws that govern water markets and water use, and a commitment to ensuring adequate water access to vulnerable populations.

14.3 DISASTERS AND HEALTH

Both natural and human-generated disasters can lead to urgent humanitarian situations (**Table 14–5**). The critical needs immediately after any humanitarian incident include (1) water supply, sanitation, and hygiene ("WASH"); (2) food security and nutrition; (3) shelter and essential nonfood items such as personal care items, clothing, bedding, cooking and eating utensils, fuel, and lighting; and (4) essential health services for communicable diseases, sexual and reproductive health, injuries, mental health, and noncommunicable diseases.[40] After attending to urgent and immediate needs, response efforts typically shift from relief activities toward recovery and reconstruction.

The players involved in a particular humanitarian response depend on the scale of the incident (**Tables 14–6** and **14–7**).[41,42] A **crisis** is a small-scale event that can easily be addressed locally, like when a tornado damages several homes in a small town and neighbors provide aid to the affected households. An **emergency** is a larger event that stresses local resources but can still be managed locally. A **disaster** occurs when the

Table 14–5 Examples of types of disasters.

Natural Disasters	Human-Generated Disasters
Weather-related disasters	Intentional
• Floods	• War
• Landslides/mudslides	• Genocide/ethnic cleansing
• Hurricanes/cyclones/typhoons	• Terrorism
• Tornadoes	• Refugee crises
• Winter storms	• Internally displaced persons (IDP) crises
Geophysical disasters	Nonintentional
• Earthquakes	• Transportation accidents
• Tsunamis	• Industrial accidents
• Volcanic eruptions	• Hazardous materials spills
Climate-related disasters	• Explosions/fires
• Droughts	• Radiation
• Extreme heat	• Structural collapses (buildings, bridges, dams, tunnels)
• Extreme cold	
• Wildfires and forest fires	
Biological disasters	
• Pandemic disease	
• Insect infestations	

Table 14–6 Scale of critical incidents.

1	crisis	capacity > demand	local response is sufficient
2	emergency	capacity = demand	local response is sufficient
3	disaster	demand > capacity	outside assistance is necessary
4	catastrophe	demand >> capacity	extensive outside assistance is necessary

Source: Information from Quarantelli EL. Just as a disaster is not simply a big accident, so a catastrophe is not just a big disaster. *J Am Soc Professional Emerg Planners*. 1996; 3: 68–71.

need for assistance exceeds local capacity. A **catastrophe** overwhelms the local response network and requires extensive outside assistance, as was the case following the earthquake in Haiti in 2010 and the tsunami in Southeast Asia in 2004.

Table 14–7 PICE (potential injury–creating event) nomenclature.

PICE Stage	Potential for Additional Casualties	Effect on Local Resources	Extent of Geographic Involvement	Projected Need for Outside Assistance	Status of Outside Help
0	static	controlled	local	little to none	inactive
1	dynamic	disruptive	regional	small	alert
2	dynamic	paralytic	national	moderate	standby
3	dynamic	paralytic	international	great	dispatch

Source: Information from Koenig KL, Dinerman N, Kuehl AE. Disaster nomenclature—a functional impact approach: the PICE system. *Acad Emerg Med.* 1996;3:723–727.

In any response, careful attention must be paid to protecting the civil, political, economic, social, and cultural rights of affected persons. In some situations, individual and collective rights must be balanced. A **nonderogable right** is a human right that is irrevocable, such as the rights to freedom from slavery and freedom from torture. But some other rights may be temporarily suspended under special circumstances when restrictions on some individual rights protect the community as a whole. For example, freedom of movement for people with highly contagious infections may be temporarily limited during an epidemic so that the right of other people to health can be protected.[43] If rights are derogated during or immediately after a critical incident, the new rules must not be discriminatory, and full rights should be restored as soon as possible. Communities engaged in civil conflicts and wars, hosting refugees and internally displaced persons, beginning postconflict recovery, or damaged by natural disasters all face special health and human rights concerns.

14.3.A Civil Conflict and War

A **complex humanitarian emergency** occurs when civil conflict or war cause mass migration of civilian populations, food insecurity, and long-term public health concerns.[44] Unlike natural disasters, which usually create an immediate period of acute need but quickly transition into recovery mode, complex humanitarian emergencies may remain in an acute phase for years or even decades. International humanitarian laws are supposed to provide protection to civilians and armed forces, but these rules are not always enforced.[45] For example, rape and sexual violence have become military tactics in many recent conflicts.[46]

Malnutrition is a primary concern during conflicts.[47] Food production tends to decrease as farms are abandoned, and it is more difficult to import affordable food during times of instability. Food supply chains—processing, transportation, storage, sales—are often interrupted by conflict and uncertainty. And large numbers of people may be migrating and in need of a daily supply of nutrients. The combination of too few calories and micronutrients plus other diseases often leads to severe undernutrition.

Outbreaks of communicable diseases also often occur during complex emergencies, in large part because of the breakdown of social services, including water and sanitation services and public health services. Diarrheal diseases are very common. Other concerns include measles (because of lack of vaccination), respiratory infections like pneumonia and tuberculosis (associated with inadequate shelter), meningitis and malaria (in endemic areas), hepatitis, and sexually transmitted infections (which may have resulted from gender-based violence and may remain untreated because of lack of access to health care).[48] Reproductive health services, including family planning and obstetric care, and psychiatric services tend to be severely inadequate during conflicts.

14.3.B Refugees and Internally Displaced People

A **refugee** is a person who has been forced to involuntarily move because of security concerns like war, civil conflict, political strife, or persecution based on race, tribe, religion, political affiliation, or membership in some other group. There were about 10 million refugees worldwide at the end of 2011.[49] At the beginning of a refugee migration, UNHCR (the office of the UN High Commissioner for Refugees) and other humanitarian organizations, both governmental and private, attempt to provide for the basic needs of refugees, including shelter, food, water, sanitation, and medical care. These services are often provided in "camps" that provide long-term shelter, especially for children, women, and the elderly. A little less than half of refugees live in camps; the rest are displaced to cities or rural areas, where they live alongside residents and other types of migrants and may not have access to special services for refugees.[50] The long-term goal is to find durable (lasting) solutions by helping refugees to repatriate if possible, or to integrate into their countries of asylum or resettlement.

To be classified as a refugee by the UN, a person must have crossed an international border. An **internally displaced person (IDP)** who fled his or her home community because of civil war, famine, natural disaster, or another crisis, but did not cross into another country is not afforded the same protection and assistance. There were estimated to be more than 26 million IDPs worldwide at the end of 2011.[51] IDPs may have many of the same health needs as refugees, but UNHCR may not be able to address their problems because they have remained in their home country. IDPs usually do not live in camps; most move to new rural areas or cities.

Refugees and IDPs share the experience of having lost their homes, jobs, social support networks, and some of their independence and sense of security. Special health concerns are associated with different stages of the **cycle of displacement**, which begins at the onset of migration and continues until a lasting solution is implemented. Emergency interventions focus on the provision of water, food, sanitation, shelter, fuel, and health care for sick, pregnant, and vulnerable individuals. Longer-term interventions include treatment of malnutrition, addressing violence and security issues, and providing therapy for mental health problems such as posttraumatic stress disorder (PTSD).

Communities that are hosting displaced people or refugees may also have special economic and health concerns related to having new members in their population.[52] One risk is that infectious disease outbreaks might occur as the host community is exposed for the first time to infectious agents carried by the migrant population. Another fear is that when a large number of displaced people move to one town or city, they may overwhelm the social service providers and strain the resources of the host community.

Later relief efforts focus on finding longer-term solutions to homelessness and displacement. IDPs and refugees who return to their home communities may face challenges related to the destruction of homes, healthcare facilities, and other community buildings like schools; the loss of farmland to environmental damage and hazards like unexploded ordnance; and the displacement of their family members, neighbors, and other members of their community. Those who settle in new areas often face challenges associated with learning new cultural practices and adapting to them (a process called **acculturation**), overcoming language and communication barriers, having limited occupational options, and potentially having limited access to health care. No matter where involuntary migrants settle, they are at risk for developing PTSD and other chronic conditions related to illnesses or injuries sustained during their displacement.

14.3.C Postconflict Areas

In addition to rebuilding political and economic systems and restoring educational and social services after a civil conflict or war, postconflict areas need to repair health systems (because of loss of infrastructure and personnel, among other issues), expand rehabilitation services (including physical rehabilitation and mental health care), and address environmental concerns. Public health work has the potential to help with the transition back to peace by creating a sense of solidarity and strengthening social connections across diverse populations.[53]

Contaminated environments may take much longer to renovate than health systems.[54] For example, landmines and other unexploded ordnance buried during wartime remain hazards to workers, children, and communities long after the conflict is over. This means, among many other problems, that large tracts of potential farmland are unable to be cultivated because of the risk of encountering a mine while clearing a field. Most people who sustain landmine injuries are civilians, and children may have elevated risk because they do not know how to recognize mines and may pick them up and even play with them. Landmines remain a concern in many parts of the world (**Figure 14–3**).[55] Although it only costs a few dollars to purchase and plant a mine, it can cost $1000 to safely remove one.[56]

14.3.D Natural Disasters

People who have survived a natural disaster like an earthquake, hurricane, tsunami, mudslide, or major flood may have an urgent need for immediate medical treatment for injuries and for basic necessities such as water, food, and shelter, especially if a large geographic area has severely damaged infrastructure. Because natural disasters are generally seen as apolitical events, it is usually fairly easy for aid agencies to assist survivors. (This is quite different from the complicated response to complex humanitarian emergencies, as governments and faction leaders engaged in armed conflicts are often disinclined to allow outsiders to assess and assist vulnerable populations.[57])

However, if the various responders do not coordinate their efforts, the result can be chaos. In the weeks after the massive earthquake in Haiti in 2010, thousands of well-intentioned volunteers flew to Port-au-Prince to assist. But many of the volunteers were unaffiliated with a Haiti-based host organization and arrived without adequate personal supplies, so they ended up being a burden rather than a help.[58] Supplies ended up being

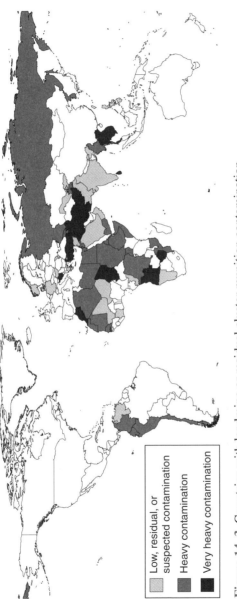

Figure 14–3 Countries with landmine or residual cluster munition contamination.
Source: Data from *Landmine monitor 2011.* International Campaign to Ban Landmines; 2011.

stockpiled at the airport because the Haitian government, local institutions, and various international governmental and nongovernmental organizations had difficulty communicating about on-the-ground needs, securing local transportation, and coordinating distribution efforts.[59] Similar logistical issues have occurred after other large-scale natural disasters, including the devastating tsunami that hit Southeast Asia in 2004.[60]

A well-managed international response to a natural disaster begins when an affected country invites the UN and other organizations to assist. A lead agency, often the UN Office for the Coordination of Humanitarian Affairs (OCHA), is designated to coordinate the response by other UN agencies, government agencies (including militaries), the national Red Cross or Red Crescent society, and nongovernmental organizations. These groups work together to meet essential needs that have been designated as humanitarian response "clusters" (Table 14–8).[61]

Table 14–8 Humanitarian response clusters.

Cluster		Lead UN Agency
Overall Coordination		OCHA
Technical Clusters	Agriculture/food security	FAO
	Camp coordination and management	UNHCR/IOM
	Early recovery	UNDP
	Education	UNICEF (and Save the Children)
	Emergency shelter	IFRC/UNHCR
	Health	WHO
	Nutrition	UNICEF
	Protection	UNHCR/OHCHR/UNICEF
	Sanitation, water, and hygiene (WASH)	UNICEF
Support Clusters	Emergency telecommunications	WFP/UNICEF
	Logistics	WFP

Source: Information from Stumpenhorst M, Stumpenhorst R, Razum O. The UN OCHA cluster approach: gaps between theory and practice. *J Public Health.* 2011;19:587–592.

This coordination—and requiring that volunteers and their host organizations complete appropriate training before traveling to the disaster site and fully provide for themselves in the field[62]—helps facilitate a relatively rapid and comprehensive response. National and local responses benefit from similar coordination strategies. In the United States, for example, the National Incident Management System (NIMS) spells out how different public and private sector organizations should work together to respond to a disaster, and the Incident Command System (ICS) is used in the field to provide a clear chain of command for responders.[63] Fifteen "essential support functions" are covered by the national response system (**Table 14–9**).[63] A coordinated response can maximize use of resources and save lives.

Table 14–9 Essential support functions.

ESF #1	Transportation
ESF #2	Communications
ESF #3	Public works and engineering
ESF #4	Firefighting
ESF #5	Emergency management
ESF #6	Mass care, emergency assistance, housing, and human services
ESF #7	Logistics management and resource support
ESF #8	Public health and medical services
ESF #9	Search and rescue
ESF #10	Oil and hazardous materials response
ESF #11	Agriculture and natural resources
ESF #12	Energy
ESF #13	Public safety and security
ESF #14	Long-term community recovery
ESF #15	External affairs

Source: Information from *National Incidence Management System*. Washington DC: U.S. Department of Homeland Security; 2008.

14.4 EMERGENCY PREPAREDNESS AND RESPONSE

Emergency response is not just about responding to problems. The emergency management cycle includes four steps, sometimes called the "4 Rs" (Figure 14–4):[64]

- *Reduction (mitigation)* of risks: Preemptive measures should be implemented to protect people and property from hazards (for example, by enforcing building codes).
- *Readiness (preparedness)*: Preparation for responding to an emergency should include the creation and refinement of emergency operations plans, the establishment of emergency communications infrastructure, and the training of public employees and emergency response volunteers.
- *Response*: The response to an imminent, ongoing, or immediately past threat should include provision of emergency medical assistance, shelter, and other critical services.
- *Recovery*: During the recovery phase, continued efforts should focus on rebuilding affected communities.

Mitigating risks and preparing for potential critical incidents before they happen are the best ways to enable a smooth response and recovery when a natural or human-generated disaster does occur.

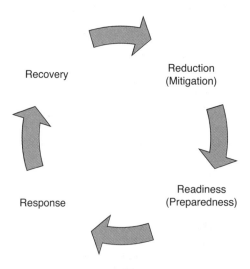

Figure 14–4 Emergency management phases.

14.5 DISCUSSION QUESTIONS

1. Read the Universal Declaration of Human Rights. Do you agree that all of the listed items are universal human rights? Why or why not?
2. What do you think should be included in a basic healthcare package that every human has access to? (In other words, what is an appropriate global "standard of health"?)
3. Who do you think should pay for a basic healthcare package for people who cannot afford to pay out-of-pocket for health services?
4. Do you think that people have the right to immediately access new medications and other health technologies at low or no cost? Why or why not?
5. The average American household spends less than 1% of its income paying for its water. What would happen in the United States if rates increased to about 20% of income, as happened in parts of Cochabamba, Bolivia?
6. What organizations in your community respond to local crises and emergencies, including those caused by natural disasters?
7. If you were being persecuted and decided that you had to leave your home to avoid torture and possible death, where would you go? How would you get there? What would you take with you? Would you try to cross a national border?
8. What natural disasters are threats where you live? How prepared are you to take care of yourself if one of these disasters occurs?

REFERENCES

1. World Health Organization (WHO). *The Constitution of the World Health Organization.* Accessed from http://whqlibdoc.who.int/hist/official_records/constitution.pdf.
2. United Nations Human Rights. *The Universal Declaration of Human Rights.* Accessed from http://www.ohchr.org/en/udhr/Pages/UDHRIndex.aspx.
3. Leckie S. Another step towards indivisibility: identifying the key features of violations of economic, social and cultural rights. *Human Rights Q.* 1998;20:81–124.
4. *Twenty-five questions & answers on health & human rights.* Health and Human Rights Publication Series, Issue 1; 2002. Geneva: WHO; 2002.
5. *International Covenant on Economic, Social and Cultural Rights.* New York: United Nations General Assembly resolution 2200A (XXI);1966.
6. Farmer P. Pathologies of power: rethinking health and human rights. *Am J Public Health.* 1999;89:1486–1496.
7. Connors EE, Gostin LO. Health care reform—a historic moment in U.S. social policy. *JAMA.* 2010;303:2521–2522.
8. Victora CG, Barreto ML, do Carmo Leal M, et al. Health conditions and health-policy innovations in Brazil: the way forward. *Lancet.* 2011;377:2042–2053.

9. Chen Z. Launch of the health-care reform plan in China. *Lancet*. 2009;373:1322–1324.

10. Balarajan Y, Selvaraj S, Subramanian SV. Health care and equity in India. *Lancet*. 2011;377:505–515.

11. Donnelly J. How did Sierra Leone provide free health care? *Lancet*. 2011;377:1393–1396.

12. Farmer P. *Pathologies of power: health, human rights, and the new war on the poor*. Berkeley CA: University of California Press; 2003.

13. Backman G, Hunt P, Khosla R, et al. Health systems and the right to health: an assessment of 194 countries. *Lancet*. 2008;372:2047–2085.

14. Paim J, Travassos C, Almeida C, Bahia L, Macinko J. The Brazilian health system: history, advances, and challenges. *Lancet*. 2011;377:1778–1797.

15. Sagan A, Panteli D, Borkowski W, et al. Poland: health system review. *Health Systems in Transition*. Copenhagen: WHO European Observatory on Health Systems and Policies; 2011.

16. Spiegelhalter DJ, Gore SM, Fitzpatrick R, Fletcher AE, Jones DR, Cox DR. Quality of life measurements in health care. III: resource allocation. *BMJ*. 1992;305:1205–1209.

17. United Nations Committee on Economic, Social and Cultural Rights. *General Comment 14: The right to the highest attainable standard of health (E/C 12/2000/4)*. Geneva: CESCR; 2000.

18. *World health statistics 2012*. Geneva: WHO; 2012.

19. Taylor AL, Hwenda L, Larsen BI, Daulaire N. Stemming the brain drain—a WHO global code of practice on international recruitment of health personnel. *N Engl J Med*. 2011;365:2348–2351.

20. Adams CP, Brantner W. Spending on new drug development. *Health Econ*. 2010;19:130–141.

21. Higgins MJ, Graham SJH. Balancing innovation and access: patent challenges tip the scales. *Science*. 2009;326:370–371.

22. 't Hoen E, Berger J, Calmy A, Moon S. Driving a decade of change: HIV/AIDS, patents and access to medicines for all. *J Int AIDS Soc*. 2011;14:15.

23. World Trade Organization (Doha WTO Ministerial 2001). Declaration on the TRIPS agreement and public health (WT/MIN(01)/DEC/2); 2001.

24. Médecins Sans Frontières. *Fighting neglect: finding ways to manage and control visceral leishmaniasis, human African trypanosomiasis and Chagas disease*. Geneva: MSF; 2012.

25. Frew SE, Liu VY, Singer PA. A business plan to help the 'global South' it its fight against neglected diseases. *Health Aff*. 2009;28:1760–1773.

26. *WHO model list of essential medicines (17th list)*. Geneva: WHO; 2011.

27. van den Ham R, Bero L, Laing R. Selection of essential medicines. In: *The world medicines report 2011*. Geneva: WHO; 2011.

28. *The pharmaceutical industry and global health: facts and figures*. Geneva: International Federation of Pharmaceutical Manufacturers & Associations (IFPMA); 2011.

29. Lu Y, Hernandez P, Abegunde D, Edejer T. Medicine expenditures. In: *The world medicines report 2011*. Geneva: WHO; 2011.

30. Bill & Melinda Gates Foundation. *Global health strategy overview*. Seattle WA: Gates Foundation; 2010.

31. Frost LJ, Reich MR. *Access: how do good health technologies get to poor people in poor countries?* Cambridge MA: Harvard Center for Population and Development Studies; 2008.

32. Gliek PH. The human right to water. *Water Policy*. 1998;1:487–503.

33. Howard G, Bartram J. *Domestic water quantity, service level and health.* Geneva: WHO; 2003.

34. Bleumel EB. The implications of formulating a human right to water. *Ecology Law Q.* 2004;31:957–1006.

35. Nickson A, Vargas C. The limitations of water regulation: the failure of the Cochabamba concession in Bolivia. *Bull Latin American Res.* 2002;21:99–120.

36. Morgan B. Water: frontier markets and cosmopolitan activism. *Soundings J Politics Nature.* 2004;28:10–24.

37. Budds J, McGranahan G. Are the debates on water privatization missing the point? Experiences from Africa, Asia and Latin America. *Environment Urbanization.* 2003;15:87–113.

38. Hundley N Jr. *Water and the West: the Colorado River Compact and the politics of water in the American West.* Los Angeles: University of California Press; 2009.

39. Glennon R. Water scarcity, marketing, and privatization. *Texas Law Rev.* 2005;83:1873–1902.

40. The Sphere Project. *Humanitarian charter and minimum standards in humanitarian response, 3rd edition.* Rugby, UK: Practical Action Publishing; 2011.

41. Quarantelli EL. Just as a disaster is not simply a big accident, so a catastrophe is not just a big disaster. *J Am Soc Professional Emerg Planners.* 1996; 3: 68–71.

42. Koenig KL, Dinerman N, Kuehl AE. Disaster nomenclature—a functional impact approach: the PICE system. *Acad Emerg Med.* 1996;3:723–727.

43. Thompson AK, Faith K, Gibson JL, Upshur REG. Pandemic influenza preparedness: an ethical framework to guide decision-making. *BMC Med Ethics.* 2006;7:12.

44. Salama P, Spiegel P, Talley L, Waldman R. Lessons learned from complex emergencies over past decade. *Lancet.* 2004;364:1801–1813.

45. Kalshoven F, Zegveld L. *Constraints on the waging of war*, 4th edition. Cambridge, UK: Cambridge University Press; 2011.

46. Kivlahan C, Ewigman N. Rape as a weapon of war in modern conflicts. *BMJ.* 2010;340:c3270.

47. Young H, Borrel A, Holland D, Salama P. Public nutrition in complex emergencies. *Lancet.* 2004;364:1899–1909.

48. Toole MJ, Waldman RJ. The public health aspects of complex emergencies and refugee situations. *Annu Rev Public Health.* 1997;18:283–312.

49. *UNHCR global report 2011.* Geneva: UNHCR; 2011.

50. Spiegel PB, Checchi F, Colombo S, Paik E. Health-care needs of people affected by conflict: future trends and changing frameworks. *Lancet.* 2010;375:341–345.

51. *Global overview 2011: people internally displaced by conflict and violence.* Geneva: Internal Displacement Monitoring Centre, Norwegian Refugee Council; 2012.

52. Brun C. Reterritorializing the relationship between people and place in refugee studies. *Geografiska Annaler: Series B, Human Geography.* 2001;83:15–25.

53. MacQueen G, Santa-Barbara J. Peace building through health initiatives. *BMJ.* 2000;321:293–296.

54. Brown VJ. BattleScars: global conflicts and environmental health. *Environ Health Perspect.* 2004;112:A994-A1003.

55. *Landmine monitor 2011.* International Campaign to Ban Landmines; 2011.

56. Machel G. *Impact of armed conflict on children* (report A/51/306). New York: United Nations; 1996.

57. Spiegel PB. Differences in world responses to natural disasters and complex emergencies. *JAMA*. 2005;293:1915–1918.

58. Jobe K. Disaster relief in post-earthquake Haiti: unintended consequences of humanitarian volunteerism. *Travel Med Infect Dis*. 2011;9:1–5.

59. Sarcevic A, Palen L, White J, Starbird K, Bagdouri M, Anderson K. "Beacons of hope" in decentralized coordination: learning from on-the-ground medical twitterers during the 2010 Haiti earthquake. *Proceedings of the ACM 2012 conference on Computer Supported Cooperative Work*; 2012 Feb 11–15; Seattle WA. New York: ACM; 2012. p. 47–56.

60. VanRooyen M, Leaning J. After the tsunami—facing the public health challenges. *N Engl J Med*. 2005;352:435–438.

61. Stumpenhorst M, Stumpenhorst R, Razum O. The UN OCHA cluster approach: gaps between theory and practice. *J Public Health*. 2011;19:587–592.

61. Krin CS, Giannou C, Seppelt IM, Walker S, Mattox KL, Wigle RL, Crippen D. Appropriate response to humanitarian crises. *BMJ*. 2010;340:c562.

63. *National Incidence Management System*. Washington DC: U.S. Department of Homeland Security; 2008.

64. McLoughlin D. A framework for integrated emergency management. *Public Admin Rev*. 1985;45(special issue):165–172.

CHAPTER 15

Global Health Progress and Priorities

Public health and medical innovations in the 20th century resulted in amazing advancements in global health, but also exacerbated health disparities. The goal of global health in the 21st century is for people and organizations from around the world to work together to develop and implement innovative and cost-effective solutions for shared health concerns.

15.1 GLOBAL HEALTH SUCCESSES

Global health has become an incredibly dynamic field. The 20th century was marked by unprecedented progress in medical science. New antibiotics were discovered along with a host of drugs for treating noncommunicable diseases (NCDs) like heart disease and cancer. Life-saving vaccines were created. Oral contraceptives transformed family planning, and assisted reproductive technologies reduced the burden of infertility. New diagnostic tools, such as electrocardiographs, CT scans, and MRIs, increased the quality of medical care. So did new therapies, like dialysis for kidney disease, insulin for diabetes, and contact lenses for vision impairments. Modern surgical techniques made joint replacements, open heart surgery, and organ transplants routine in some parts of the world.

The 20th century was also characterized by a massive intensification of health disparities. While the global rich now have access to an array of healthcare innovations that would have been nearly unimaginable 100 years ago, the global poor continue to succumb to the same diseases that have been major killers for centuries, like hunger and measles and tuberculosis (TB). Richer countries have gone through demographic transitions, epidemiologic transitions, and nutrition transitions. Poorer countries are experiencing an increasing burden from diseases of affluence, while many of their residents continue to die because they do not have access to food, hygiene, sanitation, basic health care, or other life essentials.

Yet despite these major differences in the health profiles of populations around the world, the 20th century also brought significant reminders of the common global threats to health. In particular, the emergence of HIV, virulent new strains of influenza, and drug-resistant pathogens prompted truly global research and practice efforts. Global research collaborations and global health partnerships have never been more important.

The goals of global public health in the 21st century are to continue to create innovative solutions to public health problems; to increase access to health, healthcare services, and health technologies around the world; and to expand global communication and action about shared health concerns. The first decade provides evidence that these aims can be accomplished, as progress has already been made on many fronts (**Table 15–1**).[1]

15.2 MILLENNIUM DEVELOPMENT GOALS

One of chief contributors to the global health successes to date in the 21st century is the **Millennium Development Goals (MDGs)** that were adopted by the United Nations (UN) in 2000 and have been endorsed by nearly 200 countries from across the globe. The MDGs set out eight major goals for significantly reducing global poverty by 2015 (**Table 15–2**).[2] Most of these goals have direct links to health—eradicating extreme poverty and hunger (goal 1); reducing child mortality (goal 4); improving maternal health (goal 5); combatting HIV/AIDS, malaria, and other diseases (goal 6); and ensuring environmental sustainability (goal 7)—and all relate to creating an environment in which everyone has the tools to access health. Each UN member nation has committed to working toward these goals, so the MDGs have provided a blueprint for national-level priority setting, for bilateral and multilateral aid, and for World Bank and International Monetary Fund funding. Many nongovernmental organizations (NGOs) and international partnerships have also used the MDGs to guide their work.

Eighteen targets provide benchmarks for progress toward achieving the MDGs. Many of these are also directly health related. For example, some of the targets are to halve the proportion of people who suffer from hunger (target 1C), to reduce by two-thirds the under-5 mortality rate (target 4A), to reduce by three-quarters the maternal mortality ratio (target 5A), to achieve universal access to reproductive health (target 5B), to begin to reverse the

Table 15–1 Top 10 global public health achievements in the first decade of the 21st century (2001–2010), as listed by the U.S. Centers for Disease Control and Prevention (CDC)

1	Reductions in child mortality	The number of children who die each year has been reduced by more than 2 million
2	Vaccine-preventable diseases	An estimated 2.5 million deaths were prevented
3	Access to safe water and sanitation	About 800 million people gained access to an improved drinking water source and about 570 million gained access to improved sanitation
4	Malaria prevention and control	Malaria deaths have been reduced by about 200,000 per year
5	Prevention and control of HIV/AIDS	The number of new infections and the number of deaths each year have both been reduced
6	Tuberculosis control	The case detection rate and successful treatment rate have increased
7	Control of neglected tropical diseases	The transmission rates for Guinea worm and onchocerciasis (river blindness) are much lower
8	Tobacco control	Most of the world's countries are participating in tobacco control efforts
9	Increased awareness and response for improving global road safety	Many countries have lowered their annual number of traffic-related deaths
10	Improved preparedness and response to global health threats	Global health surveillance and response networks are being developed

Source: Information from Global Public Health Achievements Team, CDC. Ten great public health achievements: worldwide, 2001–2010. *Morb Mort Wkly Rep.* 2011;60:814–818.

spread of HIV/AIDS (target 6A), to achieve universal access to treatment for HIV/AIDS for all those who need it (target 6B), to begin to reverse the incidence of malaria and other major diseases (target 6C), to halve the proportion of the population without sustainable access to safe drinking water and sanitation (target 7C), and to provide access to affordable essential drugs in developing countries, in cooperation with pharmaceutical companies (target 8E).

Table 15–2 Millennium Development Goals.

1	Eradicate extreme poverty and hunger
2	Achieve universal primary education
3	Promote gender equality and empower women
4	Reduce child mortality
5	Improve maternal health
6	Combat HIV/AIDS, malaria, and other diseases
7	Ensure environmental sustainability
8	Develop a global partnership for development

Source: United Nations. Millennium Development Goals. http://www.un.org /millenniumgoals/.

There are also 48 specific indicators that are used to assess whether the targets are being reached. These include measures of the prevalence of underweight children in their first 5 years of life (indicator 1.8), the proportion of 1-year-old children immunized against measles (indicator 4.3), the proportion of births attended by skilled health personnel (indicator 5.2), the contraceptive prevalence rate (indicator 5.3), the proportion of 15- to 24-year-olds with knowledge about HIV/AIDS (indicator 6.3), the proportion of TB cases detected and cured under directly observed therapy (DOTS) (indicator 6.10), and the proportion of the urban population living in slums (indicator 7.10). All the UN agencies are now collecting data from member states on the indicators relevant to their areas of work and are implementing programs that will support reaching the targets.[2]

One of the main reasons the MDGs have been so influential is that they provide a clear strategy for evaluation. Progress on each of the 48 indicators is collected from each participating country on an annual basis so the status of each target can be monitored and countries can determine how much progress they have made toward reaching their goals (Table 15–3).[3] The assessment data allow donors to determine whether programs are making good use of their resources and are on track toward achieving the desired outcomes. While some concerns have been raised about how well the MDGs promote equity, sustainability, local ownership of priorities, and holistic development (rather than relatively narrow, single-sector "silos" of focus), the general consensus is that the MDGs have provided a helpful framework for global cooperation toward international development.[4]

Table 15–3 MDG progress for selected countries, circa 2010.

MDG Goal	South Korea	Brazil	China	India	Kenya	Sierra Leone
1	**Achieved**	**Achieved**	**On track**	*Possible*	Off track	*Possible*
2	**Achieved**	**Achieved**	**On track**	*Possible*	**On track**	**On track**
3	*Possible*	**Achieved**	*Possible*	*Possible*	*Possible*	**On track**
4	**Achieved**	**On track**	*Possible*	Off track	*Possible*	*Possible*
5	**Achieved**	**On track**	**On track**	*Possible*	*Possible*	*Possible*
6	**Achieved**	**Achieved**	(Unknown)	(Unknown)	*Possible*	**On track**
7	(Unknown)	**On track**	(Unknown)	(Unknown)	*Possible*	Off track
8	(Unknown)	**On track**	(Unknown)	(Unknown)	(Unknown)	(Unknown)

Source: Data from *MDG Monitor country profiles 2012.* New York: UN; 2012.

15.3 CURRENT PRIORITIES

A variety of governments, international NGOs, and global health partnerships have created lists of various types of global health priorities for the coming years. For example, **Table 15–4** lists the top 10 priorities from the Disease Control Priorities Project, sponsored by the Fogarty International Center of the U.S. National Institutes of Health and collaborators such as the World Bank, the World Health Organization, and the Population Reference Bureau. In addition to the focus on infectious disease prevention and control (2, 4, 5), improved nutrition (3), and maternal and child health (1), this "top 10" list also emphasizes that every country in the world needs to begin preparing to provide health care (9, 10) to a large number of people with chronic, noncommunicable conditions (6, 7, 8).[5]

The Grand Challenges in Global Health list from the Bill & Melinda Gates Foundation takes a different approach, emphasizing the need for new scientific technologies (**Table 15–5**).[6] The Grand Challenges initiative was launched in 2003 and focused on the creation of new and improved vaccines, vector control methods, and therapies, in partnership with agencies such as the Foundation for the (U.S.) National Institutes of Health, the Wellcome Trust, and the Canadian Institutes of Health Research.

Table 15–4 Top 10 global health priorities from the Disease Control Priorities Project.

1	Ensure healthier mothers and children.
2	Stop the AIDS pandemic.
3	Promote good nutrition.
4	Stem the tide of tuberculosis.
5	Control malaria.
6	Reduce the toll from cardiovascular disease.
7	Combat tobacco use.
8	Reduce fatal and disabling injuries.
9	Ensure equal access to quality health care.
10	Forge strong, integrated, effective health systems.

Source: Information from *Investing in global health: 'best buys' and priorities for action in developing countries*. Disease Control Priorities Project; 2006.

Table 15–5 Grand Challenges in Global Health.

Improve childhood vaccines	1	Create effective single-dose vaccines
	2	Prepare vaccines that do not require refrigeration
	3	Develop needle-free vaccine delivery systems
Create new vaccines	4	Devise testing systems for new vaccines
	5	Design antigens for protective immunity
	6	Learn about immunological responses
Control insects that transmit agents of disease	7	Develop genetic strategy to control insects
	8	Develop chemical strategy to control insects
Improve nutrition to promote health	9	Create a nutrient-rich staple plant species
Improve drug treatment of infectious diseases	10	Find drugs and delivery systems to limit drug resistance
Cure latent and chronic infection	11	Create therapies that can cure latent infection
	12	Create immunological methods to cure latent infection
Measure health status accurately and economically in developing countries	13	Develop technologies to assess population health
	14	Develop versatile diagnostic tools

Source: Information from Varmus H, Klausner R, Zerhouni E, Acharya T, Daar AS, Singer PA. Grand challenge in global health. *Science*. 2003;302:398–399.

An international collaborative group exploring national and global responsibilities for health has proposed four key questions for global health that must be answered to move the field forward (**Table 15–6**).[7]

Some lists designed to promote a set of health priorities in one country apply more globally, such as the list from the U.S. Centers for Disease Control and Prevention (CDC) shown in **Table 15–7**.[8] Every country would benefit from attention to healthy living across the lifespan, improvements in the healthcare system, and the judicious adoption of new technologies.

Table 15–6 Four defining questions for global health.

1	What are the services and goods guaranteed to every person under the human right to health?
2	What responsibilities do states have for the health of their own populations?
3	What duties do states owe to people beyond their borders in securing the right to health?
4	What kind of global governance for health is needed to ensure that all states live up to their mutual responsibilities?

Source: Information from Gostin LO, Friedman EA, Ooms G, et al. The Joint Action and Learning Initiative; towards a global agreement on national and global responsibilities for health. *PLoS Med*. 2011;8:e1001031.

Table 15–7 Top 10 public health priorities in the United States, as listed by the U.S. CDC.

1	Institute a rational healthcare system (balance equity, cost, and quality)
2	Eliminate health disparities
3	Focus on children's emotional and intellectual development
4	Achieve a longer "healthspan" (healthy aging)
5	Integrate physical activity and healthy eating into daily lives
6	Clean up and protect the environment
7	Prepare to respond to emerging infectious diseases
8	Recognize and address the contributions of mental health to overall health and well-being
9	Reduce the toll of violence in society
10	Use new scientific knowledge and technological advances wisely

Source: Information from Koplan JP, Fleming DW. Current and future public health challenges. *JAMA*. 2000;284:1696–1698.

And some lists focus on just one category of disease but emphasize tools that would address a variety of health concerns, such as the NCD challenges list written by contributors from more than 50 countries and published in *Nature*, one of the leading science research journals (**Table 15–8**).[9]

Together, these lists provide insight into the common health priorities of nations and populations around the world—issues related to the major causes of disease, disability, and premature death; the socioeconomic and

Table 15–8 Top 20 challenges for noncommunicable diseases (NCDs).

Raise public awareness	1	Raise the political priority of NCDs
	2	Promote healthy lifestyle and consumption choices
	3	Foster widespread, sustained, and accurate media coverage
Enhance economic, legal, and environmental policies	4	Address the impact of government spending and taxation on health
	5	Implement policies to discourage consumption of alcohol, tobacco, and unhealthy foods
	6	Address the impacts of poor health on economic productivity
Modify risk factors	7	Deploy measures proven to reduce tobacco use
	8	Increase the availability and consumption of healthy food
	9	Promote lifelong physical activity
	10	Better understand the environmental and cultural factors that change behavior
Engage business and community	11	Make business a key partner in promoting health and preventing disease
	12	Develop and monitor codes of responsible conduct with industries
	13	Empower community resources
Mitigate health impacts of poverty and urbanization	14	Address how poverty increases risk factors
	15	Address the links between the built environment, urbanization, and NCDs
Reorient health systems	16	Allocate health systems resources based on the burden of disease
	17	Move health practice toward prevention
	18	Increase the skills of professionals who prevent, treat, and manage NCDs
	19	Integrate screening and prevention within health delivery
	20	Increase access to medications to prevent complications of NCDs

Source: Information from Daar AS, Singer PA, Persad DL, et al. Grand challenges in chronic non-communicable diseases. *Nature*. 2007;450:494–496.

environmental factors that influence health; the funding and management of health systems; and the development and accessibility of new health technologies.

15.4 THE PRICE OF GLOBAL HEALTH

Many public health intervention packages would increase the quality of life of millions of people at a relatively low cost per person. For example:

- A package of road safety interventions—enforcement of speed limits, drunk driving laws, seatbelt use in cars, and helmet use by all motorcyclists and child bicyclists—could cost considerably less than a dollar per person per year in Africa and Southeast Asia.[10]
- An integrated pharmacology package for treating neglected tropical diseases (NTDs)—albendazole or mebendazole for intestinal worms (ascariasis, trichuriasis, and hookworm), praziquantel for schistosomiasis, ivermectin or diethylcarbamazine (DEC) for lymphatic filariasis and onchocerciasis, and azithromycin for trachoma—could cost less than $1 per person per year in sub-Saharan Africa.[11]
- An NCD "best buy" package suggested by the World Health Organization—with interventions for reducing tobacco use and harmful alcohol use, promoting physical activity and a healthy diet (that reduces sodium intake to lower the risk of hypertension and replaces trans fats with polyunsaturated fats to help reduce blood cholesterol levels), preventing cervical cancer through screening and removal of lesions, providing multidrug ("polypill") therapy to people at risk of a heart attack or stroke, and providing aspirin to people having an acute heart attack—could cost about $1 to $3 per adult per year in low- and middle-income countries, a tiny fraction of the costs of NCDs to the healthcare system if the prevention package is not implemented.[12]
- An extra $2 per person per year in low- and middle-income countries could provide a package of antenatal and obstetric care that would prevent a substantial portion of stillbirths, neonatal deaths, and maternal deaths.[13]
- A mental health package for treatment of depression, bipolar disorder, schizophrenia, and alcoholism with antidepressant, mood stabilizing, and antipsychotic medications and psychosocial therapy could cost only a few dollars per adult each year in low- and middle-income countries.[14]

However, all of these interventions together add up to a lot of money, especially for low-income countries where the total amount spent on health per person per year is significantly less than $100. For example, the Roll Back Malaria partnership needs about $6 billion annually in order to make progress on the Global Malaria Action Plan (GMAP),[15] the Global Plan to Stop TB requires nearly $10 billion each year,[16] increasing access to clean drinking water and sanitation costs more than $20 billion annually,[17] and providing modern contraception and maternal and new-born health care to all who would like these services but are not currently able to access them would require about $25 billion a year.[18] Together, trillions of dollars each year would be required to implement global health strategies for all of the various causes of disease, disability, and death in every region of the world. Thus, difficult decisions have to be made about how to allocate limited resources. Cost-effectiveness analysis, considerations of sustainability, and evaluations of the costs of doing nothing can provide support for making sound decisions about how to prioritize the distribution of funds.

15.4.A Cost-Effectiveness

The goal of **cost-effectiveness analysis** is to be sure that the funds being used for a public health initiative are **effective** at achieving the planned outcomes and are making **efficient** use of financial and other resources. A variety of "best buys" in global health have been identified, including a top 10 list from the Disease Control Priorities Project (**Table 15–9**).[5] The most cost-effective global health interventions tend to be relatively inexpensive, easily distributed to lots of people, and targeted toward children and young adults (so that they can avert many potential years of life lost to long-term disability or premature death). A child can be fully immunized for about $20 (best buy #1) and an integrated management of childhood illnesses (IMCI) package of vitamin A and zinc supplementation plus management of pneumonia, malaria, and diarrhea, including provision of oral rehydration therapy, costs less than $5 per child per year in sub-Saharan Africa (best buy #2).[19] Hygiene promotion for the prevention of diarrheal diseases, deworming medications to reduce the burden from soil-transmitted helminths in endemic areas, first-aid training for emergency care, intermittent preventive treatment of malaria in pregnant women (IPTp) in endemic areas, and insecticide-treated bednets (ITNs) for malaria prevention are also

Table 15–9 Top 10 "best buys" in global health from the Disease Control Priorities Project.

	Target	Action
1	Child health	Vaccinate children against major childhood killers, including measles, polio, tetanus, whooping cough, and diphtheria
2	Child health	Monitor children's health to prevent or, if necessary, treat childhood pneumonia, diarrhea, and malaria
3	Tobacco use	Tax tobacco products to increase consumers' costs by at least one-third to curb smoking and reduce the prevalence of cardiovascular disease, cancer, and respiratory disease
4	HIV/AIDS	Attack the spread of HIV through a coordinated approach that includes: promoting 100% condom use among populations at high risk; treating other sexually transmitted infections; providing antiretroviral medications, especially for pregnant women; and offering voluntary HIV counseling and testing
5	Maternal and child health	Give children and pregnant women essential nutrients, including vitamin A, iron, and iodine, to prevent maternal anemia, infant deaths, and long-term health problems
6	Malaria	Provide insecticide-treated bednets in malaria-endemic areas to drastically reduce malaria
7	Injury prevention	Enforce traffic regulations and install speed bumps at dangerous intersections to reduce traffic-related injuries
8	TB	Treat TB patients with short-course chemotherapy to cure infected people and prevent new infections
9	Child health	Teach mothers and train birth attendants to keep newborns warm and clean to reduce illness and death
10	Cardiovascular disease	Promote use of aspirin and other inexpensive drugs to treat and prevent heart attack and stroke

Source: Information from *Investing in global health: 'best buys' and priorities for action in developing countries*. Disease Control Priorities Project; 2006.

highly cost-effective.[19] High-tech solutions, like coronary artery bypass surgery for treatment of ischemic heart disease, tend to be among the least cost-effective interventions.[19] In general, prevention is much less expensive than treatment.

Cost-effectiveness evaluations focus on how well an intervention contributes to achieving a goal. The goal may be something specific and measurable, such as reducing the incidence of malaria or increasing the number of people taking medications for HIV. Or the goal may be something less tangible and harder to quantify, such as reducing the risk of bioterrorism or promoting new trade agreements via bilateral aid that helps communities address the conditions that foment violence or support markets. No matter what the goal is, **monitoring and evaluation (M&E)**, the systematic collection of information about an ongoing project (monitoring) and the determination of whether the project is on track to achieve its objectives (evaluation), is an essential part of keeping in-progress interventions on track. If the M&E process reveals that a project or program is not fulfilling its mandate, adjustments can be made to increase the impact of the intervention. Cost-effectiveness is critical for maximizing the outcomes of the resources put into global health activities.

15.4.B Sustainability

Sustainability aims to provide for current human needs without compromising the ability of future generations to meet their needs. Sustainable health programs aim to generate long-term health benefits that endure even after specific projects end. A program that depletes natural resources and promotes overconsumption is not sustainable, just as a program that is fully dependent on outside donors and does not involve recipients in planning, decision making, and evaluation is not sustainable. Ideally, global health programs should foster capacity building and encourage the self-sufficiency of participating communities, such as by facilitating the integration of successful externally funded healthcare programs into the routine services offered by internally funded national healthcare systems.[20] New NCD initiatives around the world that increase taxes on tobacco and other unhealthy products to support prevention and management of chronic diseases are examples of how health projects can be financially sustainable as well as socially and environmentally sustainable.[21]

15.4.C Costs of Inaction

When considering the cost of solutions to global health crises, it can be helpful to compare the cost of action to the cost of inaction. Consider the economic costs of lost human life and lost productivity due to just a few common causes of disease and disability. Malaria-endemic countries have significantly reduced economic growth rates due to premature deaths, medical expenses, lost worker productivity, and other costs.[22] Nearly $400 billion is spent on treating diabetes and complications of diabetes worldwide each year.[23] The per-person cost of excessive alcohol drinking in terms of lost productivity, direct healthcare expenses, law enforcement, and other costs is more than 1% of the gross domestic product (GDP) in high- and middle-income countries, at a cost of several hundred dollars per capita.[24] Knowing the high costs of these preventable conditions makes it possible to see how spending money can, in the long term, save money. For example, the money spent on controlling malaria would likely significantly expand national economies in currently endemic areas, preventing type 2 diabetes through lifestyle changes and other measures would save huge costs to healthcare systems, and curbing excessive drinking would significantly reduce the burden of injuries and NCDs in addition to enhancing economies.

15.5 BEYOND COST-EFFECTIVENESS

A focus on cost-effectiveness is not by itself sufficient for making decisions about health priorities and health funding. One limitation is that cost–benefit analyses tend to promote interventions that have already proven to be successful (in at least one population in one part of the world) and to downplay innovations that have not yet proven to achieve reliable results. New inventions are necessary for moving global health forward, even though creative ideas can be "risky" uses of resources. For example, vaccine programs, if successful, are extremely cost-effective, but there is a chance of failure, and the up-front cost of research and development is extremely high. Still, it is important for some funding agencies and research organizations to be willing to risk failure so that new technologies and innovative approaches to global health problems can be developed.

Another shortcoming of cost-effectiveness analysis is that it often requires the analysts to make judgments about what a healthy life is worth. The calculations may require an estimate of how much it costs a disabled person to be unable to work, or an approximation of how much a year of life is worth for a 70-year-old compared to a 7-year-old. While these sorts of estimates may be helpful at the population planning level, they break down at the individual level. Estimates of lost wages do not capture the burden of lost self-sufficiency that may accompany a disability. Few families would put a price tag on grandpa and deem his year of life to be worth less than that of his grandchild.

Global health statistics, budget details, and progress reports tend to hide individual human beings behind numbers, reducing real people to nameless, faceless masses. A few million children dying from preventable diseases like diarrhea and malaria. A few million people with treatable mental health issues going untreated. A few million young adults with HIV infection gaining access to life-saving antiretroviral medications. A few million households gaining access to a reliable source of clean drinking water. But statistics cannot capture the profound grief experienced by families who lose a child, just as they cannot fully express how life-changing a new water well can be.

It is important that people involved in local health and global health never lose sight of health being about real people—people who merely want the means to be healthy enough to be able to support themselves and their families, and who hope they will be fortunate enough to see their children and grandchildren grow up. Staying attuned to the human side of global health sometimes means acting out of simple compassion or a sense of solidarity with other human beings, whether those people live next door or on the other side of the planet.[25] Global health in the 21st century has the tools and technology to discover groundbreaking new ways to promote health and prevent disease and disability, to significantly improve health standards and reduce health disparities, to tackle the problems associated with extreme poverty, and to bring together people from across the world as equals to address our common health challenges. If we choose to prioritize global health in the coming decades—both because it makes economic sense to do so and because it makes "human" sense to foster everyone's health and well-being—we have the opportunity to make unparalleled improvements in the lives of billions of people.

15.6 DISCUSSION QUESTIONS

1. What achievements would you include in a list of the top 10 global health successes of the 20th century (the 1900s)?
2. What are five specific items you would like to include in a "top 10" list of current global health priorities? Before making your list, consider the diversity of health issues (such as infectious diseases, nutrition, NCDs, mental health, and injuries) affecting various populations across the lifespan and across the globe that could be included in the list.
3. For each of the five current priorities you identified, what is one relatively cost-effective method for addressing the concern?
4. For each of the five current priorities you identified, what is one organization that is currently working to address the concern? What are the approaches each of these organizations is using to achieve its global health goals?
5. If you had $1 million to spend on improving global health, what would you do with the money?
6. If you had $25 to contribute toward improving global health, what would you do with the money?
7. How should decisions about how to spend global health funds be made? How should health concerns be prioritized? How should interventions be selected?
8. What items do you hope will be included in a list of the top 10 global health successes of the 21st century (the 2000s)?

REFERENCES

1. Global Public Health Achievements Team, CDC. Ten great public health achievements: worldwide, 2001–2010. *Morb Mort Wkly Rep.* 2011;60:814–818.
2. *The Millennium Development Goals report 2011.* New York: United Nations; 2011.
3. *MDG Monitor country profiles 2012.* New York: UN; 2012.
4. Waage J, Banerji R, Campbell O, et al. The Millennium Development Goals: a cross-sectoral analysis and principles for goal setting after 2015. *Lancet.* 2010;376:991–1023.
5. *Investing in global health: 'best buys' and priorities for action in developing countries.* Disease Control Priorities Project; 2006.
6. Varmus H, Klausner R, Zerhouni E, Acharya T, Daar AS, Singer PA. Grand challenge in global health. *Science.* 2003;302:398–399.
7. Gostin LO, Friedman EA, Ooms G, et al. The Joint Action and Learning Initiative; towards a global agreement on national and global responsibilities for health. *PLoS Med.* 2011;8:e1001031.

8. Koplan JP, Fleming DW. Current and future public health challenges. *JAMA*. 2000;284:1696–1698.

9. Daar AS, Singer PA, Persad DL, et al. Grand challenges in chronic non-communicable diseases. *Nature*. 2007;450:494–496.

10. Chisholm D, Naci H, Hyder AA, Tran NT, Peden M. Cost effectiveness of strategies to combat road traffic injuries in sub-Saharan Africa and South East Asia: mathematical modeling study. *BMJ*. 2012;344:e612.

11. Hotez PJ, Molyneux DH, Fenwick A, et al. Control of neglected tropical diseases. *New Engl J Med*. 2007;357:1018–1027.

12. *Scaling up action against noncommunicable diseases: how much will it cost?* Geneva: World Health Organization; 2011.

13. Pattinson R, Kerber K, Buchmann E, et al.; The Lancet Stillbirths Series steering committee. Stillbirths: how can health systems deliver for mothers and babies? *Lancet*. 2011;377:1610–1623.

14. Chisholm D, Lund C, Saxena S. Cost of scaling up mental healthcare in low- and middle-income countries. *Br J Psychiatry*. 2007;191:528–535.

15. *Roll Back Malaria annual report 2011*. Geneva: WHO; 2011.

16. *The global plan to stop TB 2011–2015*. Geneva: Stop TB Partnership; 2011.

17. UN-Water Global Analysis and Assessment of Sanitation and Drinking-Water. *GLAAS 2012 Report*. Geneva: WHO; 2012.

18. Singh S, Darroch JE, Ashford LS, Vlassoff M. *Adding it up: the costs and benefits of investing in family planning and maternal and newborn health*. New York: UNFPA/Guttmacher Institute; 2009.

19. Laxminarayan R, Mills AJ, Breman JG, et al. Advancement of global health: key messages from the Disease Control Priorities Project. *Lancet*. 2006;367:1193–1208.

20. Shediac-Rizkallah MC, Bone LR. Planning for the sustainability of community-based health programs: conceptual frameworks and future directions for research, practice and policy. *Health Educ Res*. 1998;13:87–108.

21. Beaglehole R, Bonita R, Horton R, et al. Priority actions for the non-communicable disease crisis. *Lancet*. 2011;377:1438–1447.

22. Sachs J, Malaney P. The economic and social burden of malaria. *Nature*. 2002;415:680–685.

23. Zhang P, Zhang X, Brown J, et al. Global healthcare expenditure on diabetes for 2010 and 2030. *Diabetes Res Clin Pract*. 2010;87:293–301.

24. Rehm J, Mathers C, Popova S, Thavorncharoensap M, Teerawattanonon Y, Patra J. Global burden of disease and injury and economic cost attributable to alcohol use and alcohol use disorders. *Lancet*. 2009;373:2223–2233.

25. Benatar SR, Daar AS, Singer PA. Global health ethics: the rationale for mutual caring. *Int Affairs*. 2003;79:107–138.

Index

379